Low-Cost Veterinary Clinical Diagnostics

Low-Cost Veterinary Clinical Diagnostics

Ryane E. Englar DVM, DABVP (Canine and Feline Practice)
Executive Director of Clinical and Professional Skills
&
Associate Professor of Practice
University of Arizona College of Veterinary Medicine
Oro Valley, Arizona, USA

Sharon M. Dial DVM, PhD, DACVP (Clinical and Anatomic Pathology)
Research Scientist
University of Arizona College of Veterinary Medicine
Oro Valley, Arizona, USA

WILEY Blackwell

Registered Offices
John Wiley & Sons, Inc., 111 River Street, Hoboken, NJ 07030, USA
John Wiley & Sons Ltd, The Atrium, Southern Gate, Chichester, West Sussex, PO19 8SQ, UK

For details of our global editorial offices, customer services, and more information about Wiley products visit us at www.wiley.com.

Wiley also publishes its books in a variety of electronic formats and by print-on-demand. Some content that appears in standard print versions of this book may not be available in other formats.

Library of Congress Cataloging-in-Publication Data applied for
Hardback: 9781119714507

Cover Design: Wiley
Cover Images: Courtesy of Robert Eisemann, DVM; © Ryane E. Englar, DVM, DABVP (Canine and Feline Practice)

Set in 9.5/12.5pt STIXTwoText by Straive, Pondicherry, India

Printed in Singapore
M109228_151122

Dedication

Isaac Newton once shared that:

"If I have seen further, it is by standing on the shoulders of giants."

He was correct in ways that I didn't even recognize the first and the second and the third time that I read his quote.

The veterinary profession is full of giants, but I'm not talking about the neurosurgeons, orthopedic surgeons, or internists.

I'm not talking about Louis J. Camuti, the first veterinarian to devote his entire practice to cats, or even Bernhard Lauritz Frederik Bang, the Danish veterinarian who discovered *Brucella abortus*.

When I speak of giants, I am recalling those individuals who are ever-present, yet underrecognized both in clinical practice and throughout veterinary medical education.

These giants are none other than our veterinary technicians.

Technicians are veterinarians' shadows – literally and figuratively – although my hope in penning this dedication is that we can extract them from the shadows and into the light, where they belong.

After all, they are the reason I have survived veterinary practice. The reason I am a good veterinarian today is because I have been lifted on the shoulders of great technicians.

Technicians are all-star people, colleagues, and friends.

In a profession where they do so much for so many, we often fail to see them for who they are and all they contribute to the team.

They are talented and motivating individuals who excel in ways that I could never hold a candle to.

They are the blood, sweat, and tears of veterinary practice.

They are skilled diagnosticians, managers, nurses, and criticalists who maintain the pace and keep us all on track.

They are our pulse in ways that we can't even begin to wrap our heads around until we've been standing knee-deep in the trenches for hours, days, weeks, years, lifetimes only to discover that they never left our sides. Through thick and thin. Through emergency C-sections and CPR codes. Through life and death. And in the aftermath of death, too, when everyone else has gone home. They're still there, too, waiting with you, beside you.

They are the only ones dedicated enough, determined enough, bold enough, and brave enough to stand with us, from dawn to dusk and from dusk to dawn, over and over and over again, putting forth all that they are and all that they strive to be, despite being continuously overworked and underpaid.

In the years that they have stood beside me, they have supported me, encouraged me, nurtured me, and taught me.

They have placed intravenous catheters when I could not; they have reassured clients when I could not.

They are the last gentle souls that my patients see when they are induced with general anesthesia, and they are the first gentle spirits that my patients awake to in recovery.

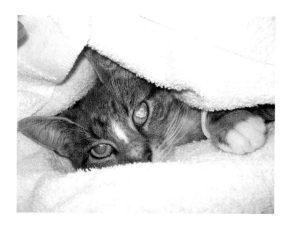

They have held my patients to quiet their fears and to provide comfort and warmth.

They have known the answers when I did not and believed in me when I did not.

Together, we have hoped and grieved, celebrated, and cried. And when I have felt too weak, too lost, too alone to carry on, they have wiped away my tears and offered a hand and helped me stand so that together we could try again.

Dominique Wilkins was once credited as saying:

> ***"You are only as good as your team."***

I am going to paraphrase this quote when I write this most essential truth of all for the veterinary profession: veterinarians are only as good as their technicians.

Veterinary technicians are extraordinary. They make us exceptional. They complete us. They make us whole.

To all the veterinary technicians out there, I see you. I appreciate you. I support you. I stand beside you.

May I never forget the sacrifices you have made on behalf of me and my patients.

You pave the way so that I can be me. You give my patients life and hope.

Thank you for being the backbone of our profession and the footprints in the sand.

You walk the walk beside us, with us, for us. And because of you, we are never ever the same.

– Ryane E. Englar

Every life is a culmination of the support and encouragement of those surrounding them. I have been remarkably fortunate to have grown up in the field of pathology surrounded by amazing individuals. As I contemplated returning to Colorado State University (CSU) to start my residency and PhD, I was told that the three most important things to consider are

1) choosing your mentor
2) choosing your mentor

And, finally

3) choosing your mentor.

I was fortunate to have been given the opportunity to work with Dr. Mary Anna Thrall (MAT) and it was the most important decision I made as I took my first steps toward being a clinical pathologist. She challenged me and my fellow residents to have an opinion and engage in lively discussion. As a PhD advisor, she provided support when, as is often the case, the research did not always go as planned. The quote she handed me when there was a difficult and unexpected outcome in our study is one that I have kept at heart since:

> ***The joy of research must be in the doing for the outcome is uncertain –Theobald Smith.***

She made sure her residents participated in annual conferences and introduced us to the remarkable people who shaped the discipline of clinical pathology. As a friend, she showed me how to enjoy life in the moment. Thank you, MAT!

– Sharon M. Dial

Contents

About the Authors

Ryane E. Englar, DVM, DABVP (Canine and Feline Practice) graduated from Cornell University College of Veterinary Medicine in 2008. She practiced as an associate veterinarian in companion animal practice before transitioning into the educational circuit as an advocate for pre-clinical training in primary care. She debuted in academia as a Clinical Instructor of the Community Practice Service at Cornell University's Hospital for Animals. She then transitioned into the role of Assistant Professor as founding faculty at Midwestern University College of Veterinary Medicine. While at Midwestern University, she had the opportunity to teach the inaugural class of 2018, the class of 2019, and the class of 2020. While training these remarkable young professionals, Dr. Englar became a Diplomat of the American Board of Veterinary Practitioners (ABVP). She then joined the faculty at Kansas State University between May 2017 and January 2020 to launch the clinical skills curriculum.

In February 2020, Dr. Englar reprised her role of founding faculty when she returned "home" to Tucson to join the University of Arizona College of Veterinary Medicine. As a dual appointment, Associate Professor of Practice and the Executive Director of Clinical and Professional Skills, Dr. Englar currently plays a lead role in the development and delivery of the pre-clinical curriculum.

Dr. Englar is passionate about advancing education for generalists by thinking outside of the box to develop new course materials for the hands-on learner. This labor of love is preceded by five sole-authored texts that collectively provide students, clinicians, and educators alike with functional, relatable, and practice-friendly tools for success:

- *Performing the Small Animal Physical Examination* (John Wiley & Sons, Inc., 2017)
- *Writing Skills for Veterinarians* (5M Publishing, Ltd., 2019)
- *Common Clinical Presentations in Dogs and Cats* (John Wiley & Sons, Inc., 2019)
- *A Guide to Oral Communication in Veterinary Medicine* (5M Publishing, Ltd., 2020)
- *The Veterinary Workbook of Small Animal Clinical Cases* (5M Books. Ltd., 2021)

Dr. Englar's students inspire her to write so that they have the resources they need to thrive in clinical practice.

When Dr. Englar is not teaching or advancing companion animal primary care, she trains in the art of ballroom dancing and competes nationally with her instructor, Lowell E. Fox.

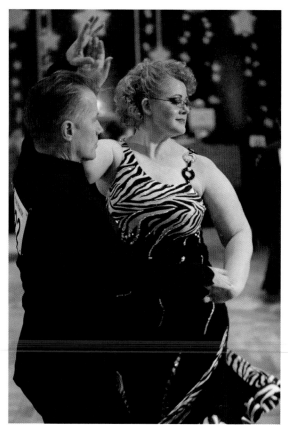

Source: Courtesy of Tony Eng, Decadance Photography.

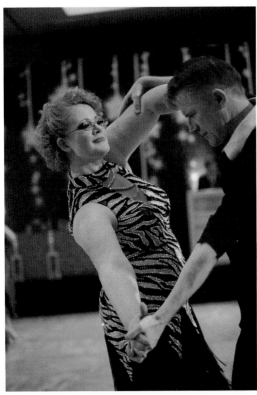

Source: Courtesy of Tony Eng, Decadance Photography.

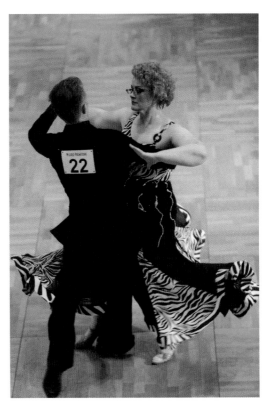

Source: Courtesy of Tony Eng, Decadance Photography.

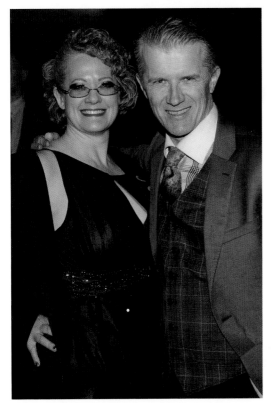

Source: Courtesy of Tony Eng, Decadance Photography.

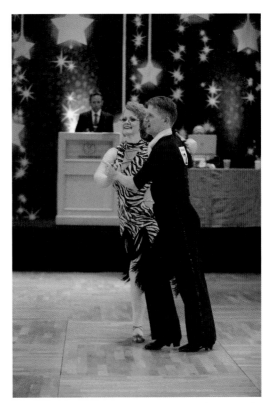

Source: Courtesy of Tony Eng, Decadance Photography.

Sharon M. Dial, DVM, PhD, DACVP (Clinical and Anatomic Pathology) received her DVM degree in 1982 from Colorado State University College of Veterinary Medicine. After practicing in a small rural community in Colorado for one year, she returned to CSU for a combined PhD and residency in clinical pathology. Her PhD research focused on using 4-methylpyrazole to treat ethylene glycol poisoning in dogs and cats. She remained at CSU and completed a National Institute of Health (NIH) National Research Service Award (NRSA) to investigate bone marrow transplantation for mucopolysaccharidosis VI in cats. Following the completion of the NRSA, she spent one year at the University of Wisconsin School of Veterinary Medicine as an instructor in clinical pathology.

In 1990, she joined the Louisiana State University (LSU) School of Veterinary Medicine faculty as an Assistant Professor in the Department of Pathology. While at LSU, she developed a passion for diagnostic pathology and teaching. It was at LSU that she developed interest in incorporating active, self-directed learning into the pedagogy of clinical pathology.

She left academia in 1994 to pursue diagnostic pathology in a large private veterinary diagnostic laboratory. Here she realized the importance of communication and "teaching in the moment" in case consultations with submitting veterinarians. After 25 years in the diagnostic world, she is excited to have returned to academia at the University of Arizona College of Veterinary Medicine (UAzCVM).

The innovative curriculum at the UAzCVM has allowed her to take the insight that she received as a working diagnostic pathologist from practicing veterinarians and apply it to educating veterinary students in the skills they need to succeed as day-one veterinarians. The students and faculty of the veterinary program provide daily inspiration for continuing her journey into active learning using team-based Learning (TBL) and peer instruction (PI) active learning methodology. She is currently working with the UAzCVM faculty development team to create Open Education Resources including clinical cases and software tools for veterinary medical education. Working on this project has prompted her interest in helping to understand how to partner with clients and manage understand managing their clients' financial resources to optimize patient care. Understanding the value and limitations of low-cost diagnostic tests is essential for veterinarians providing the spectrum of care.

When not working in academia, Sharon had dabbled in many hobbies, including quilting, weaving, woodworking, and, currently, metalsmithing. Her newest favorite pastime is hammering metal into interesting forms using a technique called fold forming. The joy is in the hammering and fire, the metal object that results is, as they say in Louisiana, lagniappe.

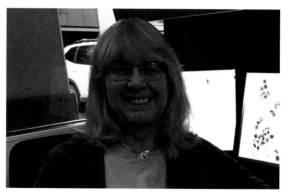

Credit line: Sharon M. Dial (Author).

About the Contributors

Jeremy Bessett is a DVM Candidate at the University of Arizona College of Veterinary Medicine and a member of the Inaugural Class of 2023.

Jeremy spent 11 years working as a technician in a rural mixed animal veterinary practice in southern Arizona. Low-cost veterinary diagnostics were paramount to patient management at this clinic. Jeremy was introduced to his passion, pathology, in his undergraduate courses at the University of Arizona. In veterinary school, Jeremy has worked to continuously expand his knowledge in veterinary pathology and plans to pursue board certification in both clinical and anatomic pathology.

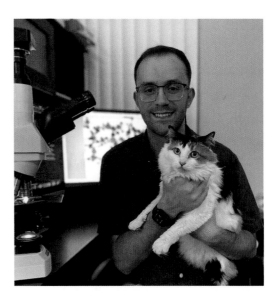

Preface

"What was it like when you were in vet school?"

It is a simple question that I am often asked by my students. A simple question with no easy answer.

The vet school experience to discover our own personal and professional identities encapsulates so many thoughts and feels, so many unique milestones and setbacks.

It is a journey that I would do all over again yet one that I frequently fast-forward when taking a walk down memory lane because mine, like many, was riddled with insecurity and the fear of never being "enough."

No one in my graduating class knew what constituted "enough," yet the one thing we collectively convinced ourselves of, on Commencement Day, is that whatever "enough" was, we did not have it!

In those days, we lived in perpetual fear of being labeled substandard. We compensated by committing facts to memory. We learned through positive punishment which answers to questions were "correct" and therefore worthy of accolades. We steered clear of those that spelled defeat.

So it was that most of my clinical year was spent reciting diagnostic plans like recipes. In truth, I did not always understand the purpose of each or how to interpret them. I simply knew how to play the game to get the answer "right."

What I learned in the years that followed was that the practice of medicine is not a game and that "why?" often matters more than "what?" But in the moment, the "what?" took precedence and at times clouded my understanding of clinical casework during my early years as a "baby vet."

When I close my eyes to reflect upon my journey through veterinary medicine, I can still place myself as a timid student in clinical year.

The year was 2008.

It was a few months shy of graduation and I was well into week two of my Emergency/Critical Care rotation at Cornell University Hospital for Animals, standing in the adrenaline-infused corridor that led to the ICU.

I had just triaged my 26th case in less than 24 hours over a holiday weekend.

I was running on no sleep and no food.

The case was a 12-year-old female spayed domestic short-haired cat that presented for acute vomiting. The patient was stable enough to sit in its carrier and watch me with trepidation as I summarized her history for the benefit of the attending resident.

I did as I was trained to do. I led with the patient's signalment, followed by a timeline of their chief complaint:

- three-day history of "ADR"
- two-day history of hyporexia
- four emetic episodes overnight
- lethargic all morning

I tacked on other pieces of data that seemed relevant to the case:

- indoor-only
- no other pets in household
- no pre-existing conditions
- no known access to or ingestion of toxins
- no current medications, including supplements and preventatives.

Keep in mind that I had yet to perform a physical exam. If you asked me today what my exam findings were for that patient on that specific day, I could not tell you. I cannot recall. What I do remember, as if it were yesterday, was what the attending clinician asked of me in follow-up:

"What is your diagnostic plan?"

I remember the question because, back in those days, my response was programmed to recite the same thing, each time, every time, regardless of whether the case presentation was diarrheic dog or a diabetic cat.

My response was always:

QATS, Blood gas analysis, CBC/Chem/UA, chest rads, and abdominal ultrasound.

I might have added in FeLV/FIV serology as a bonus for a cat or HW/L/E/A for a dog. Maybe even a thyroid panel for good measure. But the foundational plan was always the same. If nothing else, I had learned to be consistent in my test selection.

I was far less certain of the rationale – that is, why each test was vital to the patient's workup.

As a student, I was rarely asked to contemplate the "why?," as in:

- *Why should each test be run?*
- *Why is each diagnostic test of value?*
- *Why might each step of the diagnostic plan be efficacious?*
- *Why this test and not another?*
- *Why run tests simultaneously rather than sequentially?*
- *Why was there value in broadening the data set?*

It was always just assumed in the Teaching Hospital that we could ask the client for the sun, the moon, and the stars, so why not? And if for some reason our hands were tied, then we were taught that the client was not allowing us to be thorough.

It never occurred to us, as students, that we could choose to prioritize some test(s) over others – and with good reason.

What we were not taught then but needed more than ever when we graduated was the skill of clinical reasoning. Clinical reasoning requires health-care providers to be detectives. We must consider for every patient the odds that disease "x" is most likely and balance these odds against clinical uncertainties. We must problem-solve, strategize, and customize to provide patient-specific care. We must acquire and analyze data that is specific to the patient's problem list to accurately initiate, evaluate, and adapt case management as patient-specific needs evolve.

Clinical reasoning is inherently tied to critical thinking. Both are dynamic processes. They do not begin and end with diagnosis. They require an intimate understanding of contributing inputs and patient-specific factors.

To become effective at clinical reasoning, clinicians must gather and compare key pieces of data that are obtained through deliberate history-taking. Physical examination findings provide an additional layer of evidence for clinicians to interpret and formulate hypotheses about which diagnoses are most consistent with case presentation.

To test hypotheses, we must perform diagnostic tests. Which test to run is a critical component of the detective work that is required of us in veterinary practice yet the answer to this question is not inherently obvious.

The Veterinarian's Oath tasks us to act as stewards of the animal kingdom. This ethical agreement requires veterinarians to prioritize patient welfare and the prevention of disease above all other external influences, including finances. On paper, these tasks are self-explanatory and clear-cut. However, patients more often present in shades of gray that threaten our understanding of how to deliver high-quality, gold standard medicine, particularly when patient outcomes may be contingent upon cost.

What do we do when we can't do it all? What do we do when we can't run every test? What happens when our clients experience financial constraints? What happens when we lack the diagnostic equipment to proceed? What happens if we lack the client's consent?

Ryane Englar the Student was not prepared to face this clinical reality.

The student in me was not trained to brainstorm alternatives.

Instead, the student in me was trained to see alternative approaches as "lesser" or "substandard" in the same way that I was taught to view myself when I did not have all the answers.

The student in me was trained to recommend the gold standard for every patient with the understanding that this approach always provides the greatest diagnostic accuracy. In a world of ideals, the gold standard was always possible.

However, as scientific advances revolutionize the number of diagnostic tests that are available to our client, the gold standard is not always feasible. *What happens when the price of treatment exceeds the client's ability or willingness to afford the gold standard? Are we pricing people out of pet ownership?*

Beyond the question of affordability, who determines standard of care? Where is the evidence to support it?

Is a one-size-fits-all approach truly best? Or should the "best" approach be determined by the situation, the context, the patient, and the client?

It is vital that we offer our clients options. It is vital that we consider the whole patient. It is vital that we investigate clinical signs and offer a comprehensive approach to diagnostic medicine so that we find permanent solutions rather than Band-Aid approaches that offer temporary fixes.

At the same time, what constitutes comprehensive *and why do certain tests fall under that umbrella? Are we testing out of the desire for completeness, to cover all bases for the good of the patient? Or are we testing because we are expected to?*

If we are testing because we are expected to, then who is it that determines the standards? Who sets the bar? Are we testing out of peer pressure or are we testing to cover our bases in the event of litigation? If that is the case, then is testing appropriate? Is it right for the patient or right for our reputation? Does it matter? *Should it matter?*

As is typical of veterinary practice, there are no easy answers. As clinicians, we are left to determine for ourselves what constitutes "best practices." The challenge to understand "best practices" has recently precipitated discussion within our profession about a shift away from the "gold standard" toward "spectrum of care." This term implies that there is a continuum of acceptable care for each clinical scenario that is contingent on evidence-based medicine, client and provider expectations for patient outcomes, and financial constraints.

The spectrum of care philosophy is relatively new to the veterinary profession and *formal* training in "Plan B" approaches to the practice of clinical medicine is rare. Often, such approaches are anecdotal, established through trial and error, and spread through word of mouth.

It would therefore be of benefit to provide students and perhaps more importantly new graduates with a candid, pragmatic approach to diagnostic medicine.

At the end of the day, it still may be advisable to recommend the following treatment plan:

> *QATS, Blood gas analysis, CBC/Chem/UA, chest rads, and abdominal ultrasound.*

But it is only advisable if you, the clinician, can answer the question of "why?" in addition to "what?"

Testing to test achieves nothing, particularly if we do not know what it is that we are looking for.

A robot can perform tests.

A clinician, on the other hand, understands the value that comes from testing. A clinician uses clinical reasoning to prioritize which diagnostic tests are essential and why. A clinician maximizes data that is obtained and knows how and when to apply it to case management to improve patient outcomes.

The primary goal of this textbook is to train clinicians to think like clinicians so that we individually and collectively understand the wealth of information that can come from point-of-care diagnostic tests.

It is not enough to know which tests to perform. Our clients look to us for advice beyond the "what?" to include the "why" and "how" – in other words, why is this test essential and how might test results be interpreted in a way that effectively and efficiently manages patient care?

This text is intended to be a reference guide for maximizing the information that is obtained through each test that is performed in-house.

Note that the authors are not here to tell you what you can and cannot offer each client. That is an individual decision that each of us as attending clinicians must make with respect to each individual case, patient, and client.

Note also that this text is not intended to disparage the gold standard as it represents a comprehensive approach to the practice of clinical medicine. However, we must also ground ourselves in the reality that the full gamut of proposed diagnostic plans is often an impossibility in general practice. When we hit this literal and figurative obstruction, we must be prepared to flex our diagnostic approach. We must learn how to get the most out of a finite set of data that is acquired from a limited selection of tests and feel confident applying this knowledge to develop patient-specific, appropriate care plans.

This text is among the first of its kind to provide a layered approach to diagnostic medicine by highlighting point-of-care tests and the wealth of information that can be gathered from a step-by step approach to case management.

– **Ryane E. Englar**

Acknowledgments

Coaches

Richard Back once wrote that:

> *"Don't believe what your eyes are telling you. All they show is limitation. Look with your understanding. Find out what you already know and you will see the way to fly."*

And:

> *"To bring anything into your life, imagine that it's already there."*

By the time this text comes into print, I will have been dancing with Lowell Fox of Arrowhead Arthur Murray (Peoria, Arizona) for eight years. Eight years is a long time to be paired with a teacher and a coach. Eight years is a long time for you to get to know them and for them to get to know you. In those eight years of mutual respect and trust, I have come to appreciate the depth that Lowell brings to our partnership.

For as long as I have known him, Lowell has taught with the mindset of who I will become. He sees the sculpture rather than a block of marble. He sees only potential whereas I tend to see only rough spots.

Dance did not come easy to me. I was not born with raw talent, and I preferred sneakers to high heels. (I still do!) What Lowell has made me acutely aware of is that it is one thing to be talented. It is another to be skilled.

Skill is not something you come into this world with. *It is something you build.*

Skill is not something you build overnight. *It takes hours, days, weeks, months, years of determination and grit.*

Skill is investing in something and holding onto it for dear life even after your knuckles turn white because you believe in it – and in yourself – that much.

Lowell has seen me and my dance steps at their most basic, unrefined, unpolished state. I have practiced a box step in any number of dances, any number of ways badly. In many ways, our lessons are those first drafts that end up coated in so much red ink that the second draft bears strikingly no resemblance to the first.

Yet that first draft is foundational.

Lowell is foundational.

As a professional dancer, there is nothing that Lowell cannot do. I often tell him that if he went out on a competition floor alone, he would have far better success than he does when he is paired with me.

Yet the beauty of Lowell as a dancer, teacher, and coach is that he does not eclipse his student. Instead, Lowell frames us, as we wish to be seen, in our best light.

Over the years, Lowell has taught me about life as much as he has taught me about dance.

He has given me the courage to achieve what I never thought was possible, both on and off the dance floor.

He has given me the drive to set the bar higher than I ever thought I could reach because I knew that he believed I could.

I want to believe one day in me the way that he believes in me every day.

And it is the desire that he has awakened in me to be the best me that propels me to new heights.

Before I met Lowell, obstacles stopped me in my tracks. If someone discounted me or my work, their criticism drove me off course. Same-day ideas lined the next day's wastebins, literally and figuratively.

Lowell views the world through a unique lens.

Lowell sees possibility when others see defeat.

Lowell opens doors when others close them.

I say, "Why?" and he says, "Why not?"

It may seem like a simple question.

But it has changed my world.

It changed the lens through which I see the world.

And now I, too, see open doors and a lifetime of possibility.

This text is possibility turned into life and I do not know that it would have happened if I did not believe it could first.

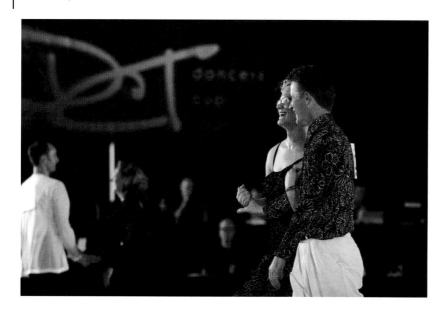

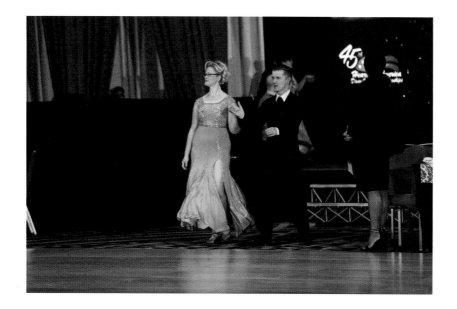

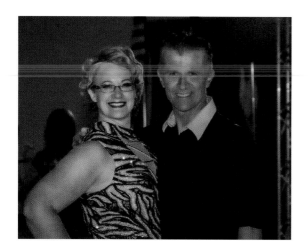

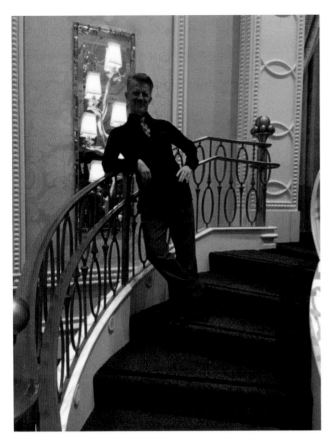

Colleagues

Richard Back once wrote that:

> *"The bond that links your true family is not one of blood, but of respect and joy in each other's life. Rarely do members of one family grow up under the same roof."*

And:

> *"Your friends will know you better in the first minute you meet than your acquaintances will know you in a thousand years."*

I first met Teresa Graham Brett when she was interviewing for the position of Senior Associate Dean of Diversity, Equity, and Inclusion (DEI) at the University of Arizona College of Veterinary Medicine.

I did not know then how closely our professional paths would intersect in our current roles of co-course coordinators for the professional skills preclinical curriculum.

I only knew then that Teresa was precisely who our program needed.

But more than that, she was precisely who I needed, too.

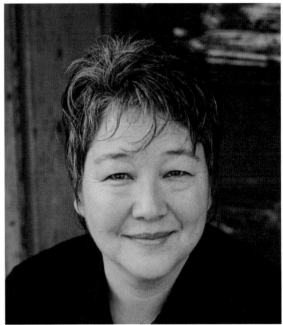

Credit line: Courtesy of Teresa-Graham-Brett

There are colleagues and then there are *Colleagues*.

The former type of colleagues share office space. They are there for you and you are there for them in a sort of symbiotic relationship. You coexist. Your paths cross. You collaborate to achieve a predetermined purpose – in this case, teaching. You begin the day and end the day together, over the same Keurig. Then you prepare to restart all over again tomorrow.

Colleagues are cut from a different cloth. They share your vision, and your heart. *Colleagues* are those who know you better than you know yourself and they go out of their way to find you when you are literally or figuratively lost. They remind you of the "why" when you lose sight of your internal compass.

When you can't find you, they can.

From the very first moment I met Teresa, I knew that she was a rare find.

I knew that Teresa had come into my life for a reason. And I knew that by her side I would grow immensely.

Teresa is, by virtue of the authenticity of her words and actions, a trio of *Colleague*, friend, and family all at once.

She provides that spark and zest for life.

She provides the extra punctuation that motivates and nourishes my soul.

She reminds me of what and who matter most.

She reminds me to persevere.

When I think of Teresa, what comes to mind most is her strength, spirit, determination, and grit.

She is a force of nature in the quiet, yet powerful way in which she conducts herself.

Her energy changes the world around her, the people around her, for the better.

All of us have colleagues, but few among us have *Colleagues*. Every day that I am fortunate enough to be in her inner circle, I find myself grateful and whole.

Teresa's opportunity to effect positive change in my life in this way calls to mind adaptations of the 1969 publication "The Star Thrower" by Loren Eiseley in *The Unexpected Universe*. It is a story that has been retold by motivational speakers again and again. An adult crosses the path of a young child on a beach, tossing starfish back into the ocean.

The starfish had been swept onto the shore by the tide and they could not return to the sea by themselves. The adult asks the child what they are doing. The child explains that the starfish will die without a helping hand. The adult responds that there are thousands of starfish along the beach and that they cannot possibly make a difference. The child tosses yet another starfish into the ocean and proclaims that they made a difference to that one.

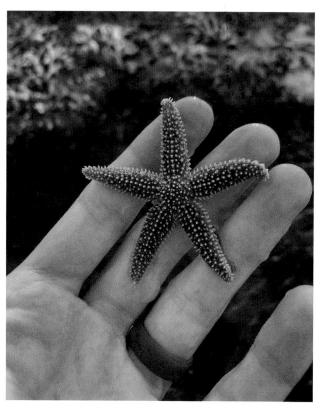

Starfish – Courtesy of Ian Hubbard

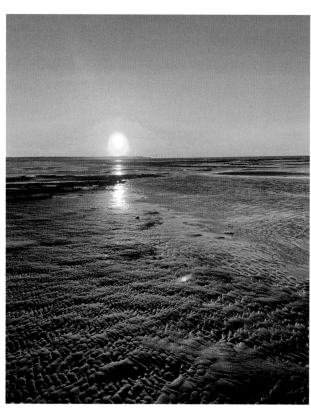

Sunset – Courtesy of Ian Hubbard

Coming back to Teresa's presence in my life, the truth is that she did not have to teach with me.

That she chose to teach with me, that she chose me, makes all the difference.

– Ryane E. Englar

One of the truths embraced by the mission of the University of Arizona College of Veterinary Medicine (UAzCVM) is that *we are all teachers and learners in our program.* This truth is evident daily as faculty members challenge students to take ownership of their education; and students challenge faculty by bringing ideas and information they gained in their studies back into the classroom for discussion. I have been exceptionally fortunate to work closely with the student Jeremy Bessett, DVM Candidate, inaugural class of 2023. Jeremy brought his long-standing passion for pathology to the CVM when he matriculated in our program. He has contributed to the development of teaching cases by collecting case material and authoring learning modules in teaching software. His dedication to providing images for the chapters in this textbook has been inspiring and essential. Jeremy wrote the cases in Part 6 from case material he collected over his years working in private practice as a veterinary technician. The cases needed minimal editing. As we reviewed the cases together, our discussions were excellent examples of the student mentoring the mentor. Jeremy's continued journey into the field of pathology will be a joy to watch.

– **Sharon M. Dial**

Part 1

Patient Care Considerations

1

The Gold Standard, Standards of Care, and Spectrum of Care: An Evolving Approach to Diagnostic Medicine

Ryane E. Englar

1.1 Defining the Gold Standard

Imagine that you are knee-deep in your fifth consecutive overnight shift at a 24-hour walk-in clinic when a four-year-old male castrated Ragdoll cat presents to you on emergency for evaluation of acute onset of stranguria. The client discloses that the patient was "fine" this morning, when they left for work; however, they returned home to find the patient frantically vocalizing while straining over the rug in the foyer. Despite 20+ trips to the litter box within the past two hours, the cat has produced only a few dribbles of urine. When the cat refused his evening meal and vomited bile, the client became concerned and transported the cat to the clinic. Physical examination discloses a painful, turgid urinary bladder and a urethral plug at the tip of the erythematous penis. Your working diagnosis is urinary tract obstruction (UTO).

How should you proceed with case management? Which paired diagnostic and therapeutic plans are most appropriate for this patient? What will you present to the client as your recommendations for next steps?

As students, we are trained to provide the gold standard when it comes to health care delivery, but what defines this approach to the practice of medicine and from where did this term originate?

The term, gold standard, is rooted in the discipline of economics [1]. Gold standard refers to an antiquated exchange rate system in which currency has a value that is directly linked to gold [1–3]. Any country that subscribed to the gold standard set a fixed price for gold [1–3]. That fixed price determined how much paper money was worth [1–3]. For example, one ounce of gold cost $20.67 in the United States and £4.24 in the United Kingdom during the late nineteenth and early twentieth centuries [2–4]. The value of the US dollar was therefore said to be roughly 1/20th of an ounce of gold [2]. If someone wished to convert one British pound to US dollars based upon this exchange rate, they could. The exchange rate between the US dollar and the British pound was calculated by $20.67/£4.247 = $4.867 to £1. This allowed for ease of comparisons between currencies in the arena of international trade.

When the gold standard first appeared within the medical literature in a 1962 anonymous commentary in *The Lancet*, it did not carry the same meaning [1]. Instead, the penned article, *Toward a Gold Standard*, was quite literal with the term, and called upon physicians to support the practice of administering gold salts to patients with rheumatoid arthritis [1].

It was not until 1979 that the term took on its present-day meaning in an editorial by Peter Rudd, M.D. that appeared in the Archives of Internal Medicine [1]. Rudd acknowledged the challenges of practicing medicine in the face of noncompliance when he shared that [5]:

> With the help of strong societal pressures, we are learning to acknowledge several nontraditional factors in medicine. We must now consider relative costs, absolute effectiveness, and "informed" patient-consumers. These new concerns form part of a larger trend to translate more directly the dramatic scientific advances of recent years into the practical arena. Amid cries for parsimonious medicine and maximized benefit, compliance has emerged as a major issue.

Rudd went on to state that [5]:

> The problem of noncompliance is hardly new. But its recognition and acknowledgment have come haltingly, apparently since few health professionals considered it worthy of attention and, probably more importantly, because few of them believed in their responsibility.

Low-Cost Veterinary Clinical Diagnostics, First Edition. Ryane E. Englar and Sharon M. Dial.
© 2023 John Wiley & Sons, Inc. Published 2023 by John Wiley & Sons, Inc.

Rudd tasked the medical profession with developing a gold standard for compliance that would facilitate case management [5]. The term has since appeared in over 10 000 publications since 1995 [1] despite concerns from some that "because the phrase smacks of dogma its use should be discontinued in medical science. After all, the financiers gave up the idea of a gold standard decades ago" [6].

P. Finbarr Duggan, who expressed this sentiment in 1992, explained that he was "taken back" by the use of this term since [6]:

> As a practising [sp] biochemist for nearly 40 years I had never heard these words used to describe any biological test. Because the subject is in a state of perpetual evolution gold standards are, by definition almost, never reached.

1.2 Limitations of the Gold Standard

Fast-forward to the present day in both human and veterinary healthcare. There is ongoing debate about the realities and practicalities of the gold standard approach to practicing medicine. Gold standard care implies that which is the best available under reasonable circumstances. Likewise, a gold standard diagnostic test refers to the most accurate assessment that can be performed without restrictions.

On paper, the gold standard implies that patient care is comprehensive. For instance, in his 2005 article in Veterinary Clinics of North America: Small Animal Practice, Benjamin Colmery III, DVM, outlined the gold standard of veterinary oral health care to include [7]:

- thorough physical examination and history
- preoperative blood profiles, including blood gases
- inhalation anesthesia with sevoflurane
- regional and local nerve blocks
- concurrent intravenous fluid therapy
- blood pressure, electrocardiography (ECG), pulse oximetry, respiratory monitors, and body temperature monitors
- intraoral dental radiology
- air-driven high-speed dental equipment and complete hand instrumentation
- trained dental operator
- complete dental charting
- home care
- rechecks.

Oral health care that is in alignment with this gold standard is deemed complete. Colmery's list is precisely that which we might aspire to provide to our patients.

However, we veterinarians are often restricted in terms of what we can provide by way of patient care. Delivering the gold standard may work well when we speak of theoretical cases, yet this level of care is not always within reach when we replace theoretical clients with actual ones [8]. Cost of care is a frequent barrier [8]. Even in the absence of financial constraints, our client may not comply with patient care recommendations [8]. Even if compliance is not an issue for our client, we may not be able to offer the industry standard. Maybe we do not have access to equipment for intraoral dental radiography, or maybe our team has not been adequately trained in procedural analgesia, including nerve blocks.

In these situations, it may feel as though our deviation from the gold standard offers a lower level of care, as if we are providing an economy experience instead of first class [9]. Even though we may feel that we are doing right by our client or patient, we may feel "trapped by the language we use" [9]. In this respect, "gold standard feels more like a marketing term than one suitable for patient welfare" [9].

This concern has led to a proposition that we shift the way that we approach care. Davidson explains it best when writing that [9]:

> Once we introduce real clients and patients then "the best available option" needs to be put into context of their needs and abilities. This is the skill of a medical care provider; not offering every possible combination of treatments, but listening to the client and assessing the patient.

1.3 Returning to the Case of the Cat with Stranguria: a Different Perspective on Standards of Care

Let's return now to the case that was introduced at the start of this chapter: a four-year-old male castrated Ragdoll cat presents to you on emergency for evaluation of acute onset of stranguria. Based upon history and physical exam findings, the patient's working diagnosis is UTO.

Gold standard care dictates that the following measures be taken to effectively manage the patient [10]:

- complete blood count (CBC)
- blood chemistry profile
- urinalysis (UA) with evaluation of the sediment
- urine culture
- intravenous (IV) catheter placement
- IV fluid therapy

- blood gas analysis
- sedation
- pulse oximetry
- blood pressure monitoring
- electrocardiogram (ECG)
- epidural nerve block during indwelling urinary catheter placement with closed collection system
- pharmacotherapy
- abdominal imaging: radiography or ultrasonography
- blood chemistry profile recheck
- electrolyte recheck
- blood gas analysis recheck
- follow-up urine culture after urinary catheter removal

Is this the only means of case management?
No.
Might other means of case management be appropriate?
Yes.

The case of urethral obstruction in a male cat is one of many clinical scenarios in veterinary practice in which a variety of treatment options are available [10].

Depending upon the situation, we might choose to proceed with one of the following approaches instead of the gold standard [10]:

- conservative management
  - ○ sedation
  - ○ analgesia
  - ○ urinary catheter placement
  - ○ subcutaneous fluid therapy
  - ○ anti-spasmodic pharmacotherapy (e.g. prazosin)
  - ○ discharge home with open-ended tomcat urinary catheter.
- hospitalization without urinary catheter placement
  - ○ sedation
  - ○ analgesia
  - ○ cystocentesis
  - ○ observation of cat until urination occurs.

Neither of these approaches is considered the gold standard.

Neither of these approaches is accepted as the universal standard of care [10]. In the eyes of the law, standard of care has been defined as that which is "required of and practiced by the average reasonably prudent, competent veterinarian in the community" [10]: in other words, standards outline that which constitutes legally acceptable care by competent healthcare providers [11]. Outside of the legal lens, standards can be considered guidelines or protocols that are evidence-based [11]. These protocols have defined steps that can be optimized and sequenced in such a way as to afford predictable outcomes [11].

Standards exist so that veterinarians, veterinary organizations, associations, and specialty colleges can hold each other accountable to deliver the same consistent quality of health care [11]. Yet not all standards are upheld [11]. Not all clients can afford all standards of care, just as not all practices can afford to implement them [11].

To muddy the waters further, not all clinicians agree upon the same standards of care, regardless of what overseeing bodies promote [11]. For example, the Advisory Panel of the American Association of Feline Practitioners (AAFP) advises that the feline leukemia (FeLV) vaccine be administered to all kittens regardless of lifestyle [12, 13]. However, not all veterinarians follow through with this recommendation. Some exclude indoor-only, single-pet households from this guideline out of concern for adverse effects associated with vaccination, specifically the risk of injection-site sarcoma. Does this mean that those unvaccinated kittens are receiving substandard care? Undoubtedly not. It means that the practice of medicine must allow for some degree of flexibility by offering incremental care options with the understanding that not all standards are appropriate for all patients in all circumstances [11].

Optimal care is not necessarily gold standard care. It is best defined within the context of real clients and their animals, based upon their needs and abilities. Within the context of this case, the male cat with UTO, either approach to care may be medically defensible, reasonable, and successful even though neither approach met the so-called "standard" [10].

1.4 Limitations to Standards of Care

Standards are intended to facilitate care, yet sometimes they have the opposite effect. As one colleague shared in a 2016 article, *Is the Gold Standard the Old Standard?* [14]

> Our profession sometimes emphasizes the 'best' care, and that sometimes turns into an insistence that all pet owners need to do this. . . Assuming the choices are medically appropriate, I think our profession has a responsibility to offer different levels of care.

Another colleague agreed that options, rather than edicts, are essential to veterinary practice [14]:

> Sometimes you don't have to even finish the 'I' at the end of MRI to know a client isn't going to pursue a neurologist consultation for a dog that suddenly does not have the use of the back legs. But it's with options C and D that a great veterinarian really shines. You have offered the standard practice, and

it's been declined by the owner. You're left with the moral and ethical task of doing your best, and sometimes it is in these moments a general practitioner can shine with problem-solving skills.

Rather than insist upon a universally accepted medical definition of standard of care, we might instead consider that there is for every clinical scenario an acceptable continuum of care [10, 11]. This continuum is born out of the understanding that limiting the scope to standard of care hinders our ability to deliver health care [10]. A recent survey shared that roughly one out of every four pet owners in the United States has experienced an obstacle to veterinary care, and that barrier is often financial [15, 16]. If clinicians only offer standard of care, then we may price people out of owning pets [14].

Instead of tying the clinicians' hands by saying that they either rise to meet the standard or fall below it, we must recognize that there are multiple paths to achieve the same patient outcome. These multiple forks in the proverbial road are evidence-based and factor into the equation all players and their perspectives including [16, 17]:

- the anticipated patient outcome
- the provider's knowledge
- the provider's skillset
- the practice's resources, including team members and equipment
- the provider's comfort and confidence with procedural medicine
- the safety and efficacy of available treatments
- best-practice guidelines
- quality-of-life measures, coupled with treatment effectiveness
- practice-specific goals
- client's access to care
- client's goals and values
- client's expectations for care, including the diagnostic and therapeutic timeline
- client's ability to comply with health care recommendations
- client's ability to finance care

There is value to the customization of the practice of medicine so that we ultimately deliver client-driven, pet-specific care.

1.5 Spectrum of Care

There is an added layer of value to learning how to modify preexisting treatment protocols. This is not a skill that is typically prioritized by the traditional model of veterinary education in the United States and Canada [18]. Students are classically trained in best practices, which leads to a disconnect between the so-called ivory tower medicine and the real world. Students therefore only acquire a sample of the knowledge and skills they need to succeed in practice [18].

When students transition from clinical year to general practice, they may not always feel comfortable offering Plan B, Plan C, or Plan D approaches to care. They may feel that care is all or none. Either they can refer a canine patient with a broken leg to an orthopedic surgeon for open reduction/internal fixation or they are faced with the reality of euthanizing the patient [18]. This is a gut-wrenching ethical dilemma that is commonly faced in general practice. In fact, in a 2018 survey by Kipperman et al., 52% of respondents acknowledged that they experienced an ethical dilemma as DVMs at least once per week [19].

"No one should have to euthanize their pet because it can't be provided some level of care" [18]. Yet, this is a frequent occurrence among veterinarians and their clients. According to Stull et al., the challenge is that [16]:

> Given the highly sophisticated nature of procedures commonly taught and observed in veterinary colleges, veterinarians (most notably recent graduates) may be unaware of, and lack the knowledge and skills to offer, a wide spectrum of care options for a given condition and therefore may be unable to communicate to clients the relative effectiveness and costs of options along this spectrum.

Veterinary educators must shift their approach to preparing students for general practice by broadening evidence-based options for diagnostic and treatment plans [18]. Rather than prescribing one gold standard or one standard of care, instructors can demonstrate a continuum of acceptable care options that can meet the needs of a diverse clientele [18]. Spectrum of care is not just about overcoming financial constraints [18]. It is about applying evidence-based medicine to clinical casework in a way that incorporates the client's perspective so that we can be responsive to a broad range of needs [18].

If we were to apply gold standard care, then a middle-aged vomiting dog can be managed only one way [18]:

- CBC
- blood chemistry profile
- UA
- pancreatic-specific lipase immunoreactivity
- abdominal imaging
- IV fluid therapy
- hospitalization

- observation
- pharmacotherapy.

Yet, experienced practitioners all know that a vomiting dog can be managed in many ways [18]:

> An alternative approach, for example, would be to check the dog's [hematocrit] and total protein concentration to evaluate hydration status, submit a blood sample for biochemical testing to rule out diabetic ketoacidosis and uremia, and administer fluids SC. If the owner declines this approach, another option could be to administer fluids SC and send the dog home with instructions for the owner to give the dog nothing to eat except ice chips for the first 24 hours and to offer small amounts of water and a homemade, low-fat diet of boiled chicken and rice over the next 24 hours if vomiting subsides, but to return for additional diagnostic testing if vomiting continues.

Spectrum of care training opens the door to dialogue concerning which management approaches are appropriate for each patient – and why [18]. As explained by Fingland et al., spectrum of care training gives students "the knowledge needed to discuss with owners the degree of diagnostic certainty, likelihood of a favorable or unfavorable outcome, possible need for additional testing or treatment, and costs associated with each option" [18].

Spectrum of care, in this respect, values all parties and tailors the approach to meet the specific needs and circumstances in the moment.

It is out of respect for these principles that this text proceeds. Parts 2 through 5 of this text will outline how to maximize each diagnostic test that is performed in-house, particularly when a step-by-step approach to case management is employed. Part 6 will provide sample cases to test your clinical acumen as you apply what you have learned about diagnostic testing to real-life case vignettes.

References

1 Claassen, J.A. (2005). 'Gold standard', not 'golden standard'. *Ned Tijdschr Geneeskd.* 149 (52): 2937.

2 Roosevelt's Gold Program. Federal Reserve History [Internet]. (2013). https://www.federalreservehistory.org/essays/roosevelts-gold-program#:~:text=The%20law%20required%20the%20Federal,per%20ounce%20of%20pure%20gold.

3 Historical Gold Prices – 1833 to Present: National Mining Association (NMA). (2016). https://nma.org/wp-content/uploads/2016/09/historic_gold_prices_1833_pres.pdf.

4 Press A. (2020). Commentary: The gold standard and why the U.S. left it behind: Finance & Commerce; (2020). https://finance-commerce.com/2020/11/commentary-the-gold-standard-and-why-the-u-s-left-it-behind.

5 Rudd, P. (1979). In search of the gold standard for compliance measurement. *Archives of Internal Medicine* 139 (6): 627–628.

6 Duggan, P.F. (1992). Time to abolish "gold standard". *British Medical Journal* 304: 1568–1569.

7 Colmery, B. 3rd. (2005). The gold standard of veterinary oral health care. *Veterinary Clinics of North America: Small Animal Practice* 35 (4): 781–787. v.

8 Hicks, M. (2019). Striving for the gold standard in animal welfare. *Canadian Veterinary Journal* 60 (11): 1145–1146.

9 Davidson J. (2021) Defining gold-standard care. vettimes [Internet]. www.vettimes.co.uk/defining-gold-standard-care.

10 Block, G. (2021). A different perspective on standard of care. In: *Pet-Specific Care for the Veterinary Teams* (ed. L.J. Ackerman), 715–717. Hoboken, NJ: Wiley.

11 Ackerman, L.J. (2021). Standards of care. In: *Pet-Specific Care for the Veterinary Teams* (ed. L.J. Ackerman), 711–714. Hoboken, NJ: Wiley.

12 Scherk, M.A., Ford, R.B., Gaskell, R.M. et al. (2013). 2013 AAFP Feline Vaccination Advisory Panel report. *Journal of Feline Medicine and Surgery* 15 (9): 785–808.

13 Stone, A.E., Brummet, G.O., Carozza, E.M. et al. (2020). 2020 AAHA/AAFP Feline Vaccination Guidelines. *Journal of Feline Medicine and Surgery* 22 (9): 813–830.

14 Is the gold standard the old standard? dvm360 [Internet]. (2016). https://www.dvm360.com/view/gold-standard-old-standard.

15 Brown, C.R., Garrett, L.D., Gilles, W.K. et al. (2021). Spectrum of care: more than treatment options. *Journal of the American Veterinary Medical Association* 259 (7): 712–717.

16 Stull, J.W., Shelby, J.A., Bonnett, B.N. et al. (2018). Barriers and next steps to providing a spectrum of effective health care to companion animals. *Journal of the American Veterinary Medical Association* 253 (11): 1386–1389.

17 Block, G. (2018). A new look at standard of care. *Journal of the American Veterinary Medical Association* 252 (11): 1343–1344.

18 Fingland, R.B., Stone, L.R., Read, E.K., and Moore, R.M. (2021). Preparing veterinary students for excellence in general practice: building confidence and competence by focusing on spectrum of care. *Journal of the American Veterinary Medical Association* 259 (5): 463–470.

19 Kipperman, B., Morris, P., and Rollin, B. (2018). Ethical dilemmas encountered by small animal veterinarians: characterisation, responses, consequences and beliefs regarding euthanasia. *Veterinary Record* 182 (19): 548.

2

Consultation Room Communication Strategies that Facilitate Dialogue on the Diagnostic Approach to Patient Care

Ryane E. Englar

2.1 Emergence of Communication as a Clinically Relevant Skill in Human Health Care

Prior to the 1990s, the content area of communication was largely excluded from programs designed to educate human healthcare providers. The soft sciences that supported relationship-centered care through the exploration of human interactions and other intangibles, such as thoughts and feelings, took a backseat to hard sciences of biology, chemistry, anatomy, and physiology. Clinicians were trained to apply clinical reasoning skills and evidence-based medicine to case management, but they were not taught how to communicate clinical findings, diagnoses, prognoses, or treatment recommendations to patients.

Healthcare educators assumed that experiences gained through on-the-job training would lead to competency in provider–patient communication. However, research that explored postgraduate clinical acumen identified deficiencies in clinician performance. Byrne and Long critically examined the consultation and expressed concern that "doctors become fixed in their style of interviewing soon after qualifying" [2]. The resultant publication, *Doctors Talking with Patients*, was among the first to suggest that doctors would benefit from continuing education that provided formalized feedback on how they conducted medical interviews.

Ten years later, a publication in the *British Medical Journal* confirmed that the traditional approach to education fell short in teaching medical students how to take a comprehensive patient history [3]. The investigators, Maguire et al., reassessed the communication styles of 36 clinicians 5 years after medical school and concluded that many seemed reluctant to expand upon patient history during the medical interview. In particular, the clinicians hesitated to explore psychosocial concerns in physically ill patients. In addition, Maguire et al. noted that closed-ended questions dominated the medical interview and patient statements were not always clarified to check for mutual understanding.

In a second publication, Maguire et al. reported on a cohort of 40 clinicians, who were also reassessed 5 years after graduating from medical school. Each clinician was observed to interview three patients. They were then tasked with disclosing the following pieces of information to each patient: physical exam and diagnostic findings, diagnosis, and prognosis. Although most provided the patient with the clinical findings and treatment options, few solicited the patient's perspective. In addition, few explained the etiology of the diagnosis or the anticipated patient outcome [4]. This led Maguire et al. to conclude that [4]:

> Some young doctors do discover for themselves how best to give patients information and advice, but most remain extremely incompetent. This is presumably because they get no training as students in this important aspect of clinical practice. This deficiency should be corrected, and competence tested before qualification to practice.

What concerned Maguire et al. most was that the clinicians in this second study were weakest in demonstrating skills that are of greatest importance to patients when they consider their overall satisfaction with health care [4–7]. Patients expected to be heard. They expected to be asked to share their perspectives concerning their diagnoses and their expectations for how care should proceed [5–7].

This expectation of patient-centered care represented a significant change from the historic approach of medical paternalism. As health care modernized, patients saw themselves as essential members of their healthcare teams who had to advocate for their rights to be determinants in their case outcomes [8].

Research demonstrates that shared decision-making in health care contributes to improved clinical outcomes, including, but not limited to patient satisfaction and increased connectivity to the provider, a greater likelihood that the patient will listen to and comply with the provider's treatment recommendations, better prognosis and management of an illness, fewer patient care costs, and a lower likelihood that a patient will initiate litigation against a provider [8–14].

Regulatory bodies for medical institutions began to see this correlation between improved clinical outcomes and the interpersonal elements of case management. This inspired curricular revision to promote the value of teaching clinical communication to student clinicians [8, 15]. The 1990s experienced the biggest wave of curricular reform designed to embed interpersonal skills within healthcare education. The Institute for International Medical Education (IIME), General Medical Council (GMC), Liaison Committee on Medical Education, Committee on Accreditation of Canadian Medical Schools (CACMS), Association of American Medical Colleges (AAMC), and the Association of Canadian Medical Colleges (ACMC) developed guidelines for effective communication training [15–18].

In addition, several regulatory bodies, including the Accreditation Council for Graduate Medical Education (ACGME), adjusted their prerequisites for new graduates, requiring them to demonstrate competence in communication [15, 16]. The ACGME has taken it a step further by outlining specific communication skills that are considered essential for clinical practice [18, 19]. These include effective listening, questioning to gather individualized data about the patient, delivery of information when explaining and planning in the consultation, counseling of patients, and decision-making that considers patient preference. Furthermore, communication is also assessed as a core competency on the United States Medical Licensing Examination (USMLE) [8, 15].

Because communication is no longer an optional component of medical curricula, human healthcare educators have been tasked to integrate this content area into student training. However, how best to deliver the content and where within the curriculum to do so has been the subject of debate, resulting in immense variability among programs [9, 20–22].

2.2 The Evolution of Communication in Veterinary Health Care

Effective communication is not just essential to building the provider–patient relationship in human health care. Veterinarians also need to connect with clients to expedite patient care through shared decision-making [23].

Dialogue facilitates next steps in case management. Clients who feel heard and accepted as essential members of the healthcare team are more likely to understand the need for diagnostic tests, invest in patient care, and comply with treatment recommendations [12–14, 24].

Missteps in communication are obstacles to patient care and a leading cause of client-initiated complaints to veterinary state licensing boards throughout the United States. Ineffective communication also has been associated with a high incidence of veterinary negligence claims in the United Kingdom [21] and Canada [25]. The risk of litigation is greatest among recent graduates. Up to 10% of newly licensed veterinarians have a claim filed against them within their first year of practice [21].

New graduates experience a steep learning curve as they transition from veterinary college into clinical practice [26]. To facilitate their success during this "make or break" period [26], veterinary educators once concentrated on book knowledge and technical skills [27]. Much like human healthcare educators, veterinary professors had not emphasized life skills or communication [28].

It was assumed that veterinarians only needed knowledge to deliver effective, expedient health care. However, many recent graduates reported feeling unprepared for the relationships that they needed to foster with clients to effectively practice medicine [29]. Many expressed concerns about connecting with clients, particularly those who challenged their recommendations. Specific content areas that seemed particularly problematic were the delivery of bad news [30, 31] and how to navigate clinical cases in which cost of care was prohibitive.

New graduates were not the only members of the veterinary profession to express concerns about deficiencies in interpersonal skills. Employers of new graduates also expressed concern that many entered clinical practice without understanding how to relate to and bond with their clients. This was especially troubling to employers who ranked interpersonal skills over knowledge when asked what they were looking for in associate veterinarians and which attributes translated into successful veterinary practice [32, 33]. Pet owners agree that it matters less how much a veterinarian knows and more that they are perceived to care. When considering whether to partner with a new veterinarian, pet owners prioritize interpersonal skills, specifically their ability to communicate [20, 34].

Concerns about the readiness of new graduates to deliver relationship-centered care have not gone unnoticed by veterinary educators or accrediting bodies. In the late 1990s, some veterinary educators inserted opportunities for student role-play into the curriculum to practice communication skills. This was in large part a response to the push for curricular reform by the American Veterinary Medical Association (AVMA), the American Animal

Hospital Association (AAHA), and the American Association of Veterinary Medical Colleges (AAVMC) [34].

In 2000, the Ontario Veterinary College (OVC) was among the first to incorporate simulated clients (SCs) within the curriculum [35, 36]. The United Kingdom and Ireland followed suit shortly thereafter [21, 37]. Simulated clients are trained actors that reproduce real-life clinical scenarios within mock consultation rooms to facilitate communication training.

Communication is now a part of the core curriculum in the British Isles and the Netherlands [21, 38, 39], and veterinary students can no longer graduate from the OVC or the Royal Veterinary College of Veterinary Surgeons without competence in communication [37, 39, 40]. Other universities, including the Atlantic Veterinary College of the University of Prince Edward Island, have incorporated communication training into electives [41].

In 2002, the North American Veterinary Medical Education Consortium was launched by the AAVMC to develop guidelines for communication training [42, 43]. This momentum paved the way for US-based colleges of veterinary medicine, including Colorado State University, Michigan State University, Washington State University, and Western University of Health Science's College of Veterinary Medicine to modify preexisting programs [44–46].

The AVMA Council on Education (COE) now requires that communication be taught in all accredited colleges of veterinary medicine. However, there is inconsistency in terms of which content is offered by each college and how that content is delivered. For the past 15 years, veterinary educators have experimented with faculty and guest lectures, small group discussions, Web-based video learning, peer-assisted learning, role-play with SCs, communications-based objective structured clinical examinations (OSCEs), clinical evaluation exercises, and video review of consultations with clients [47–54].

While there is no universal approach to communication training, many veterinary educators have found value in experiential learning because it promotes personal and professional growth through opportunities to formulate, deliver, and receive feedback, and reflect upon one's performance [42, 55, 56]. Receiving feedback from colleagues inspires self-awareness as learners consider their strengths as well as specific opportunity areas for growth [42, 50, 55, 57–60].

2.3 Communication Skills That Are Essential to Diagnosis-Making

As students transition from their preclinical to clinical year and then graduate from clinical year into clinical practice, they quickly find that a new breed of client awaits them in the consultation room. Today's clients are informed. They have access to information at their fingertips that past generations never had, and they apply what they know now to what they carry forward into the future as opinions, thoughts, ideas, and perspectives.

Our clients are perhaps our best resource in the consultation room. We may be the experts about medicine, but our clients are experts when it comes to their pets. We are dependent upon our clients to relay key historical details about the patient. We are responsible for interpreting the patient history and physical exam findings to develop a patient-specific plan, but our clients determine whether diagnostic and treatment plans move forward. Clients are partners in health care delivery. To achieve expected patient outcomes, clients must buy into, comply with, and adhere to our recommendations. This requires us to communicate recommendations in a way that inspires shared decision-making and relationship-centered care.

A variety of consultation models have been developed to identify key communication skills that facilitate case management. The Calgary–Cambridge model identifies over 70 communication skills and is widely used to train present-day medical students [16, 36, 51, 61, 62] (Figure 2.1).

This model subdivides the consultation into the following sequential tasks [64, 65]:

- initiating the session
- gathering information
- explaining and planning
- closing the session.

Two additional tasks span all stages of the consultation [51, 61, 66]:

- building the relationship
- providing structure.

These tasks are essentially bookends: they package the consultation into an experience that blends medicine with social and psychological elements [66]. Building the relationship acknowledges the importance of connectivity between provider and patient. Providing structure reiterates that both physicians and patients benefit from knowing what to expect during the consultation in terms of how the consultation will flow.

As of 2014, the Calgary–Cambridge model has served as the backbone of communication training for over half of medical programs in the United Kingdom [67, 68]. The model (Figure 2.2) is also popular in Canada and the United States and has been translated for use in undergraduate and postgraduate education throughout Europe in an expanded format [67].

The expanded framework as depicted in Figure 2.2 integrates the process – what is happening in a consultation, in

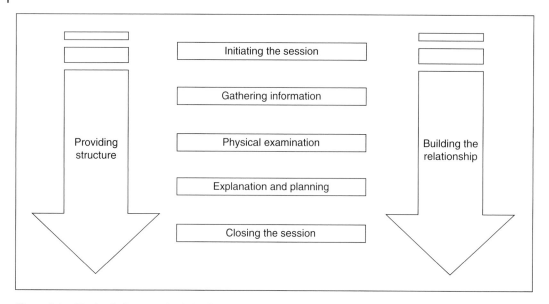

Figure 2.1 The basic framework of the Calgary-Cambridge Guides. *Source:* Reprinted with permission from the original work: Kurtz et al. [62]. Reprinted with permission from the most recent work: Adams and Kurtz [63, p. 25].

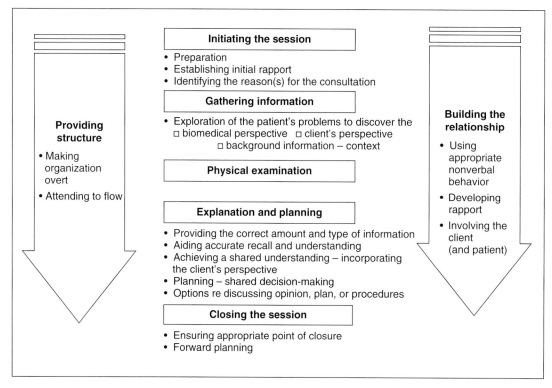

Figure 2.2 The expanded framework of the Calgary-Cambridge Guides. *Source:* Reprinted with permission from: Adams and Kurtz [63, p. 26].

the moment – with appropriate objectives for each task. Each objective can be achieved through one or more communication skills. Those skills that consistently apply to introducing, obtaining consent for, and proceeding with the diagnostic plan include:

- using easy-to-understand (nonmedical) language
- checking in

- assessing knowledge
- signposting
- addressing cost of care.

These same skills can be applied to the practice of veterinary medicine. In fact, the Calgary–Cambridge model was adapted for use by veterinarians by Radford et al. in 2002 [16, 36, 69].

2.4 Concepts of Health Literacy and Compliance

Human patients and veterinary clients cannot make informed decisions about their health without health literacy, that is, "the capacity to obtain, process, and understand basic health information and services" [70]. This capacity is shaped by educational background, cognition, critical thinking, language, speech, speech comprehension, culture, value systems, social identities, social skills, socioeconomic backgrounds, emotional states, and visual and auditory acuity [71, 72].

Collectively, these attributes facilitate the understanding and processing of health-related information and services so that human patients and veterinary clients make thoughtful decisions with respect to their needs, goals for patient care, and anticipated outcomes [71]. In this respect, health literacy is the bridge between making medical recommendations and implementing them [73].

Providers and clients must be able to share information in a way that is mutually accessible and understood. If clinicians overestimate health literacy and make assumptions that their explanations are clear, then clients may leave the consultation room without fully understanding the present situation or its implications [74–76].

Clinicians may overestimate health literacy based on the client's appearance or educational attainment when in fact the highest grade level achieved in school is an inaccurate measure [74, 77–80].

Health literacy is a global concern, even among developed countries [81, 82]. Over one-third of adults in the United States are estimated to have average to below-average health literacy [74, 83, 84]. Roughly one out of every four Americans read at or lower than a fifth-grade level [85]. The average American reads at an eighth-grade level [74, 86]. Yet over 75% of medical brochures are written at the level of a high school or undergraduate reader [74, 85].

Furthermore, what might be considered simple tasks by healthcare providers may challenge even those with intermediate health literacy. For example, many human patients incorrectly interpret what it means when they are told to take medications at mealtimes [74, 87]. They also may not be able to determine from a drug label what potential adverse reactions to watch out for [74].

When health literacy is poor, human patients (and presumably veterinary clients) lack the information they need to advocate for themselves [81]. They may not make use of available health information or services; they may not even know that these services exist [81]. Poor health literacy is associated with poor health outcomes [88]. Those with poor health literacy are more likely to [71, 74, 85, 88–91]:

- skip immunizations, recheck appointments, and cancer screenings
- misread medical forms and informed consent documents
- misunderstand prescription use, appointment, and discharge instructions
- experience acute illness and/or develop chronic disease
- confuse basic principles about their health conditions and treatment recommendations
- exhibit poor compliance and adherence to medical plans
- experience relapse or recurrence of medical ailments
- present to emergency rooms and/or be admitted to the hospital
- experience medical errors.

The use of medical jargon compounds these challenges [88]. Patients do not always understand medical terms, or they may misinterpret them. For example, patients who sustain traumatic injuries often ask the medical team if they have sustained a fracture or a break [88, 92]. A 1994 study by Peckham disclosed that most patients see these two conditions as distinct, and nearly three out of four patients believe that fractures are associated with better outcomes than breaks [92].

More than a decade later, little has changed [88, 93]. About 84% of patients still believe that breaks are not synonymous with fractures, and 68% believe that fractures are less serious [93].

As providers, the disconnect between what we know and what our patients know is problematic. Pamphlets may be handed out that define key terms; however, few patients read what has been provided and those that do often fail to retain takeaway knowledge [93]. To improve print literacy, we need to address readability. We can do so by addressing font size and style, layout, clarity, and visual appeal [88, 94].

Healthcare providers need to work harder to overcome the limitations of oral literacy. Oral literacy is particularly challenged by situations that require urgent care. Patients that present for triage at emergency rooms benefit more from an expert-in-charge than a guide-on-the-side in their immediate time of need. Life-saving interventions take precedence over partnership and clear, methodical dialogue exchange between provider and patient. Emergency and critical care scenarios are also often emotionally charged. These emotional undercurrents may cloud the patient's understanding of the situation or their ability to process complex words. Patients may not understand that hemorrhage is synonymous with bleeding or that myocardial infarction is the same as a heart attack [95]. Hearing that they have a contusion might incite panic when in fact it just means that they have a bruise.

Language comprehension also impacts oral literacy [85, 88]. Those for whom English is a second language may not understand what is being shared with them, yet they may be embarrassed by what they don't know or they may be unable to formulate clarifying questions [88, 96].

When patients do not understand what has been presented to them, they may fill in the blanks with what they believe to be true. They may also unknowingly consult inaccurate sources of medical information in a day and age where virtually anything can be found on the World Wide Web [88]. This information may misdirect patients as to whether they should seek medical attention or if they should comply with healthcare provider recommendations [88].

Veterinary clients are no different from human patients. When clients do not receive information in a way that they can understand or relate to, they will seek it elsewhere [97]. The Internet is frequented by pet owners who seek knowledge [98]. A 2012 study by Kogan et al. found that one-quarter of Internet users search at least once per month for information about pet health [99]. Just under 14% conduct weekly pet health-related searches [99]. One-third of these searches are attempts by pet owners to clarify information that was shared with them by the veterinary team [100].

Veterinarians report that two-thirds of clients bring Internet-based resources into the consultation room [98]. Veterinarians are concerned that much of the material that is accessed by clients online is inaccurate and may confuse them further [98]. Despite this, team members rarely direct or redirect clients to vetted sites [100, 101]. Yet the validity of information that is accessible by clients on the Internet is often questionable or incomplete [102]. Consider, for instance, the topic of breed-related risks by dogs undergoing anesthesia. A 2008 study by Hofmeister et al. found that nearly one-third of web sites about veterinary anesthesia disclosed breed sensitivities yet warnings were not evidence-based [102]. They were purely anecdotal [102]. Even so, these claims prompted clients to believe that Boxers, Afghan Hounds, Anatolian Shepherd Dogs, Border Terriers, and Tibetan Spaniels were more susceptible to anesthetic reactions [102].

Inaccurate, yet accessible information, is concerning to veterinarians, particularly when it delays patient care. Clients are apt to consult the Internet before contacting the clinic to establish if a sick or injured pet needs to be seen [101].

Clients may also conduct Internet searches so that they can be better informed [98]. If clients do not find information that supports the veterinary team's recommendations, then they are less likely to comply with the prescribed care plan. Compliance breakdowns are common in veterinary practice and often due to information cramming: veterinarians often feel that they must deliver an exceptionally large amount of information to clients in a limited time frame [103].

2.5 Using Easy-to-Understand (Nonmedical) Language

Health literacy influences the language that we use to deliver patient care recommendations to clients [104]. Using medical jargon to explain case management does little to promote our cause [104]. Instead, jargon may deter clients from engaging in open dialogue about treatment options [104]. Clients may ultimately decline care based upon lack of understanding rather than informed decision-making [104].

Consider how the following phrases, spoken by veterinary team members, challenge the client's comprehension when they client is not fluent in medical jargon:

- "We are going to perform venipuncture."
- "We are going to perform a comprehensive blood count."
- "We are going to perform a serum biochemistry profile."
- "We are going to take radiographs."
- "We are going to run an electrocardiogram."
- "We are going to perform echocardiography."

If these terms are meaningless to the client, then how does the client determine which test to authorize and assess the merit of each? We are essentially asking the client to make a choice about case management that is a shot in the dark.

It is no different than when I present my car to a mechanic for automobile issues only to be told that the camshaft, sway bar link, or intake manifold gasket needs to be replaced. No matter how hard I try to picture the problem, I have no frame of reference to assist with decision-making. I either must proceed with blind trust or decline care on the basis that I do not understand what is being asked of me and therefore it cannot be that critical. Jargon makes information-sharing less relatable and therefore less believable [104].

Rather than risk the client questioning the veracity of the information that has been shared, why not incorporate easy-to-understand language into the consultation? Let us revisit the previous list of diagnostic recommendations and reword each item in a way that may be more easily understood:

- Original: "We are going to perform venipuncture."
  - Revision A: "We are going to perform bloodwork."
  - Revision B: "We are going to draw blood."
- Original: "We are going to perform a comprehensive blood count."
  - Revision A: "We are going to take a look at Bailey's red and white blood cell counts."
  - Revision B: "We are going to perform a blood test that looks at Bailey's red and white blood cell counts."

- Original: "We are going to perform a serum biochemistry profile."
  - Revision A: "We are going to evaluate Lowell's liver and kidney values as well as his electrolytes."
  - Revision B: "We are going to perform a blood test that looks at Lowell's liver and kidney values as well as his electrolytes."
- Original: "We are going to perform a fecal float."
  - Revision: "We are going to examine Draco's stool."
- Original: "We are going to take radiographs."
  - Revision A: "We are going to image Darcy's chest."
  - Revision B: "We are going to take x-rays of Darcy's chest."
- Original: "We are going to run an electrocardiogram."
  - Revision: "We are going to run an ECG, a non-painful test that measures the electrical activity of Pemberly's heart."
- Original: "We are going to perform echocardiography."
  - Revision: "We are going to ultrasound Dolly's heart."

These revisions demonstrate how changes in word choice make health care more accessible [104]. If the client more clearly understands what is being talked about, then the client is set up for success in decision-making.

In addition to incorporating easy-to-understand language into the consultation, why not also include a rationale for each diagnostic test? In other words, why are you advising that this test be performed? What information might this test reveal that will be benefit the patient? How will test results help us to better understand the patient's condition and increase the likelihood of a positive patient outcome?

If clients do not understand why a diagnostic test is necessary, then they may be more likely to decline that assessment. It's not enough to say, "Do this test because I am advising you to." Clients expect to play a central role in decision-making. For clients to make a choice that aligns with our recommendations, they must first understand why that diagnostic or therapeutic approach is best for the patient.

Instead of assuming that clients know why tests are being performed, give them a brief overview of what type of information each test will yield. For example:

- "We are going to draw blood to get a better sense of how Nina's organs are functioning."
- "We are going to perform a CBC, which means that we will examine Bailey's red and white blood cell counts. This will tell us whether Bailey is anemic or fighting off an infection."
- "We are going to perform a chemistry panel. This type of bloodwork will tell us if Lowell's kidneys and liver can tolerate the medication that I would like to prescribe to reduce his pain and improve his mobility."

- "We are going to examine Draco's stool. This will let us know if Draco would benefit from being dewormed because there are a lot of parasites that pups can get that could cause him a lot of problems. It would be good to know which, if any, are present so that we can prescribe medicine to eliminate them from his body."
- "We are going to take X-rays of Darcy's chest. This will help us to determine if there is an underlying reason that could be causing her cough, such as an enlarged heart."
- "We are going to run an ECG, which means that we will be looking at the electrical activity of Pemberly's heart. This will help us to evaluate the rhythm of Pemberly's heart and whether it is beating adequately."
- "We are going to ultrasound Dolly's heart. This means that we will get a more complete picture of Dolly's heart. If Dolly's heart is enlarged, then we will be able to see how this change is impacting blood flow. That will help us to determine if Dolly would benefit from medication to increase her heart's efficiency and reduce the stress on it as it pumps."

Being clear about your recommendations helps clients understand the value of diagnostic testing [104]. They begin to consider the utility of each test rather than assuming they are unnecessary add-ons that pad the bill.

Explaining diagnostic procedures to clients clearly may challenge healthcare students. In the classroom, student doctors are trained to use medical jargon when discussing clinical cases with colleagues. Yet the same training that teaches them to replace the word *vomit* with *emesis* detracts from their ability to connect with clients. Student doctors must learn how to flex between doctor-speak and client-friendly language that better suits the consultation room. To facilitate this transition, educators might task students with relaying diagnostic recommendations to simulated clients who can then provide feedback. Students require practice with word choice to discover their own unique phraseology. Their words must be accurate and authentic, yet easy to understand by clients who expect to play a role in case management.

2.6 Checking in

Checking in is a way to assess the client's understanding of what you have shared so that you can clarify anything that may be unclear [105]. Think of a "check in" as an intentional break in the exchange of information to see if the client is still with you [105]. This prevents us from reaching the end of the consultation, only to have the client say, "I didn't follow that. Can you start over?" [105]

The simplest form of "checking in" is a thoughtful pause [105].

Let's see what that might look like in practice:

Background Information:

> You are an associate veterinarian. You have just been presented with an eight-year-old male castrated Labrador retriever named Dilbert whose owner reports weight gain despite no apparent changes in feeding or caloric intake. Dilbert has preexisting osteoarthritis secondary to unilateral cranial cruciate ligament rupture that was never repaired surgically.

Clinical Conversation:

VETERINARIAN: "Given what you have shared with me about Dilbert – that he is gaining weight even though there have been no changes in diet – I am concerned about his thyroid. Dogs of his age are at greater risk of developing hypothyroidism, that is, a sluggish thyroid. If his thyroid is not working at full capacity, that could account for his weight gain. I agree that he is already having mobility issues because of his painful joints, so any additional weight is going to make it that much harder for him to get around. I think it's time that we consider assessing his thyroid function."

You pause.

The client nods to demonstrate understanding before you move on to the next segment of the consultation.

VETERINARIAN: "We need to first confirm my suspicions through bloodwork. Several blood tests together will tell us if Dilbert does in fact have hypothyroidism. If he does, the good news is that we can manage him successfully with medication."

You pause again.

The client nods to demonstrate understanding before you move on to discuss cost of care.

Incidentally, this same skill of checking in can be employed in clinical practice to disclose other case management recommendations, including, but not limited to treatment options [105]. Let us fast-forward the case of Dilbert and assume that diagnostic tests confirmed that the patient is hypothyroid. Let us explore how checking in may facilitate a conversation about treatment options.

Clinical Conversation:

VETERINARIAN: "If we do not treat Dilbert's sluggish thyroid, then he will continue to gain weight even though you are not overfeeding him. As you've already shared with me today and as was evident during my physical exam, he is already having mobility issues due to painful joints. Any additional weight is going to make it that much harder for him to get around. That tells us that we need to start treating his condition right away."

You pause.

The client nods to demonstrate understanding before you move on to the next segment of the consultation.

VETERINARIAN: "We cannot cure Dilbert's hypothyroidism, but we can give him medication that better regulates his metabolism. That will help to keep his thyroid in check."

You pause again and wait for the client to respond with oral or nonverbal feedback.

In this way, pausing spaces out the conversation into a series of bite-sized chunks that the client can more easily follow.

Check-ins sometimes require more than a pause [105]. At times, a phrase or statement may feel more natural to you. "Check-in" statements include [105]:

- "Does that make sense?"
- "How does that sound?"
- "Is that reasonable?"
- "Are you with me?"

Let us revisit the same clinical scenario of the hypothyroid dog, Dilbert, to demonstrate effective use of check-in statements.

Clinical Conversation:

VETERINARIAN: "If we do not treat Dilbert's sluggish thyroid, then he will continue to gain weight even though you are not overfeeding him. As you've already shared with me today and as was evident during my physical exam, he is already having mobility issues due to painful joints. Any additional weight is going to make it that much harder for him to get around. That tells us that we need to start treating his condition right away. Does that make sense?"

CLIENT: "Yes."

VETERINARIAN: "We cannot cure Dilbert's hypothyroidism, but we can give him medication that speeds up his metabolism to overcome these issues. The medication is a way of keeping his thyroid in check. How does that sound to you?"

CLIENT: "That sounds reasonable to me. Where do we begin? What's next for Dilbert?"

Check-ins are a valuable tool to assess the client's level of understanding with regards to your recommendations. Check-ins allow the client to speak up if something is not making sense [105]. For instance, let us revisit the conversation concerning treatment options for Dilbert.

> VETERINARIAN: "We cannot cure Dilbert's hypothyroidism, but we can give him medication that better regulates his metabolism. That will help to keep his thyroid in check.". How does that sound to you?"

Let us assume that the client is not on the same page and needs further assistance. A check-in offers the client an opportunity to say, "Hold on a second, time-out, what are you saying? Help me to understand." [105]

For instance, Dilbert's owner may respond to your recommendation that you treat the dog's condition medically with one of the following statements:

> CLIENT: "Are you saying that this is something we're going to have to manage forever?"
> CLIENT: "So you're saying that once he starts this medication, he can't go off it?"
> CLIENT: "Hold up. Are you saying that Dilbert must take this medication for the rest of his life?"

Allowing the client to speak up gives you a chance to hear their perspective [105, 106]:

- What concerns the client most?
- What is on the client's mind?
- What is their reaction to the news that you have just shared?
- What lingering questions might they have about your recommendations?
- What questions might they have about following through on your recommendations?
- Are they on board with your recommendations? Why or why not?
- Is the client reluctant to proceed with your proposed diagnostic and/or treatment plan? If so, what reservations might they have?

As you explain your diagnostic recommendations to the client, incorporate check-ins so that the client has time to process and question the plan [105]. The client may ask you to reword or re-explain a concept if it did not make sense to them on the first go-around [105]. The client may paraphrase what you shared in a way that resonates with them to check for mutual understanding [105]. The client may get figuratively stuck on a concept and need your help to extract themselves [105]. The client may simply need to reiterate the plan to be sure they understand it fully [105].

Any of these outcomes is possible. Client questions may take the form of [105]:

- "Are you saying that we have to do this test first or else. . .?"
- "Are you saying that we need to prioritize this test because. . .?"
- "So, you're saying that we need to start with this blood test, but that we may have to do additional testing?"
- "So, you're saying that we need to test the urine because if we don't, then we could miss something?"
- "So, you're saying that we have lots of options available to us, but that if Dilbert were your dog, then you would. . .?"

Some veterinarians have a knee-jerk reaction to questions from clients. They may feel that the client is questioning their knowledge or expertise. In most cases, the client is simply asking clarifying questions to better understand the situation and the options that have been presented to them.

Learn to not only accept the client's line of questioning, but to welcome it. Check-ins offer an ideal space in the consultation for free exchange of dialogue so that everyone can be heard.

2.7 Assessing the Client's Knowledge

The veterinary client represents a wealth of information and is therefore an integral member of the team, but what specific knowledge do they bring to the table?

On the surface, knowledge may seem easy to discern. Either someone knows something, or they do not. But is it ever as simple as that? There are many layers of knowledge, as demonstrated in Figure 2.3 below.

Sometimes what we think we know, we may not. Sometimes what we think others might know, they may not. On the other hand, sometimes we think that others should *not* know something, yet they do, or they expect us to know something that we do *not*.

These shades of gray make it difficult to know where knowledge begins and ends. Yet we need to consider our client's knowledge – what they know, what they perceive they know, and what they do not know – to navigate the consultation effectively and efficiently.

Not all clients come to us with the same background information [107]. Some clients may be well-versed when it comes to routine health care, wellness, and preventive medicine. Maybe they have owned and raised animals before. Maybe they are familiar with certain diagnostic tests such as annual heartworm and fecal testing or

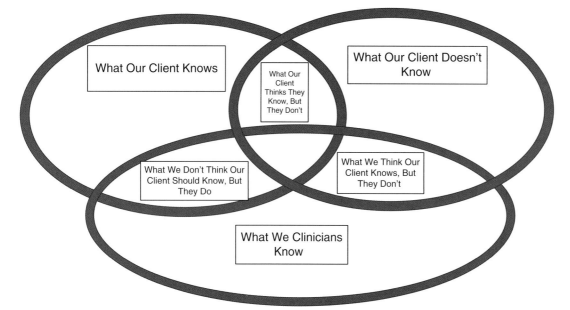

Figure 2.3 Intricacies of knowledge in the consultation room: a consideration of what the client and clinician bring to the table and where their knowledge overlaps.

pre-anesthetic screens prior to their pet undergoing dental prophylaxis.

Other clients may have never owned pets. Or maybe they have, but a different species than the one that they are presenting to you today. Or maybe they have never encountered this clinical presentation. Maybe they have never dealt with a vomiting dog or a cat in respiratory distress. Maybe this is all new territory for them to discover, and they need you to be their guide. In this case, what might seem obvious to us as veterinarians may not be so apparent to them. It is up to us to figure out what they know and how to apply that knowledge to the situation at hand because what clients have experienced in the past influences their approach to patient care [107].

Assessing your client's knowledge is a skill. You should assess your client's knowledge every time that you present a diagnostic or therapeutic recommendation, or any time that a diagnosis is made [107]. Consider the following phrases that assist us with this communication skill [107]:

- "Are you familiar with [insert diagnostic procedure]?"
  - Example: "Are you familiar with CT scans?"
- "Have you heard of [insert diagnostic procedure]?"
  - Example: "Have you heard of MRIs?"
- "Did you know that we can [insert diagnostic procedure]?"
  - Example: "Did you know that we can ultrasound the heart to look for abnormal patterns of blood flow?"
- "What do you know about [insert organ] function and the blood tests we can run to evaluate [insert organ] health?"

- Example: "What do you know about kidney function and the blood tests we can run to evaluate kidney health?"

Assessing the client's knowledge provides us with a starting point for clinical conversations. This skill also allows us to check our client's knowledge against our own [107]. Clients may think they know more about something than they do. Maybe the client has incorrect or misguided information that requires clarification or correction.

If we take the time to assess the client's knowledge, then we can correct information before true misunderstandings arise [107]. For example, maybe a client thinks that the only test needed to diagnose diabetic ketoacidosis (DKA) in a cat is blood glucose. By assessing the client's knowledge, we can learn what the client thinks they know and correct it so that the client does not feel blindsided when we expand our diagnostic arsenal to incorporate urinalysis. Assessing the client's knowledge paves the way for an exchange of information that clarifies what needs to be done for the patient and why. This allows everything to be out on the table and discussed freely so that critical questions can be asked before you both elect to proceed with diagnostics.

2.8 Signposting

Consultations are rarely simple. Clients often present patients to us with more than one presenting complaint. Patient histories are frequently complex, and clinical signs may be unrelated. This may result in a convoluted exchange of dialogue with a client who departs the clinic feeling unsure or even overwhelmed. Clients may grapple with several questions as they are asked to weigh in on decision-making and consent to diagnostic testing [108]:

- What information do we know about the patient?
- What information will we gain from diagnostic testing?
- Which diagnostic tests should be performed and in what order?
- Is it appropriate to stage diagnostic tests? Why or why not?
- Which diagnostic tests should be performed *now*?
- Which diagnostic tests can be performed *later*?
- What is the time frame in which a decision should be made?
- What is the *short-term* impact on the patient if a decision is delayed?
- What is the *long-term* impact on the patient if a decision is delayed?
- What can the client afford to do *today*?
- What can the client afford to do *tomorrow*?
- What happens to the patient if financial constraints preclude testing?
- Are there any other options available to the client?

These questions are difficult to answer, and clients look to us to guide decision-making. We can assist our clients in their journey through the consultation by creating a roadmap that outlines what they can expect to encounter along the way [108]. After all, we understand how to make sense of the patient's clinical signs and formulate an approach to case management that will clarify the patient's diagnosis [108]. We know what to test for, when to test, in what order to test, how to test, and why to test.

Mapping out the consultation through signposting is a communication skill that provides clients with the sense of direction they may need to move forward [108]. Signposting provides structure that clients may need to hold onto, particularly during challenging conversations about complex medical maladies [108]. Think of it as outlining the diagnostic plan in the order in which tests should happen.

Because they prioritize the plan, mapping statements often begin with ordinal numbers [108]:

- "First. . ."
- "Second. . ."
- "Third. . .".

For example, consider the case of a three-year-old male castrated Standard Poodle, Gizmo, who presents to you for evaluation of a third bout of waxing/waning diarrhea over the course of the past two months. During episodes, Gizmo exhibits depression, lethargy, and inappetence. Stressful situations, such as being kenneled in a boarding facility or being moved cross-country, appear to trigger the episodes. The first two crises were managed with supportive care; however, this third episode has piqued your interest in performing a diagnostic work-up for hypoadrenocorticism.

Let us explore how you might utilize signposting to share your diagnostic recommendations:

- "*First*, we will draw blood to evaluate Gizmo's baseline organ function and electrolytes. Because I am suspicious that Gizmo may have Addison's disease, I suspect that he might have an elevated potassium and low sodium. In addition, I might expect to see slight increases in his kidney values."
- "*Second*, if our suspicions are correct, then we will need to perform an ACTH-stimulation test – a blood test – to measure cortisol levels. Cortisol is a stress hormone that is not produced in sufficient amounts in dogs with Addison's disease."
- "*Third*, we'll chat about any abnormal findings. If Gizmo truly has Addison's, then I would expect to see undetectable or very low cortisol levels."

Signposting may also include the use of transitional words or phrases to describe the diagnostic plan [108]:

- "Initially. . ."
- "Next. . ."
- "Then. . .".

For example:

- "*Initially*, we will draw blood to evaluate Gizmo's baseline organ function and electrolytes. Because I am suspicious that Gizmo may have Addison's disease, I suspect that he might have an elevated potassium and low sodium. In addition, I might expect to see slight increases in his kidney values."
- "*Next*, if our suspicions are correct, then we will need to perform an ACTH-stimulation test – a blood test – to measure cortisol levels. Cortisol is a stress hormone that is not produced in sufficient amounts in dogs with Addison's disease."
- "*Then* we'll chat about any abnormal findings. If Gizmo truly has Addison's, then I would expect to see undetectable or very low cortisol levels."

Other appropriate transitional words or phrases that structure the chronology of the consultation include [108]:

- Before
- After
- Afterward
- At the end.

For example:

- "*Before* we get ahead of ourselves, we need to start by evaluating Gizmo's baseline organ function and electrolytes. Because I am suspicious that Gizmo may have Addison's disease, I suspect that he might have an elevated potassium and low sodium. In addition, I might expect to see slight increases in his kidney values."
- "*After* reviewing the results of Gizmo's baseline blood tests, we may need to perform an additional study. This requires another blood draw so that we can run an ACTH-stimulation test to measure cortisol levels. Cortisol is a stress hormone that is not produced in sufficient amounts in dogs with Addison's disease."
- "*Afterward*, we'll chat about any abnormal findings. If Gizmo truly has Addison's, then I would expect to see undetectable or very low cortisol levels."
- "*At the end* of testing, we can initiate treatment if Gizmo is truly Addisonian. He will need to stay on medication for life; however, I am confident that we can manage his condition well."

Signposting is an effective way to structure dialogue so that clients have a very clear picture in their minds about next steps [108]. In order for clients to agree to our diagnostic plan, they need to first see for themselves how the plan will unfold and in what order [108].

2.9 Addressing the Cost of Care

Most pet owners in both the United States and Canada do not have pet health insurance; therefore, they pay out of pocket for veterinary care [34, 109, 110]. As a result, cost of care often influences decision-making surrounding case management [34, 109, 110]. Cost of care may limit a client's ability to present their pet to the veterinary clinic for evaluation, decrease options for care, reduce quality of care, and necessitate economic euthanasia [111, 112].

Financial constraints stress practitioners and clients alike. Practitioners are conflicted because they have taken an oath to preserve animal health and welfare and alleviate suffering yet cannot deliver services free of charge [111]. At the same time, pet owners expect animal health to be prioritized over cost of care but find themselves unable to receive care in the face of financial constraints [113].

Clients look to the veterinary team to initiate conversations about cost; however, discussions of costs in the consultation room infrequently take place within companion animal practice [113]. It is not uncommon for clients to depart the exam room uninformed about veterinary care costs [111]. In a 2009 study by Coe et al., only 58 out of 200 (29%) appointments addressed cost of care, and only 28 out of 200 (14%) referenced a written estimate [109]. Discussions about cost were more likely to occur when decisions were required concerning diagnostic testing [109]. Cost-focused discussions were associated with longer appointment times [109].

Surveyed veterinarians have acknowledged the following reasons for failing to initiate conversations about cost [111]:

- time constraints
- forgetfulness/out of sight, out of mind
- fear that the client might feel pressured
- the client did not initiate the conversation
- lack of relevance to the presenting complaint (e.g., the patient presented for a wellness visit)
- perceptions that discussing cost would not change delivery of care or the case outcome.

Reluctance to broach the topic of cost leads to clients with unmet needs that may detract from the veterinarian–client–patient relationship (VCPR) [113, 114]. A 2007 study by Coe et al. reported that even experienced veterinary clients who are familiar with costs of routine care expect upfront discussions about pricing [113]. When costs are not acknowledged or addressed, clients may get in over their heads. As one survey respondent shared, "People do not know what they're getting into in a lot of cases before it is past what they can afford" [113]. Emotionally charged cases complicate decision-making because "when you're emotionally upset. . ., it's easy to get pulled into things" [113]. Another respondent affirmed that ". . .people get caught in that emotional side of it and they get into financial situations that they can't handle because it wasn't really explained to them well enough" [113].

Clients expect to discuss cost in a meaningful context [113]. This requires veterinarians to share cost in tandem with prognosis. Furthermore, veterinarians must elicit the client's perspective when it comes to personal beliefs, values, expectations, and constraints. As one pet owner shared [113]:

> For my wife and I, we have got to be realistic. Like, we can't re-mortgage the house, can't do this, can't take out all the [registered retirement savings plan] just for a cat.

Veterinarians need to be open to hearing what clients can and cannot afford as well as what clients expect in terms of care:

- What are the client's expectations about diagnosis?
- What are the client's expectations about prognosis?
- Are the client's expectations realistic?
- Are the client's expectations reasonable?
- What are potential barriers to meeting those expectations?

- Have barriers to care been discussed with the client?
- If barriers arise, can they be overcome? If so, how?
- If barriers complicate treatment and cannot be overcome, then how will the care team (including the client) respond?

A frank dialogue is required before clients commit to care. Decision-making requires clients to be informed, and in order for clients to provide informed consent, they must know all likely outcomes. That includes how a patient might respond to diagnostic and/or therapeutic recommendations in best- and worst-case scenarios. If a client is going to consent to "x" dollars of diagnostic testing, then they need to be aware if follow-up tests may be indicated. For instance, in the case of a suspected foreign body ingestion, clients need to be prepared that one set of abdominal radiographs may not necessarily be diagnostic. Additional films may be indicated. In other words, taking one set of films *today* does not mean that radiographs will not be required *tomorrow*. Client preparedness is key to developing and maintaining trust in the VCPR. If clients know what to expect or what might transpire, then they are better able to budget or otherwise plan for potential patient outcomes.

Addressing cost of care is not easy. Veterinarians often express concern that clients think they are in this field because they are driven by money [113]. The reality is that many veterinarians feel undervalued by those who expect to receive cheap care. One DVM respondent in Coe's (2007) study shared that "our vaccine visits are undercharged, our spays and neuters are grossly undercharged, and then we've trained [clients] that they don't need pet health insurance because veterinary medicine is so cheap" [113].

Yet the more veterinarians steer away from conversations about cost of care, the more questions arise from the client's point of view. Clients may question if fees are being hidden or if veterinary recommendations are motivated by income [113]. If the connection is not made by the veterinary team that recommendations are in the best interests of the pet, regardless of cost, then clients may be less likely to consent to care whether they can afford it or not.

Initiate conversations about financing care. Be proactive. Address the elephant in the room. Acknowledge cost of care. Outline recommendations and explain their value [113]. Share why recommendations have been made and how they will contribute to delivery of health care. If a patient will benefit from a CBC, explain how. We know the answer to that question, but do our clients? Openly share rationales for diagnostic tests with clients: "The CBC will help us out by. . ."

Provide estimates. In some states, estimates are required by law. These written summaries ballpark what care is expected to cost and how costs may vary depending upon the patient's response to care. Estimates allow clients to see the full scope of what is being asked of them, and estimates can go hand in hand with discussions about the value of each test.

Elicit each client's perspective concerning the estimate:

- "What are your thoughts about what I have shared with you today?"
- "What, if any questions, might you have based upon what I have shared with you just now?"
- "Do you understand the diagnostic tests that I am recommending and how they will help Dobby?"
- "Are there any follow-up questions you might have to clarify why I'm advising that we begin with these tests?"
- "What are your thoughts about cost of care?"
- "Is this approach to Dobby's care within your budget?"
- "Are you comfortable with this approach to Dobby's care?"
- "Are you comfortable with how I have outlined the cost to manage Dobby in this manner?"
- "Based upon what I have shared with you, what can you afford today to manage Dobby's care?"
- "Is there a price point that we need to keep the bill for Dobby's care below?"
- "What concerns you most about cost of care?"
- "What can I do to assist with cost of care?"

Veterinarians often hear from clients, "I don't care what it costs," when typically "they're the ones that do" [113]. It pays to ask questions now before you get into conflict with clients later. When clients share that cost is no concern, address the comment head-on:

- "I appreciate your willingness to treat Petunia at all costs. I still want to outline my recommendations for her care along with pricing so that you can see what kinds of costs we are looking at."
- "I appreciate your commitment to Petunia's care. I still wish to provide you with an estimate so that you can see upfront what my recommendations will cost. I would feel more comfortable if you know what kinds of costs we are looking at and how these may add up over time."

Anticipate that gold standard care may not be feasible. Acknowledge and normalize this from the start and be prepared to provide alternative approaches to case management. Demonstrate empathy and regard. Withhold judgment and maintain an open mind so that you can engage in transparent dialogue:

- "I know that you weren't expecting to bring Patches in to see us today, so these costs may come as a surprise to you. Help me to know what is within reason for you to spend today so that we can come up with a plan that meets Patches' needs as well as your own."

- "How might we be able to customize care to address Patches' needs and your budget?"
- "What is within reason for us to achieve today?"

Financial discussions challenge veterinarians and clients alike because they may complicate delivery of health care. Yet they are essential to have before proceeding with care so that expectations are addressed out in the open and both sides know what, if any limitations, they are operating under. It may feel awkward to discuss cost of care, particularly if the veterinarian has prior experience with the client

declining care [113]. However, it is not appropriate to stop offering diagnostic or treatment options based upon our assumptions that what is affordable to a client remains static over time [113]. Assumptions pave the way to misunderstandings and fracture VCPRs.

Use each consultation as an opportunity to customize care. The only way we can do so is if we initiate conversations about cost in the exam room so that we better understand the needs of our clients and how best to prioritize care in alignment with budgetary constraints, if and when they arise.

References

1 Show, A. and Englar, R.E. (2018). Evaluating dog and cat owner preferences for Calgary-Cambridge communication skills: results of a questionnaire. *Journal of Veterinary Medical Education* 1–10.

2 Byrne PS. Doctors talking to patients: a study of the verbal behaviour of general practitioners consulting in their surgeries. Long BEL, Great Britain. Department of Health and Social S editors. London: H. M. Stationery Off.1976.

3 Maguire, P., Fairbairn, S., and Fletcher, C. (1986). Consultation skills of young doctors: I – Benefits of feedback training in interviewing as students persist. *British Medical Journal (Clinical Research Ed)* 292 (6535): 1573–1576.

4 Maguire, P., Fairbairn, S., and Fletcher, C. (1986). Consultation skills of young doctors: II – Most young doctors are bad at giving information. *British Medical Journal (Clinical Research Ed)* 292 (6535): 1576–1578.

5 Brody, D.S. (1980). The patient's role in clinical decision-making. *Annals of Internal Medicine* 93 (5): 718–722.

6 Haynes, R.B., Taylor, D.W., and Sackett, D.L. (1979). *Compliance in Health Care*. Baltimore: Baltimore: Johns Hopkins University Press.

7 Becker, M.H., Radius, S.M., Rosenstock, I.M. et al. (1978). Compliance with a medical regimen for asthma: a test of the health belief model. *Public Health Reports* 93 (3): 268–277.

8 Englar, R.E. (2020a). What do our clients understand? In: *The Evolution of the Doctor–Patient Relationship, Patient Autonomy, and Health Literacy. A Guide to Oral Communication in Veterinary Medicine*, 3–26. Sheffield, U.K.: 5m Publishing.

9 Kurtz, S.M., Silverman, J., Draper, J., and Silverman, J. (2005). *Teaching and Learning Communication Skills in Medicine*, 2e. Abingdon, Oxon, UK: Radcliffe Medical Press.

10 Little, P., Williamson, I., Warner, G. et al. (1997). Open randomised trial of prescribing strategies in managing sore throat. *BMJ* 314 (7082): 722–727.

11 Stewart, M., Brown, J.B., Donner, A. et al. (2000). The impact of patient-centered care on outcomes. *The Journal of Family Practice* 49 (9): 796–804.

12 Kaplan, S.H., Greenfield, S., and Ware, J.E. (1989). Assessing the effects of physician–patient interactions on the outcomes of chronic disease. *Medical Care* 27 (3): S110–S127.

13 Rost, K.M., Flavin, K.S., Cole, K., and McGill, J.B. (1991). Change in metabolic control and functional status after hospitalization. Impact of patient activation intervention in diabetic patients. *Diabetes Care* 14 (10): 881–889.

14 Fallowfield, L.J., Hall, A., Maguire, G.P., and Baum, M. (1990). Psychological outcomes of different treatment policies in women with early breast cancer outside a clinical trial. *British Medical Journal* 301 (6752): 575–580.

15 Rider, E.A., Hinrichs, M.M., and Lown, B.A. (2006). A model for communication skills assessment across the undergraduate curriculum. *Medical Teacher* 28 (5): e127–e134.

16 Englar, R.E., Williams, M., and Weingand, K. (2016). Applicability of the Calgary-Cambridge guide to dog and cat owners for teaching veterinary clinical communications. *Journal of Veterinary Medical Education* 43 (2): 143–169.

17 Batalden, P., Leach, D., Swing, S. et al. (2002). General competencies and accreditation in graduate medical education. *Health Affair (Millwood)* 21 (5): 103–111.

18 Duffy, F.D., Gordon, G.H., Whelan, G. et al. (2004). Assessing competence in communication and interpersonal skills: the Kalamazoo II report. *Academic Medicine* 79 (6): 495–507.

19 Travaline, J.M., Ruchinskas, R., and D'Alonzo, G.E. Jr. (2005). Patient–physician communication: why and how. *Journal of the American Osteopathic Association* 105 (1): 13–18.

20 Shaw, J.R., Adams, C.L., and Bonnett, B.N. (2004). What can veterinarians learn from studies of physician–patient communication about veterinarian–client–patient

communication? *Journal of the American Veterinary Medical Association* 224 (5): 676–684.

21 Radford, A.D., Stockley, P., Taylor, I.R. et al. (2003). Use of simulated clients in training veterinary undergraduates in communication skills. *Veterinary Record: Journal of the British Veterinary Association* 152 (14): 422–427.

22 Chun, R., Schaefer, S., Lotta, C.C. et al. (2009). Didactic and experiential training to teach communication skills: the University of Wisconsin-Madison School of Veterinary Medicine collaborative experience. *Journal of Veterinary Medical Education* 36 (2): 196–201.

23 Gattellari, M., Butow, P.N., and Tattersall, M.H.N. (2001). Sharing decisions in cancer care. *Social Science & Medicine* 52 (12): 1865–1878.

24 Schulman, B.A. (1979). Active patient orientation and outcomes in hypertensive treatment: application of a socio-organizational perspective. *Medical Care* 17 (3): 267–280.

25 Robinson, R. (2005). Miscommunication. . . always review the medical history Internet2005 Vol. 21 No. 3. https://cvo.org/CVO/media/College-of-Veterinarians-of-ontario/Resources%20and%20Publications/Newsletters/UpdateSeptember2005.pdf.

26 Gilling, M.L. and Parkinson, T.J. (2009). The transition from veterinary student to practitioner: a "make or break" period. *Journal of Veterinary Medical Education.* 36 (2): 209–215.

27 Heath, T. (2006). The more things change, the more they should stay the same. *Journal of Veterinary Medical Education* 33 (2): 149–154.

28 Heath, T. (1996). Teaching communication skills to veterinary students. *Journal of Veterinary Medical Education* 23 (1): 2–7.

29 Routly, J.E., Dobson, H., Taylor, I.R. et al. (2002). Support needs of veterinary surgeons during the first few years of practice: perceptions of recent graduates and senior partners. *Veterinary Record* 150 (6): 167–171.

30 Tinga, C.E., Adams, C.L., Bonnett, B.N., and Ribble, C.S. (2001). Survey of veterinary technical and professional skills in students and recent graduates of a veterinary college. *Journal of the American Veterinary Medical Association.* 219 (7): 924–931.

31 Coe, J.B., Adams, C.L., and Bonnett, B.N. (2008). A focus group study of veterinarians' and pet owners' perceptions of veterinarian–client communication in companion animal practice. *Journal of the American Veterinary Medical Association* 233 (7): 1072–1080.

32 Russell, R. (1994). Preparing veterinary students with the interactive skills to effectively work with clients and staff. *Journal of Veterinary Medical Education* 21 (2): 1–5.

33 Osborne, D. (1996) Report on the 1996 OVMA Mentor Survey (year 1).

34 Brown, J.P. and Silverman, J.D. (1999). The current and future market for veterinarians and veterinary medical services in the United States. *Journal of the American Veterinary Medical Association* 215 (2): 161–183.

35 Nogueira Borden, L.J., Adams, C.L., and Ladner, L.D. (2008). The use of standardized clients in research in the veterinary clinical setting. *Journal of Veterinary Medical Education.* 35 (3): 420–430.

36 Adams, C.L. and Ladner, L.D. (2004). Implementing a simulated client program: bridging the gap between theory and practice. *Journal of Veterinary Medical Education* 31 (2): 138–145.

37 Gray, C.A., Blaxter, A.C., Johnston, P.A. et al. (2006). Communication education in veterinary in the United Kingdom and Ireland: the NUVACS project coupled to progressive individual school endeavors. *Journal of Veterinary Medical Education* 33 (1): 85–92.

38 van Beukelen, P. (2004). Curriculum development in the Netherlands: introduction of tracks in the 2001 curriculum at Utrecht University, The Netherlands. *Journal of Veterinary Medical Education* 31 (3): 227–233.

39 A. S. Communication skills training at the Royal Veterinary College (RVC): a review of undergraduate teaching and learning methods 2010 (2010). http://docplayer.net/11792503-Communication-skills-training-at-the-royal-veterinary-college-rvc-a-review-of-undergraduate-teaching-and-learning-methods.html.

40 College DSGotOV. Professional competencies of Canadian veterinarians: a basis for curriculum development 1996. http://ovc.uoguelph.ca/sites/default/files/users/ovcweb/files/professional-competencies-of-canadian-Veterinarians_a-basis-for-curriculum-development.pdf.

41 Shaw, D.H. and Ihle, S.L. (2006). Communication skills training at the Atlantic Veterinary College, University of Prince Edward Island. *Journal of Veterinary Medical Education* 33 (1): 100–104.

42 Meehan, M.P. and Menniti, M.F. (2014). Final-year veterinary students' perceptions of their communication competencies and a communication skills training program delivered in a primary care setting and based on Kolb's Experiential Learning Theory. *Journal of Veterinary Medical Education* 41 (4): 371–383.

43 Roadmap for veterinary medical education in the 21st century: responsive, collaborative, flexible2011. http://www.aavmc.org/data/files/navmec/navmec_roadmapreport_web_booklet.pdf.

44 Medicine FoV (2017) "You can't do good medicine without good communication skills": actors and veterinarian-coaches help vet me students become great communicators 2017. http://vet.ucalgary.ca/home/news/

you-cant-do-good-medicinewithout-good-communication-skills.

45 Department of Clinical Sciences CoVMaBS. Communication Curriculum Ft. Collins: Colorado State University2016. http://csu-cvmbs.colostate.edu/academics/clinsci/veterinary-communication/Pages/communication-curriculum.aspx.

46 University WS (n.d.). Clinical Communication Program Pullman: The University. http://ccp.vetmed.wsu.edu.

47 Latham, C.E. and Morris, A. (2007). Effects of formal training in communication skills on the ability of veterinary students to communicate with clients. *Veterinary Record* 160 (6): 181–186.

48 Directors NBo (2011). The North American Veterinary Medical Education Consortium (NAVMEC) looks to veterinary medical education for the future: "roadmap for veterinary medical education in the 21st century: responsive, collaborative, flexible". *Journal of Veterinary Medical Education.* 38 (4): 320–327.

49 Hafen, M. Jr., Rush, B.R., and Nelson, S.C. (2009). Utilizing filmed authentic student–client interactions as a communication teaching tool. *Journal of Veterinary Medical Education* 36 (4): 429–435.

50 Root Kustritz, M.V., Lowum, S., Flynn, K. et al. (2017). Assessing communications competencies through reviews of client interactions and comprehensive rotation assessment: a comparison of methods. *Journal of Veterinary Medical Education* 44 (2): 290–301.

51 Kurtz, S. (2006). Teaching and learning communication in veterinary medicine. *Journal of Veterinary Medical Education* 33 (1): 11–19.

52 Walsh, D.A., Osburn, B.I., and Christopher, M.M. (2001). Defining the attributes expected of graduating veterinary medical students. *Journal of the American Veterinary Medical Association* 219 (10): 1358–1363.

53 Strand, E.B., Johnson, B., and Thompson, J. (2013). Peer-assisted communication training: veterinary students as simulated clients and communication skills trainers. *Journal of Veterinary Medical Education* 40 (3): 233–241.

54 Hafen, M., Drake, A.A.S., Rush, B.R., and Nelson, S.C. (2013). Using authentic client interactions in communication skills training: predictors of proficiency. *Journal of Veterinary Medical Education* 40 (4): 318–326.

55 Kolb, D. (1984) Experiential Learning: Experience As The Source Of Learning And Development1984.

56 Estes, C.A. (2004). Promoting student-centered learning in experiential education. *The Journal of Experiential Education* 27 (2): 141–160.

57 Silverman, J. (2005). *Skills for Communicating with Patients*, 2e (ed. S.M. Kurtz and J. Draper). Oxford San Francisco: Oxford San Francisco: Radcliffe Pub.

58 Hulsman, R.L., Ros, W.J.G., Winnubst, J.A.M., and Bensing, J.M. (1999). Teaching clinically experienced physicians communication skills. A review of evaluation studies. *Medical Education* 33 (9): 655–668.

59 Adams, C.L., Nestel, D., and Wolf, P. (2006). Reflection: a critical proficiency essential to the effective development of a high competence in communication. *Journal of Veterinary Medical Education* 33 (1): 58–64.

60 Adams, C.L. and Kurtz, S. (2012). Coaching and feedback: enhancing communication teaching and learning in veterinary practice settings. *Journal of Veterinary Medical Education* 39 (3): 217–228.

61 Silverman, J., Kurtz, S., and Draper, J. (2008). *Skills for Communicating with Patients*. Oxford, UK: Radcliffe Medical Press.

62 Kurtz, S., Silverman, J., Benson, J., and Draper, J. (2003). Marrying content and process in clinical method teaching: enhancing the Calgary-Cambridge guides. *Academic Medicine* 78 (8): 802–809.

63 Adams, C.L. and Kurtz, S.M. (2017). *Skills for Communicating in Veterinary Medicine*. Oxford, United Kingdom: Otmoor Publishing and Dewpoint Publishing (pages 25, 26).

64 Kurtz, S.M. and Silverman, J.D. (1996). The Calgary-Cambridge Referenced Observation Guides: an aid to defining the curriculum and organizing the teaching in communication training programmes. *Medical Education* 30 (2): 83–89.

65 Riccardi, V.M. and Kurtz, S.M. (1983). *Communication and Counselling in Health Care*. Springfield, Illinois: Charles C. Thomas.

66 Denness, C. (2013). What are consultation models for? *InnovAiT* 6 (9): 592–599.

67 Burt, J., Abel, G., Elmore, N. et al. (2014). Assessing communication quality of consultations in primary care: initial reliability of the Global Consultation Rating Scale, based on the Calgary-Cambridge Guide to the Medical Interview. *BMJ Open* 4 (3): e004339.

68 Gillard, S., Benson, J., and Silverman, J. (2009). Teaching and assessment of explanation and planning in medical schools in the United Kingdom: cross sectional questionnaire survey. *Medical Teacher* 31 (4): 328–331.

69 Radford, A., Stockley, P., Silverman, J. et al. (2006). Development, teaching, and evaluation of a consultation structure model for use in veterinary education. *Journal of Veterinary Medical Education* 33 (1): 38–44.

70 Ratzan, S.C. and Parker, R.M. (2000). *Introduction*. Bethesda, Maryland: National Institute of Health.

71 (2004). *Health Literacy: A Prescription to End Confusion*. Washington, DC: Institute of Medicine.

72 Baker, D.W. (2006). The meaning and the measure of health literacy. *Journal of General Internal Medicine* 21 (8): 878–883.

73 Kirsch, I.S. (2001). The framework used in developing and interpreting the International Adult Literacy Survey (IALS). *European Journal of Psychology of Education* 16 (3): 335–361.

74 Hersh, L., Salzman, B., and Snyderman, D. (2015). Health literacy in primary care practice. *American Family Physician* 92 (2): 118–124.

75 Kelly, P.A. and Haidet, P. (2007). Physician overestimation of patient literacy: a potential source of health care disparities. *Patient Education and Counseling* 66 (1): 119–122.

76 Rogers, E.S., Wallace, L.S., and Weiss, B.D. (2006). Misperceptions of medical understanding in low-literacy patients: implications for cancer prevention. *Cancer Control* 13 (3): 225–229.

77 Weiss, B.D. (2007). *Health Literacy and Patient Safety: Help Patients Understand*. Chicago, Illinois: American Medical Association Foundation.

78 Chew, L.D., Bradley, K.A., and Boyko, E.J. (2004). Brief questions to identify patients with inadequate health literacy. *Family Medicine* 36 (8): 588–594.

79 Baker, F.M., Johnson, J.T., Velli, S.A., and Wiley, C. (1996). Congruence between education and reading levels of older persons. *Psychiatric Services* 47 (2): 194–196.

80 Meade, C.D. and Byrd, J.C. (1989). Patient literacy and the readability of smoking education literature. *American Journal of Public Health* 79 (2): 204–206.

81 Nutbeam, D. (2008). The evolving concept of health literacy. *Social Science & Medicine* 67 (12): 2072–2078.

82 Dewalt, D.A., Berkman, N.D., Sheridan, S. et al. (2004). Literacy and health outcomes: a systematic review of the literature. *Journal of General Internal Medicine* 19 (12): 1228–1239.

83 Beckman, H.B. and Frankel, R.M. (2003). Training practitioners to communicate effectively in cancer care: it is the relationship that counts. *Patient Education Counseling* 50 (1): 85–89.

84 Paasche-Orlow, M.K., Parker, R.M., Gazmararian, J.A. et al. (2005). The prevalence of limited health literacy. *Journal of General Internal Medicine* 20 (2): 175–184.

85 Safeer, R.S. and Keenan, J. (2005). Health literacy: the gap between physicians and patients. *American Family Physician* 72 (3): 463–468.

86 Wallace, L.S. and Lennon, E.S. (2004). American Academy of Family Physicians patient education materials: can patients read them? *Family Medicine* 36 (8): 571–574.

87 Kutner, M.A. (2006). *The Health Literacy of America's Adults: Results from the 2003 National Assessment of Adult Literacy*. Washington, DC: U.S. Department of Education and the National Center for Education Statistics.

88 Kyle, S. and Shaw, D. (2014). Doctor–patient communication, patient knowledge, and health literacy: how difficult can it all be? *Annals of The Royal College of Surgeons of England (Suppl)* 96: e9–e13.

89 Coulter, A. and Ellins, J. (2007). Effectiveness of strategies for informing, educating, and involving patients. *BMJ* 335 (7609): 24–27.

90 Wolf, M.S., Davis, T.C., Tilson, H.H. et al. (2006). Misunderstanding of prescription drug warning labels among patients with low literacy. *American Journal of Health System Pharmacy* 63 (11): 1048–1055.

91 Williams, M.V., Baker, D.W., Honig, E.G. et al. (1998). Inadequate literacy is a barrier to asthma knowledge and self-care. *Chest* 114 (4): 1008–1015.

92 Peckham, T.J. (1994). 'Doctor, have I got a fracture or a break'? *Injury* 25 (4): 221–222.

93 Kampa, R.J., Pang, J., and Gleeson, R. (2006). Broken bones and fractures – an audit of patients' perceptions. *Annals of The Royal College of Surgeons of England* 88 (7): 663–666.

94 Krass, I., Svarstad, B.L., and Bultman, D. (2002). Using alternative methodologies for evaluating patient medication leaflets. *Patient Education and Counseling* 47 (1): 29–35.

95 Lerner, E.B., Jehle, D.V., Janicke, D.M., and Moscati, R.M. (2000). Medical communication: do our patients understand? *American Journal of Emergency Medicine* 18 (7): 764–766.

96 Bagley, C.H., Hunter, A.R., and Bacarese-Hamilton, I.A. (2011). Patients' misunderstanding of common orthopaedic terminology: the need for clarity. *Annals of The Royal College of Surgeons of England* 93 (5): 401–404.

97 Murphy, S.A. (2006). Consumer health information for pet owners. *Journal of the Medical Library Association* 94 (2): 151–158.

98 Kogan, L.R., Schoenfeld-Tacher, R., Gould, L. et al. (2014). Information prescriptions: a tool for veterinary practices. *Open Veterinary Journal* 4 (2): 90–95.

99 Kogan, L.R., Schoenfeld-Tacher, R., and Viera, A.R. (2012). The Internet and health information: differences in pet owners based on age, gender, and education. *Journal of the Medical Library Association* 100 (3): 197–204.

100 Kogan, L.R., Schoenfeld-Tacher, R., Simon, A.A., and Viera, A.R. (2010). The Internet and pet health information: perceptions and behaviors of pet owners

and veterinarians. *Internet Journal of Veterinary Medicine* 8 (1).

101 Kogan, L.R., Schoenfeld-Tacher, R., Gould, L. et al. (2014). Providing an information prescription in veterinary medical clinics: a pilot study. *Journal of the Medical Library Association* 102 (1): 41–46.

102 Hofmeister, E.H., Watson, V., Snyder, L.B., and Love, E.J. (2008). Validity and client use of information from the World Wide Web regarding veterinary anesthesia in dogs. *Journal of the American Veterinary Medical Association* 233 (12): 1860–1864.

103 American Animal Hospital Association (2003). *The Path to High Quality Care: Practical Tips for Improving Compliance*. Lakewood, Colorado: American Animal Hospital Association.

104 Englar, R.E. (2020b). *Defining Supplemental Communication Skills: Reducing Medical Jargon. A Guide to Oral Communication in Veterinary Medicine*, 169–189. Sheffield, UK: 5m Publishing.

105 Englar, R.E. (2020c). *Communication Skills that Facilitate Client Comprehension: Summarizing and Checking in with the Client. A Guide to Oral Communication in Veterinary Medicine*, 245–260. Sheffield, UK: 5m Publishing.

106 Englar, R.E. (2020d). *Eliciting the Client's Perspective to Enhance Relationship-Centered Care. A Guide to Oral Communication in Veterinary Medicine*, 202–210. Sheffield, UK: 5m Publishing.

107 Englar, R.E. (2020e). *Enhancing Relationship-Centered Care by Assessing the Client's Knowledge. A Guide to Oral Communication in Veterinary Medicine*, 224–231. Sheffield, UK: 5m Publishing.

108 Englar, R.E. (2020f). *Mapping out the Clinical Consultation. A Guide to Oral Communication in Veterinary Medicine*, 232–244. Sheffield, UK: 5m Publishing.

109 Coe, J.B., Adams, C.L., and Bonnett, B.N. (2009). Prevalence and nature of cost discussions during clinical appointments in companion animal practice. *Journal of the American Veterinary Medical Association* 234 (11): 1418–1424.

110 (2001). *Paws and Claws: A Syndicated Study on Canadian Pet Ownership*. Toronto.

111 Kipperman, B.S., Kass, P.H., and Rishniw, M. (2017). Factors that influence small animal veterinarians' opinions and actions regarding cost of care and effects of economic limitations on patient care and outcome and professional career satisfaction and burnout. *Journal of the American Veterinary Medical Association* 250 (7): 785–794.

112 Nett, R.J., Witte, T.K., Holzbauer, S.M. et al. (2015). Risk factors for suicide, attitudes toward mental illness, and practice-related stressors among US veterinarians. *Journal of the American Veterinary Medical Association* 247 (8): 945–955.

113 Coe, J.B., Adams, C.L., and Bonnett, B.N. (2007). A focus group study of veterinarians' and pet owners' perceptions of the monetary aspects of veterinary care. *Journal of the American Veterinary Medical Association* 231 (10): 1510–1518.

114 Neuberger, J. (2000). The educated patient: new challenges for the medical profession. *Journal of Internal Medicine* 247 (1): 6–10.

Part 2

Quick Assessment Tests (QATS) Involving Blood

3

Packed Cell Volume

Sharon M. Dial

3.1 Procedural Definition: What Is this Test About?

Whole blood has both fluid and formed elements (red blood cells, leukocytes, and platelets). The packed cell volume (PCV) test determines the proportion of blood that is composed of red blood cells (RBCs). Packed cell volume is determined by centrifuging a microhematocrit tube to "pack" the erythrocytes into a solid column beneath a thin layer of white blood cells and platelets. Once centrifuged, the packed column of blood is used to measure, as a percentage of the total blood column, the height of the erythrocyte column. Packed cell volume represents the percent of whole blood that is composed of erythrocytes. It is an indirect measurement of the oxygen carrying capacity of a patient's blood and considered the gold standard test for measuring RBC mass. The PCV usually correlates closely with the hematocrit (HCT) reported on automated hemograms. The HCT in an automated hemogram is a calculated value rather than a direct measurement and is based on the RBC count and mean cell volume (MCV) of the erythrocytes. The PCV is a good "internal control" for automated instrumentation and should not vary more than a few percentage units from the calculated HCT. It is important to remember that the HCT is usually slightly lower than the PCV since some trapping of plasma occurs during centrifugation of the sample.

3.2 Procedural Purpose: Why Should I Perform this Test?

Packed cell volume and plasma protein determination (see Chapter 4) are valuable in-house tests that are used to assess both healthy patients prior to elective anesthesia and surgery and ill patients. When automated hematology instrumentation is unavailable, the PCV, total protein, and blood film evaluation (see Chapter 6) can provide sufficient information for the evaluation of a patient's hematological status.

The PCV is used to assess for both decreased red cell mass (anemia) and increased red cell mass (erythrocytosis). It is a quick and easily performed test that requires instrumentation that is readily available in most veterinary clinics.

Changes in erythrocyte mass are the most common hematological changes seen in the dog and cat. Both primary and secondary diseases of the hematopoietic system are common in veterinary medicine and can affect the PCV.

A PCV or HCT should be done on most ill patients especially those that present with:

- pale mucous membranes
- icteric mucous membranes
- hepatomegaly
- splenomegaly
- clinical evidence of hypoxia
  - tachycardia
  - tachypnea
  - exercise intolerance
- systolic murmur
- clinical evidence of bleeding
  - external hemorrhage
  - hemorrhagic body cavity effusions
  - petechia
  - ecchymoses.

3.3 Equipment

The following equipment is used for this test:

- whole blood in a blood collection tube with anticoagulant (usually ethylenediaminetetraacetic acid or EDTA, but may use heparin)

Low-Cost Veterinary Clinical Diagnostics, First Edition. Ryane E. Englar and Sharon M. Dial.
© 2023 John Wiley & Sons, Inc. Published 2023 by John Wiley & Sons, Inc.

- gloves
- microhematocrit centrifuge
- hematocrit tubes without anticoagulant
- hematocrit reader
- sealant.

3.4 Procedural Steps: How Do I Perform this Test?

1) Collect all materials needed (see Figure 3.1).
2) Mix the blood sample by either inverting it several times (5–8 inversions) or placing it on a blood tube rocker for 5–8 rotations (see Figure 3.2a and b).
3) Fill two microhematocrit tubes at least to three-fourth of the length of the tube when possible.
   a) Uncap the blood tube and introduce the hematocrit tube at slightly off the horizontal position to allow capillary action to fill the tube (see Figure 3.3).
   b) Once the hematocrit tube is adequately filled, place one finger at the end of the microhematocrit tube to prevent loss of blood from the microhematocrit tube when it is removed from the blood collection tube (see Figure 3.4).

(a)

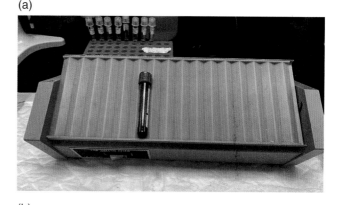

(b)

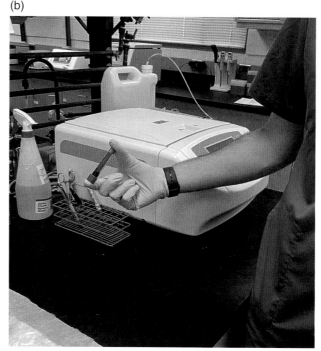

Figure 3.2 Blood tube can be mixed on a rocker (a) or manually (b). *Source:* Courtesy of Jeremy Bessett.

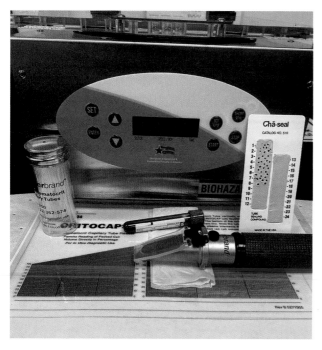

Figure 3.1 Equipment needed to perform a PCV include whole blood in a blood collection tube with anticoagulant, gloves, microhematocrit centrifuge, hematocrit tubes without anticoagulant, sealant, and hematocrit reader. *Source:* Courtesy of Jeremy Bessett.

c) Wipe the exterior surface of the tube with a gauze or "KimWipe" to remove any blood remaining on the surface (see Figure 3.5).
d) Keeping your finger at the end of the microhematocrit tube, plunge the free end of the tube into the sealant several times until you have about 2–3 mm of sealant at the end of the tube (see Figure 3.6) Alternatively, you can switch the microhematocrit tube to your other hand by placing a finger at the end that the blood was drawn into, allowing you to plunge the blood-free end of the microhematocrit tube into the sealant and keeping it from being contaminated with blood (see Figure 3.7a and b).

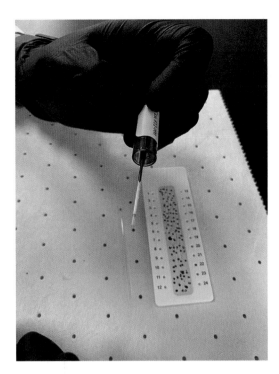

Figure 3.3 Microhematocrit tube is filled by placing it into the blood collection tube at an angle just off the horizontal plane and allowing the blood to flow into the microhematocrit tube by capillary action. *Source:* Courtesy of Jeremy Bessett.

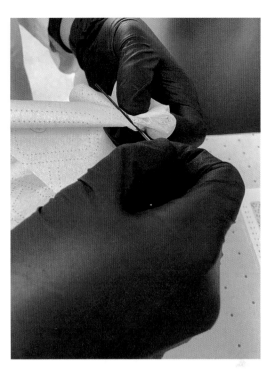

Figure 3.5 Wipe off any excess blood on the exterior of the microhematocrit tube before you seal it. *Source:* Courtesy of Jeremy Bessett.

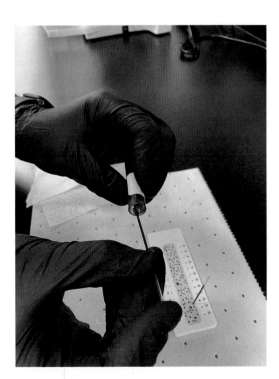

Figure 3.4 Once filled, a finger is placed at the end of the microhematocrit tube to hold the blood in the tube as you remove it from the blood collection tube. *Source:* Courtesy of Jeremy Bessett.

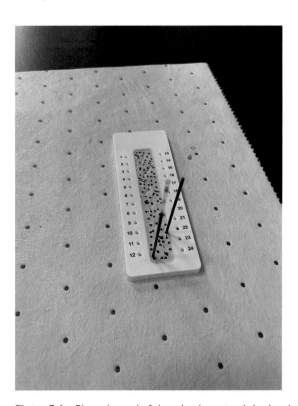

Figure 3.6 Place the end of the microhematocrit in the clay sealant to seal the end. Notice the numbered small indentations along the edge of the sealant tray. These slots can be used to keep track of individual samples when multiple blood samples are being processed. *Source:* Courtesy of Jeremy Bessett.

(a)

(b)

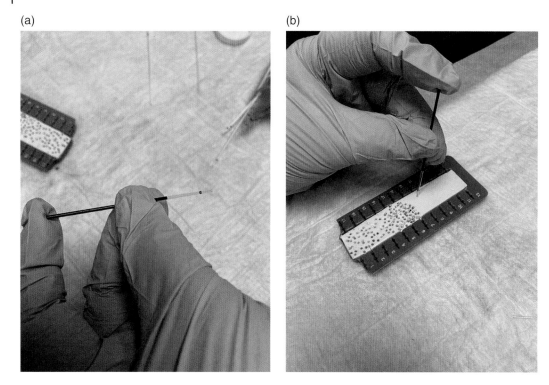

Figure 3.7 (a) To keep the sealant clay clean, the microhematocrit tube can be switched between hands to allow (b) placing the blood-free end into the clay. *Source:* Courtesy of Jeremy Bessett.

4) Place the microhematocrit tubes into a microhematocrit centrifuge in slots opposite each other with the sealant away from the center of the centrifuge. If multiple samples are being prepared at once, be sure to record which sample is in which slot (see Figure 3.8).

   If there was only enough blood to fill one microhematocrit tube, be sure to fill a separate tube with water, seal it, and place it in the opposite slot to keep the centrifuge balanced. If you run the centrifuge without balancing it, the instrument will vibrate excessively, damaging the mechanism.

5) Place the interior lid over the microcentrifuge tube prior to closing the exterior centrifuge lid. If the interior lid is not secured properly, the microhematocrit tubes will break and glass dust will contaminate the interior of the centrifuge (see Figure 3.9).

6) Set the timer to five minutes and start the centrifuge.

7) Allow the centrifuge to stop completely. Do not use the centrifuge break to stop the rotation. Use of the break for nonemergency stops will cause damage to the breaking mechanism over time.

8) Open the exterior centrifuge lid and remove the interior centrifuge lid, remove the microhematocrit tube from the centrifuge, and record the color of the plasma.

9) Place the microhematocrit tube on the microhematocrit reader, aligning the top of the clay sealant with the

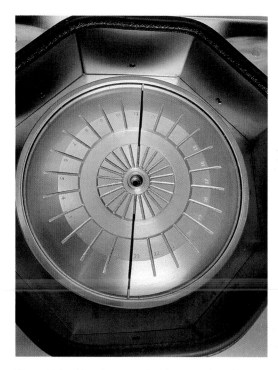

Figure 3.8 Microhematocrit tubes are placed in the centrifuge while ensuring to balance the centrifuge by placing each tube opposite the other. The microhematocrit tubes are placed with the sealed end to the outside. *Source:* Courtesy of Jeremy Bessett.

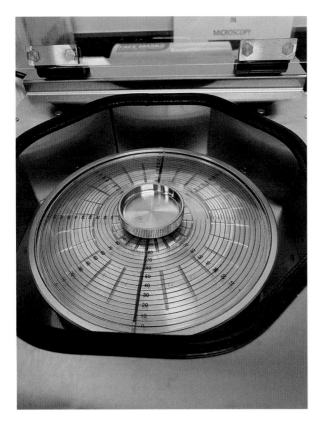

Figure 3.9 Place and secure the interior lid on the centrifuge before closing the exterior lid. *Source:* Courtesy of Jeremy Bessett.

baseline (zero line) and the top of the plasma with the topline (100). Record the value at the interface of the red cell column with the buffy coat (white layer overlying the red cell column) (see Figure 3.10a and b).

3.5 Time Estimate to Perform Test

Fifteen minutes.

3.6 Procedural Tips and Troubleshooting

The PCV procedure is commonly done on blood collected with anticoagulant using a microhematocrit tube without anticoagulant (indicated by a blue color). However, the procedure can be done with whole blood collected directly from a small vein or capillary sample using a heparinized microhematocrit tube (see Figure 3.11).

The most important component of this procedure is to be consistent in the length of time a sample is centrifuged. The standard time is five minutes. Centrifuging the sample for a shorter time will result in an erroneously high PCV, while centrifuging it for a longer time will result in an erroneously low PCV. As with all venipuncture, a good technic

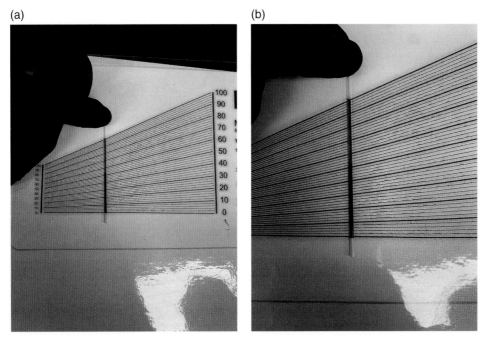

(a)   (b)

Figure 3.10 (a) Microhematocrit tube is placed on the hematocrit reader by aligning the top of the sealant at the baseline (zero) and the top of the plasma column at the topline (100); (b) reading for the packed cell volume (PCV) is the level of the interface between the red cell column and the buffy coat, the white layer just above the top of the red cell column. In this case, the PCV reading is 52% (each dark red line is 10 units). In this sample, there is significant hemolysis evident in the plasma that can make it difficult to find the red cell–buffy coat interface. *Source:* Courtesy of Jeremy Bessett.

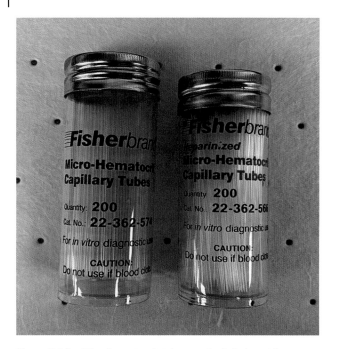

Figure 3.11 Microhematocrit tubes on the left do not have any anticoagulant and would be used with whole blood collected in a blood collection tube with anticoagulant. The microhematocrit tubes on the right are heparinized and would be used when collecting blood into the microhematocrit tube directly from a small vein or capillary sample. *Source:* Courtesy of Jeremy Bessett.

is necessary to prevent artifactual hemolysis, which can make it difficult to read the interface between the buffy coat and the red cell column.

The PCV should be read immediately after centrifugation. If reading is delayed, the tubes may need to be recentrifuged and hemolysis may occur. It is also important to remember that RBCs can swell after collection. They are usually stable if the sample is refrigerated (4 °C). In a busy practice, it may be more efficient to perform the PCV determinations in batches, storing the samples in the refrigerator until needed. If this is done, the samples will need to be thoroughly mixed before filling microhematocrit tubes.

Firmly sealing microhematocrit tubes is very important to prevent "blow out" of the blood. Sealant that is contaminated with blood does not seal as well. Using the alternative method of introducing the sealant will eliminate this problem. It is common practice to repack the sealant in its tray. This may result in the mixing of blood into the sealant. It is better practice to use as much of the sealant as possible without repacking.

Many sealant trays have numbered slots for tubes. When performing this test on multiple samples at one time, numbered slots can be used to record the position of each sample. This same numbering system can be used as the samples are placed in the centrifuge.

If the PCV and HCT values on an automated hemogram differ more than 3%, there may be a technical issue with the instrument or an abnormality in the sample that is preventing appropriate packing of the erythrocytes. If the EDTA blood collection tube is not filled to its proper amount, the excess EDTA can cause shrinkage of the RBCs resulting in a significant difference between the PCV and HCT. In this case, the HCT will be more accurate than the PCV because the RBCs will return to normal volume when an isotonic diluent is added to the sample for counting in the instrument. Any artifact that interferes with the RBC count or MCV measurement will affect the HCT value as well. Contact the instrument technical representative if the HCT and PCV of blood samples are persistently different.

When recording the PCV, do not forget to record plasma color and clarity and size of the buffy coat. Both of these findings are essential when reviewing the hemogram.

3.7 Interpreting Test Results

As a rule of thumb, the reference interval for the PCV of canine blood is 35–57% and feline blood is 30–45% [1]. In dogs, there are some breed differences in reference intervals with the Greyhound being the most well-known. The Greyhound has a significantly higher PCV compared with other breeds (52–60%) [2]. Breed differences have also been found in the cat. A reference interval determined for the Maine Coon cat was 37–48%, higher than most feline reference intervals [3]. These potential differences from the commonly published reference intervals for PCV are a good reason to obtain and monitor baseline data in wellness checks in the dog and cat.

A decreased PCV indicates decreased red cell mass or number indicative of anemia. Additional tests are necessary to classify an anemia and to assist in determining the cause. Anemia can be regenerative indicating that the bone marrow is responding by releasing young erythrocytes (reticulocytes) or nonregenerative indicating that the bone marrow is not responding with the adequate release of reticulocytes.

Causes of regenerative anemia include:

- external and internal hemorrhage
  plasma total protein will be low with external hemorrhage and is usually within reference interval with internal hemorrhage (hemorrhage into body cavities).

  Acute hemorrhage will not present as regenerative anemia because it takes at least 3–5 days before the bone marrow response is evident. In addition, it may take up to 1–3 days for the PCV to accurately reflect the degree of blood loss. This is how long it takes for fluid to shift into the vasculature to reestablish blood volume and pressure.

- Immune-mediated red cell destruction or lysis
  - ○ primary immune-mediated anemia (autoimmune)
  - ○ secondary immune-mediated anemia
    - idiosyncratic drug reaction
    - infectious disease including erythroparasites
    - neoplasia
- Nonimmune red cell destruction or lysis
  - ○ oxidative injury associated with drugs and toxins
    - acetaminophen
    - zinc
    - copper
    - moth balls
  - ○ oxidative injury associated with plants
    - onions
  - ○ fragmentation hemolysis due to vasculitis or disseminated intravascular hemolysis
  - ○ hereditary enzymopathies, membrane abnormalities.

Note: Intravascular hemolysis is often acute and may not present with significant evidence of regeneration. Extravascular hemolysis is often chronic and usually presents with significant evidence of regeneration.

Causes of nonregenerative anemia include:

- lack of production due to primary bone marrow suppression and myelophthisis or myelofibrosis
- lack of erythropoietin production associated with chronic renal disease
- immune-mediated disease directed at erythrocyte precursors in the bone marrow
- anemia of chronic inflammation (mild)
- endocrinopathies
- some infectious agents if there is concurrent inflammation
- acute hemorrhage (see hemorrhage above)

An increase in PCV indicates increased red cell mass or number indicative of erythrocytosis. Additional tests are necessary to classify erythrocytosis as either absolute (increased production of red cells by the bone marrow) or relative (increased loss of plasma water or increased red cells from splenic contraction). The most common cause of erythrocytosis in small animals is relative erythrocytosis. Absolute erythrocytosis is either primary, such as Polycythemia vera, a neoplastic condition, or secondary, due to hypoxia.

3.8 Clinical Case Example(s): Can We Link to the Cases in Chapter 5?

See Part 6, Case #2, #3, #15.

3.9 Add-On Tests That You May Need to Consider and Their Additive Value

1) Reticulocyte count

   While the degree of polychromasia seen on the blood film can indicate regeneration, not all young erythrocytes (reticulocytes) are polychromatophilic. The degree of regeneration can be underestimated without a true reticulocyte count.

2) Blood film review (see Chapter 6).

   Evaluation for polychromatophilia will assist in determining if the anemia is regenerative; however, a reticulocyte count will be necessary for a full interpretation of the degree of regeneration (see above). The presence of spherocytes, ghost cells, eccentrocytes, Heinz bodies, schistocytes, and erythroparasites will assist in determining the cause of anemia. Identification of inflammatory leukocytosis would support possible anemia of chronic inflammation. Identification of a thrombocytopenia would provide a possible cause for blood loss as the underlying mechanism of the anemia.

3) Plasma total protein (see Chapter 4)

   External blood loss (hemorrhage) results in the loss of both cellular elements and plasma. A decreased plasma total protein in the anemic patient supports hemorrhage as the cause of anemia if there are no clinical or diagnostic findings suggestive of underlying causes of protein loss attributable to the renal system (proteinuria) or gastrointestinal system. If both the plasma protein and PCV are low, a thorough clinical evaluation for evidence of external blood loss, such as hemoptysis, hematemesis, melena, and hematuria should be done.

4) Urine color (see Chapter 12), reagent strip reactions for heme and protein (see Chapter 14) and sediment examination (see Chapter 15).

   Urinalysis is an essential part of evaluation of the PCV. In the anemic patient with evidence of hemolysis/hemoglobinemia on evaluation of plasma color, a positive heme reaction and red discoloration of the urine supernatant (hemoglobinuria) supports true hemoglobinemia. Lack of hemoglobinuria supports iatrogenic or artifactual hemolysis of the blood sample. A positive heme reaction and the presence of significant numbers of erythrocytes in the urine sediment may support blood loss into the urinary system. The presence or absence of significant proteinuria will assist in the interpretation of hypoproteinemia in an anemic patient. Proteinuria would suggest an additional differential for hypoproteinemia, renal protein loss.

5) Serum chemistry profile

A serum chemistry profile to further assess organ system function will assist in refining the underlying cause of anemia. Analytes that can directly assist in evaluating an anemic patient include bilirubin, albumin, renal function (blood urea nitrogen or BUN, creatinine, electrolytes), and serum total protein.

6) Coagulation profile

If there is clinical evidence of hemorrhage into body cavities or prominent ecchymosis or bruising, a coagulation profile would assist in determining if the anemia is due to a bleeding diathesis as a result of coagulation factor deficiency, either inherited or acquired.

3.10   Key Takeaways

- Performing the test:
  - fill two microhematocrit tubes per sample whenever possible.
  - fill tubes at least three-fourth whenever possible.
  - balance all samples within the centrifuge.
  - be consistent in the time the sample is being centrifuged (five minutes is recommended).
- Interpretation of the test:
  - PCV should be interpreted in consideration of the clinical presentation and ancillary tests. Determining the cause of a change in PCV requires at least blood film examination, serum or plasma total protein and color, and a urinalysis. A complete serum chemistry profile may be needed for further interpretation of the PCV.

References

1 https://www.merckvetmanual.com/special-subjects/reference-guides/hematologic-reference-ranges

2 Torres, A.R. et al. (2014). Hematologic differences between Dachshunds and mixed breed dogs. *Veterinary Clinical Pathology* 43 (4): 519–524.

3 Spada, E. et al. (2015). Haematological and biochemical reference intervals in adult Maine coon cat blood donors. *Journal of Feline Medicine and Surgery* 17 (12): 1020–1027.

4

Total Protein as Measured by Refractometry

Sharon M. Dial

4.1 Procedural Definition: What Is This Test About?

Plasma total protein using refractometry is determining protein concentration by measuring the degree to which the protein in the plasma changes the refractive index of the plasma. In the past, the term "total solids" was used in the place of total protein because older refractometers were not calibrated to only reflect protein concentration in the plasma. Instead, those scales reported the concentration of all solids in the plasma, which include proteins and nonprotein substances. The newer refractometers are calibrated to remove the effect of nonprotein solids and their scales provide a more accurate value for the amount of protein in the sample.

Plasma total protein by refractometer is an essential part of a complete blood count. By definition, plasma total protein by refractometry measures all plasma protein in whole blood, including those involved in coagulation. In contrast, serum total protein is obtained from a sample drawn into a blood collection tube without an anticoagulant that has been allowed to clot allowing the separation of the formed elements of the blood (red blood cell [RBC], leukocytes, and platelets) and coagulation proteins from the remaining fluid components of the blood (serum). Plasma total protein by refractometry is usually higher than serum total protein because it includes the coagulation proteins that are used up in the formation of clots.

Plasma total protein is performed in conjunction with the determination of the PCV and the initial part of the procedure for obtaining the plasma total protein value is the same as that for centrifuging a blood sample for determining the PCV. An important part of determining plasma protein is the concurrent evaluation of plasma color. Abnormal plasma color can indicate the presence of substances in the blood that can preclude obtaining an accurate value and assist in the interpretation of the values obtained when evaluated in conjunction with the PCV.

4.2 Procedural Purpose: Why Should I Perform this Test?

The differential diagnosis list for anemia, hypo/hyperproteinemia, and proteinuria is greatly informed by the results obtained for each of these relatively quick and inexpensive tests when viewed as a set rather than individually. In addition, the values obtained for these essential in-house tests will help determine the choice of the most appropriate additional diagnostic tests. A good understanding of the method for using a refractometer, possible interference in obtaining a valid result, and the interpretation of plasma protein along with plasma color is necessary to fully use this in-house diagnostic test.

Because hemorrhage results in the loss of both the formed elements of blood (RBCs, leukocytes, and platelets) and the plasma or fluid portion of the blood, determination of plasma protein is essential in supporting the diagnosis of anemia due to hemorrhage. Hypoproteinemia may be present before the appearance of significant reticulocytosis that is indicative of a regenerative anemia, the hallmark of anemia due to hemorrhage.

It is important to keep in mind the following points when interpreting clinical signs associated with abnormal plasma protein concentration. Plasma proteins are the primary blood components that determine plasma oncotic pressure. The liver makes almost all plasma proteins except most gamma globulins. In addition, immunoglobulin, a component of the globulin portion of total protein, will increase with chronic inflammatory diseases.

As such, plasma protein concentration can assist in refining the differential list for the following presentation:

- pleural and abdominal effusions
- peripheral edema
- small bowel diarrhea

Low-Cost Veterinary Clinical Diagnostics, First Edition. Ryane E. Englar and Sharon M. Dial.
© 2023 John Wiley & Sons, Inc. Published 2023 by John Wiley & Sons, Inc.

- proteinuria
- chronic weight loss
- chronic infections
- icteric and pale mucous membranes.

Dehydrated patients should have normal or high plasma total protein. The plasma total protein in dehydrated patients can be used to monitor rehydration during therapy. High plasma protein is not specific for dehydration; increased serum albumin is much more specific for dehydration since total plasma protein can be increased due to inflammation and neoplasia such as plasma cell tumors (myeloma). Of the plasma proteins, albumin is present in the highest concentration, approximately one-half of the total protein concentration. Plasma and serum total protein as an individual test can provide insight into underlying pathophysiological mechanisms related to the clinical findings in an ill patient. However, total protein is best interpreted in conjunction with serum albumin and globulin concentration. If the plasma total protein is outside of the reference interval, it is necessary to obtain serum total protein, albumin, and globulin concentrations to determine the likely causes of the abnormality. The ratio of albumin to globulin (A : G ratio) is useful in refining the mechanism underlying changes in total protein.

Note: Total protein and albumin are directly measured when analyzing a serum sample. Globulin concentration is calculated by subtracting the albumin concentration from the total protein concentration.

The color/transparency of plasma should always be recorded when testing for plasma total protein. While the color and transparency do not directly relate to alterations in protein concentration, the gross character of the plasma can be important to assist in the interpretation of other diagnostic tests. For instance, a patient with red plasma indicates the presence of free hemoglobin in the plasma. This may provide support for intravascular hemolysis if the patient is anemic. Urinalysis showing hemoglobinuria is necessary to confirm *in vivo* hemolysis. Hemolysis and lipemia can make it difficult to get a precise plasma total protein reading. Hemolysis will obscure the line of interference in the refractometer (it will make getting an exact reading difficult). Lipemia (cloudy/white plasma) can artificially increase plasma protein since lipid will contribute to the change in refractive index. Icteric plasma (yellow) should increase the suspicion of hyperbilirubinemia. This information can be helpful in determining the cause of anemia. Knowing the plasma characteristic will also help interpret serum chemistry values since methods used to measure several analytes in a chemistry profile may be affected by these three plasma/serum color changes. The reference laboratory should indicate if these are interfering substances in their methods.

4.3 Equipment

Blood in a blood collection tube with anticoagulant (usually ethylenediaminetetraacetic acid, but may use heparin) as well as the following:

- gloves
- microhematocrit centrifuge
- hematocrit tubes without anticoagulant
- sealant
- refractometer.

4.4 Procedural Steps: How Do I Perform this Test?

1) Gather all materials needed for the procedure (see Figure 4.1). The refractometer is a relatively simple instrument to use. It does require an understanding of the parts that are used when performing a total plasma protein (see Figure 4.2a and b).
2) Follow steps 1–8 for the procedure to fill and centrifuge a microhematocrit tube, as mentioned in Chapter 3.
3) Record the PCV and the color of the plasma.

   Plasma color can be recorded as:
   - colorless
   - yellow (icteric)

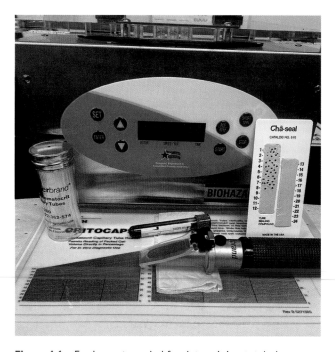

Figure 4.1 Equipment needed for determining total plasma protein by refractometry include whole blood in an anticoagulant blood collection tube, gloves, microhematocrit centrifuge, microhematocrit tubes without anticoagulant, and a refractometer. *Source:* Courtesy of Jeremy Bessett.

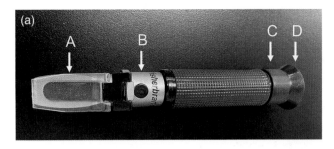

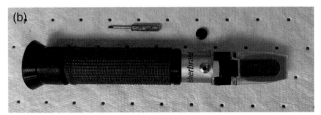

Figure 4.2 (a) The features of the refractometer: (A) the cover over the prism platten; (B) the calibration screw with its cover; (C) the focusing ring; (D) the eyepiece; (b) a small screwdriver is usually provided to allow calibration of the refractometer if needed. This image shows the screwdriver and calibration screw with the cap off. *Source:* Courtesy of Jeremy Bessett.

- red
- white opacity.

4) Check the calibration of the refractometer before performing the test on a sample. The calibration check can be done daily prior to running the samples for that day. Lift the prism cover on the refractometer and place a drop of distilled water on the prism surface (see Figure 4.3a and b).

5) Replace the cover to allow the water to spread underneath the cover by capillary action (see Figure 4.4).

6) Hold the refractometer up to the light, lightly press down on the cover and focus using the eyepiece to bring the interface line into focus.

Read the scale for urine specific gravity, usually the scale on the far right, but the location varies in different models of refractometer. The scale for specific gravity will be from 1.000 to 1.050. The interface line should be at the 1.000 value since the specific gravity of water is 1.000. Do not be concerned that the interface line is not lined up at the 0 reading on the total protein scale. If the refractometer reads 1.000 for water on the urine specific gravity scale, it will correctly read the total protein (see Figure 4.5a–c).

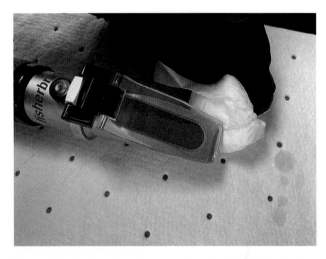

Figure 4.4 Replace the prism cover to allow the distilled water to spread out over the prism and use a wipe to remove any overflow. *Source:* Courtesy of Jeremy Bessett.

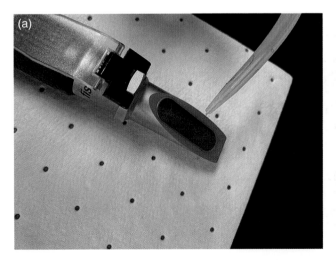

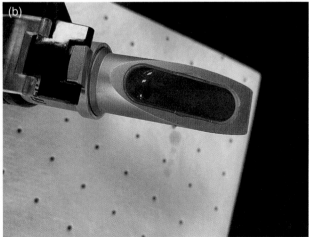

Figure 4.3 (a) Open the prism cover to expose the clean surface of the prism and, using a pipette, place a drop of distilled water onto the prism platten; (b) a drop of distilled water on the prism platten. *Source:* Courtesy of Jeremy Bessett.

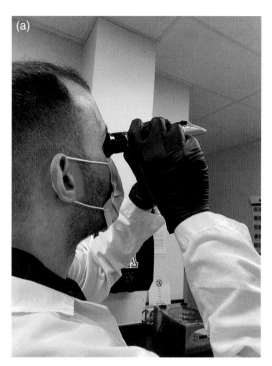

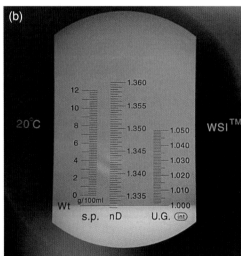
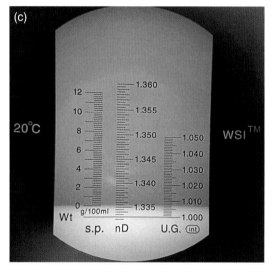

Figure 4.5 (a) Hold the refractometer up to a light and read the scale for urine specific gravity on the far right; (b) the interface line is on the 1.000 value in this image indicating the refractometer is appropriately calibrated; (c) in this image, the interface line is above the 1.000 value indicating the refractometer needs to be calibrated. *Source:* Courtesy of Jeremy Bessett.

If the interface line is not at 1.000, while looking in the refractometer, adjust the calibration knob or screw until it does read 1.000. The location of the calibration knob or screw will differ based on different models of refractometer (see Figure 4.6a and b).

7) Score the hematocrit tube just above the buffy coat using a glass scoring pen, or the edge of a glass slide (see Figure 4.7a and b).

8) Holding the microhematocrit tube close to the area that has been scored, gently snap the tube and discard the red cell portion (see Figure 4.8).

A paper towel or KimWipe can be used to prevent shards of glass from falling onto the bench by lightly wrapping the microhematocrit tube before breaking. Be careful to keep the towel or KimWipe from touching the opened end of the tube because it will draw out the plasma and can alter the reading.

9) Open the prism cover to reveal the glass surface of the refractometer's prism and gently shake out the plasma onto the prism (see Figure 4.9a–c).

You may need to use two or more microhematocrit tubes if the patient is dehydrated and has a significant

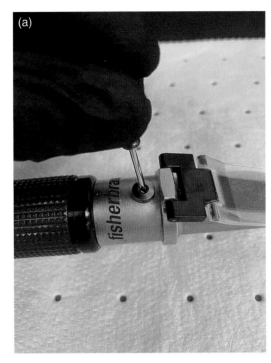

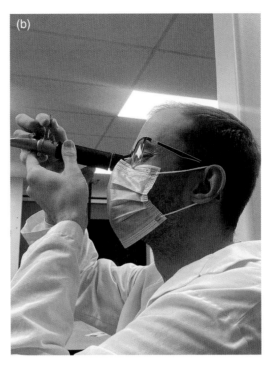

Figure 4.6 (a) Place a small screw driver in the calibration screw just behind the prism cover hinge; (b) holding the refractometer up to the light, turn the calibration screw driver until the interface line moves back to the 1.000 mark. *Source:* Courtesy of Jeremy Bessett.

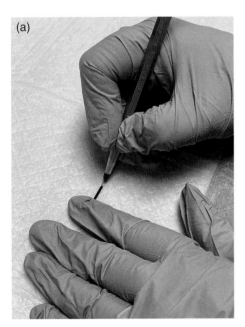

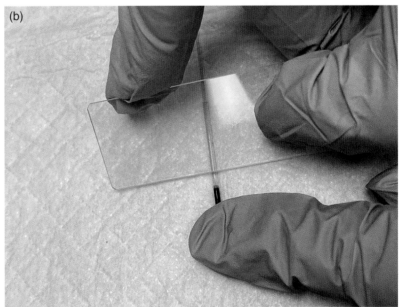

Figure 4.7 The microhematocrit tube can be scored just above the buffy coat layer using a (a) glass scoring pen or (b) the edge of a glass slide. *Source:* Courtesy of Jeremy Bessett.

increase in the PCV (erythrocytosis). Be careful not to allow the end of the microhematocrit tube to touch and mark the glass surface. A small rubber bulb can be used to express the plasma onto the prism platten rather than trying to shake it out (see Figure 4.10).

10) As when you check the calibration, look through the eyepiece as you hold the refractometer up to the light, pressing down on the cover, and using the eyepiece to help bring the interface line into focus.

11) Unlike the calibration method, the plasma total protein is read from the total protein scale, usually on the left indicated by the g/100 ml units. Record the value indicated by the interface line. The scale for total protein is usually from 0 to 12 g/100 ml or deciliter (dl) (see Figure 4.11).

4.5 Time Estimate to Perform Test

Fifteen minutes including centrifuging the sample.

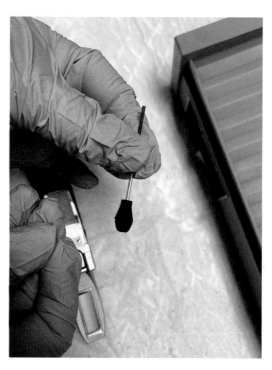

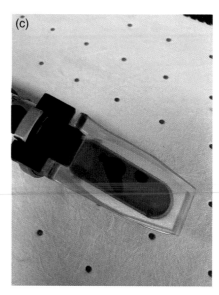

Figure 4.8 Gently break the microhematocrit tube and discard the portion containing the RBCs and buffy coat retaining the plasma portion. *Source:* Courtesy of Jeremy Bessett.

Figure 4.10 A small bulb has been placed onto the microhematocrit tube containing the plasma. This makes it much easier to express the plasma without accidently marring the prism surface. *Source:* Courtesy of Jeremy Bessett.

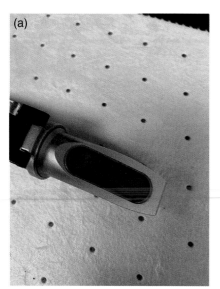
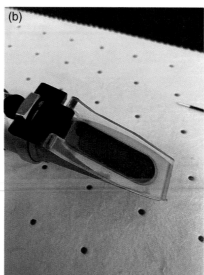
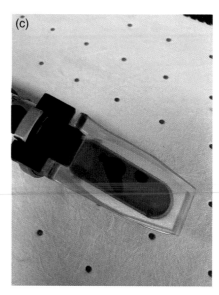

Figure 4.9 (a) Platten cover is opened and drops of the plasma have been shaken onto the prism platten; (b) cover is closed and the plasma is allowed to spread out appropriately; (c) if the plasma does not spread properly as indicated in this image, the interface line will not be clear enough to read. *Source:* Courtesy of Jeremy Bessett.

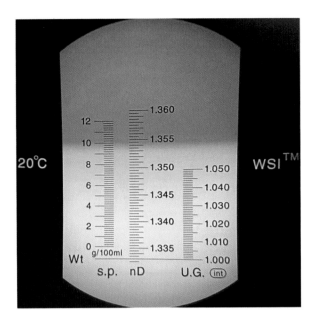

Figure 4.11 The interface line in this image indicates a plasma protein of 9.8 g/dl. You will notice the line is slightly hazy and there is a slight red color due to a hemolyzed plasma sample. *Source:* Courtesy of Jeremy Bessett.

4.6 Procedural Tips and Troubleshooting

- Both lipemia and hemolysis can affect the accuracy of the plasma total protein reading.
  o Hemolysis will make the interface line indistinct (fuzzy or blurred).
  o Lipemia can artifactually increase total protein reading.
  o Icterus does not affect plasma total protein by refractometry.
- Overtime, RBCs become fragile and can lyse during centrifugation resulting in artifactual changes in the PCV and will make an accurate reading of the plasma protein difficult.
- If the patient is dehydrated, it may be necessary to spin two or more microhematocrit tubes to obtain enough plasma for a determination.
- Checking the calibration of the refractometer is an important part of the procedure to ensure the reading is accurate.

4.7 Interpreting Test Result

Plasma total protein in the dog and cat is usually between 6.0 and 7.5 g/dl [1]. The liver is responsible for the production of the majority of protein in the plasma, including albumin, carrier proteins, such as transferrin, and acute phase inflammatory proteins, such as C-reactive protein. The only major serum proteins the liver does not produce are the immunoglobulins produced by lymphocytes (B-cells, plasma cells).

Hypoproteinemia, plasma total protein concentration below the reference interval, can be caused by external loss or lack of production of plasma proteins.

The causes of external loss of plasma protein include:

- external hemorrhage
- protein-losing gastrointestinal disease
  o neoplasia – lymphoma
  o infectious
    ▪ fungal disease – histoplasmosis, pythium
    ▪ viral disease
    ▪ parasitism
  o inflammatory bowel disease
  o primary intestinal lymphangiectasia (rare)
  o intestinal obstruction
- protein-losing renal disease
  o glomerulonephritis (most common cause) – often associated with inflammatory or infectious disease including
    ▪ dogs
      • inflammatory, noninfectious
        o chronic inflammatory diseases of the gastrointestinal tract
        o chronic immune-mediated diseases
        o chronic dental disease
      • inflammatory, infectious
        o Rickettsial disease
        o dirofilariasis
        o chronic bacterial diseases
    ▪ cats
      • inflammatory, noninfectious (relatively rare)
      • infectious
        o feline leukemia virus
        o feline immunodeficiency virus
        o feline infectious peritonitis virus
  o renal amyloidosis (relatively rare)
    ▪ breed associated (familial)
      • Abyssinian cat
      • Shar Pai dog
    ▪ systemic reactive amyloidosis – chronic inflammatory diseases.

Note: The importance of interpreting total protein in the context of albumin and globulin concentrations is illustrated by the fact that with hemorrhage and gastrointestinal loss, both albumin and globulins are decreased. In contrast, with renal protein loss where the loss of protein is more selective with albumin being the primary protein lost in the urine. The importance of interpreting hypoproteinemia in concert with a urinalysis is illustrated by the fact that if there is no proteinuria present, renal protein loss can be eliminated as a differential.

The causes of decreased production of proteins include:

- decreased production of protein by the liver (both albumin and non-immunoglobulin proteins)
  - ○ chronic end-stage liver disease
  - ○ portosystemic shunt
  - ○ starvation (requires weeks for the total protein to decrease due to starvation alone)
- decreased production of immunoglobulins
  - ○ inherited deficiencies
  - ○ inadequate colostrum intake in the neonate

Note: With hypoproteinemia associated with liver disease or starvation, hypoalbuminemia is the most prominent change.

Hyperproteinemia, total protein above the reference interval, is most commonly caused by dehydration or chronic inflammation. However, lymphoid neoplasia, such as myeloma, can result in hyperproteinemia due to the production of monoclonal immunoglobulin proteins and a moderate to marked increase in the globulin portion of serum proteins.

- Causes of hyperproteinemia include:
  - ○ dehydration – both albumin and globulins are increased
  - ○ inflammation – decreased albumin (it is a reverse phase reactant) and increased globulins (inflammatory proteins and immunoglobulins)
  - ○ monoclonal gammopathy – increased production of a single type of immunoglobulin by neoplastic lymphoid cells (usually neoplastic plasma cells).

Note: The clinical hydration status of the patient is important when evaluating total protein. If you have a clinically dehydrated patient, the total protein should be increased. Both albumin and globulin should be increased as well. If the clinically dehydrated patient has a normal total protein, the total protein may be decreased to below the reference interval with appropriate fluid therapy. If the dehydrated patient has a low total protein prior to rehydration, the effect of rehydration on further decreasing the total protein (and thus the oncotic pressure) must be taken into account as fluid therapy is instituted.

4.8 Clinical Case Example(s)

See Part 6 cases #4, #5, #9, #10, #15.

4.9 Add-On Tests That You May Need to Consider and Their Additive Values

- A full chemistry profile is warranted in assessing any patient with an abnormal plasma total protein.
  - ○ Serum total protein and albumin – As mentioned above, to fully evaluate the protein status of the patient and determine the cause of changes in plasma total protein, serum total protein, albumin, and globulin must be done.
  - ○ Alanine aminotransferase, alkaline phosphatase, bilirubin, glucose, BUN, cholesterol – since the liver is central to maintaining normal serum protein concentration, evaluation of analytes in the chemistry profile related to the liver dysfunction should be done.
  - ○ BUN, creatinine, electrolytes, cholesterol – since renal disease can result in significant loss of protein, evaluation of analytes in the chemistry profile related to renal dysfunction should be done.
- A urinalysis to identify possible renal protein loss is warranted.
- Serum protein electrophoresis is an important tool in determining the cause of a significant increase in globulins. This is a reference laboratory test that uses electrophoresis to separate proteins by both charge and size. Serum protein electrophoresis can differentiate between an increase of globulins due to inflammation, a polyclonal expansion of immunoglobulins (polyclonal gammopathy), from an increase due to neoplasia, a monoclonal expansion of immunoglobulins (monoclonal gammopathy). The majority of monoclonal gammopathies are due to lymphoid neoplasia. However, there are a few infectious agents that have been associated with a monoclonal gammopathy. These include *Ehrlichia* spp. in dogs and feline infectious peritonitis in cats.

4.10 Key Takeaways

- Plasma total protein is an essential component of compete blood count. It is necessary for the evaluation of the anemic patient or the patient with erythrocytosis.
- Plasma total protein is a quick inexpensive test with excellent value in the dehydrated patient for both assessment of degree of dehydration and for monitoring fluid therapy.
- Plasma total protein should be interpreted in the context of the patient's dehydration status. A dehydrated patient with a normal total protein may become hypoproteinemic once rehydrated.

- If abnormalities in plasma total protein are identified, a serum chemistry will be necessary to fully evaluate the underlying cause of the plasma total protein changes.

- Lipemia and hemolysis can alter the plasma total protein by refractometer, but icterus will not.

Reference

1 https://www.merckvetmanual.com/special-subjects/reference-guides/hematologic-reference-ranges

Suggested References

Stockham, S.L. and Scott, M.A. (2008). *Fundamentals of Veterinary Clinical Pathology*, 2e. Ames, Iowa: Blackwell Pub.

Villiers, E. and Risticì, J. (ed.) (2016). *BSAVA Manual of Canine and Feline Clinical Pathology*, 3e. Gloucester, Gloucestershire: British Small Animal Veterinary Association.

5

Gross and Microscopic Evaluation of the Buffy Coat
Sharon M. Dial

5.1 Procedural Definition: What Is This Test About?

Evaluation of a buffy coat has in the past been mostly associated with evaluating or staging canine mast cell tumors or systemic mastocytosis in the cat. It is now known that inflammatory diseases of the gastrointestinal or reproductive tract and hypersensitivity reactions are the most common causes of circulating mast cells in the dog and reviews of buffy coat preparation are less frequently done. Because of the focus on mast cell disease and buffy coat examination, the use of buffy coat evaluation for detection of blood-borne infectious agents and to concentrate atypical cells present in low numbers on the blood film for further evaluation has been neglected.

This procedure allows the concentration of leukocytes and platelets for further evaluation. Atypical cells and blood-borne infectious agents that are often present in low numbers on a routine blood film will be concentrated in the buffy coat layer of the hematocrit tube. Circulating microfilaria will be concentrated just above the buffy coat and can be easily visualized by microscopy prior to breaking the tube and preparing the buffy coat film. Gross evaluation of the buffy coat can quickly provide visual information on the number of leukocytes and/or platelets present.

5.2 Procedural Purpose: Why Should I Perform this Test?

The buffy coat is the small layer of leukocytes and platelets that concentrates above the red blood cell (RBC) column when whole blood is centrifuged in a microhematocrit tube. Gross inspection of the buffy coat should be a part of the evaluation of any blood sample centrifuged for a PCV and plasma protein evaluation. The preparation of a buffy coat slide is done when other tests suggest that close evaluation of leukocyte populations for atypical cells or infectious agents may be helpful or for submission of a sample for infectious disease polymerase chain reaction (PCR) or immunofluorescent tests. Buffy coat samples can be useful in dogs suspected of having canine distemper and cats for confirmation of persistent infection with feline leukemia virus.

When the buffy coat appears grossly abnormal (larger or smaller than expected), performing this procedure in conjunction with the PCV and plasma TP will save time and inform the interpretation of the complete blood count as a whole. Visual inspection of the height of the buffy coat, the plasma just above the buffy coat, and preparation of a buffy coat film are all useful tests to assist in the interpretation of the complete blood count in an ill patient. Visual inspection of the height of the buffy coat can provide a heads up that the patient may have significant changes in leukocyte and platelet numbers prompting submission of a blood sample for an automated complete blood count and close evaluation of the blood film.

The height of the buffy coat is a rough estimate of the combined leukocyte and platelet mass and can indicate significant leukocytosis or leukopenia and thrombocytosis or thrombocytopenia. Examination of the buffy coat enhances the chance of identifying atypical hematogenous and non-hematogenous cells, hemoparasites, and other blood-borne infectious agents. They are also excellent preparations to submit for more specific tests for infectious agents (PCR, fluorescent antibody tests).

Since air-dried buffy coats retain their staining quality for days to weeks when stored properly, a buffy coat film prepared at the same time as recording the PCV and TP can be stored for future testing if needed, based on history, clinical exam findings, complete blood count, and other diagnostic tests. It is important to remember that any test that depends on the recognition of a specific antigen on the cells may have a limited storage time since some antigen proteins can degrade over time.

Low-Cost Veterinary Clinical Diagnostics, First Edition. Ryane E. Englar and Sharon M. Dial.
© 2023 John Wiley & Sons, Inc. Published 2023 by John Wiley & Sons, Inc.

Examples of the infectious agents that can be difficult to find because they are present in low numbers on a blood film but will be concentrated in the buffy coat will be discussed below. Buffy coat preparations in patients with relatively low numbers of atypical cells can be used for further evaluation using special diagnostic tests, such as immunocytochemistry, cytochemistry, and PCR testing, where a concentrated sample will provide sufficient cells for interpretation.

Note: While it is tempting to perform a differential cell count on a buffy coat when the patient is leukopenic, the results will not be valid. The distribution of leukocytes in the buffy coat will be affected by the centrifugation process and how well the cells are distributed in making the slide. A more appropriate method of performing a differential cell count on a leukopenic sample is to place a temporary coverslip on the blood film and, using the 10× and 40× objectives, find and identify at least 50 or more cells.

5.3 Equipment

- Whole blood in a blood collection tube with anticoagulant (usually ethylenediaminetetraacetic acid, if heparin is used it will alter staining quality of the slide)
- Gloves
- Microhematocrit centrifuge
- Hematocrit tubes without anticoagulant
- Sealant
- Glass microscope slides
- Quick Romanowski stain set up
- Distilled water in a wash bottle.

5.4 Procedural Steps: How Do I Perform this Test?

Preparing the buffy coat slide.

- Gather all equipment needed for the procedure (see Figure 5.1).
- Mix the blood sample by either inverting it several times (5–8 inversions) or placing it on a blood tube rocker for 5–8 rotations as described in Chapter 3.
- Fill two microhematocrit tubes and centrifuge them as described in Chapter 3.
- Allow the centrifuge to stop completely. Remember, use of the break for nonemergency stops will cause damage to the breaking mechanism over time.
- Examine the height of the buffy coat. The buffy coat should be about 1% of the blood column in a normal dog or cat. Make a note in the record if the buffy coat appears

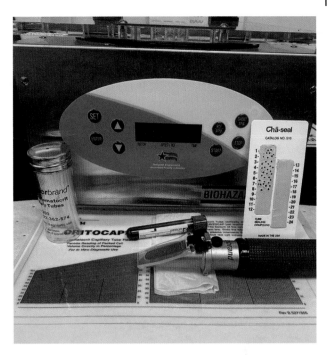

Figure 5.1 The equipment for preparing a buffy coat preparation includes whole blood with EDTA anticoagulant, gloves, microhematocrit tube without anticoagulant, sealant, glass microscope slides. (not shown is the Romanowski stain set up and distilled water). *Source:* Courtesy of Jeremy Bessett.

significantly less or greater than expected (see Figure 5.2).

- In regions where heartworm disease is endemic or suspected in a case, place the microhematocrit on the microscope stage and view the plasma at its interface with the buffy coat on 4× or 10×. Focus up and down on this area to identify any circulating microfilaria. The motility of the organisms will make them relatively easy to see.
- Score the hematocrit tube just into the RBC column below the buffy coat using a glass scoring pen or the edge of a glass slide as described in Chapter 4 (see Figure 5.3).
- Gently break the microhematocrit tube and discard the portion containing the RBCs and retain the portion with the buffy coat (see Figure 5.4).
  - A paper towel or KimWipe can be used to prevent shards of glass from falling onto the bench by lightly wrapping the microhematocrit tube before breaking.
- Gently expel the buffy coat and a small amount of plasma onto a labeled glass slide as described in Chapter 4 (see Figure 5.5).
- Make a "pull" preparation similar to those made for fine needle aspiration cytology or a blood film type preparation.
- The pull preparation is made by placing a second glass slide on top of the slide with the specimen and quickly pulling them apart (see Figure 5.6a and b).

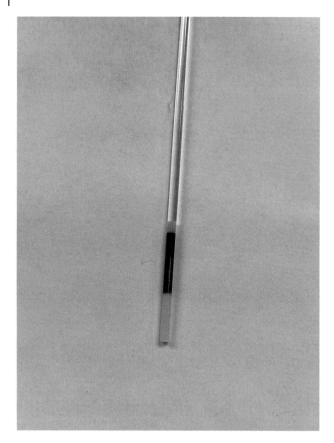

Figure 5.2 The buffy coat in this case is increased in size (greater than 1% of the RBC column). This sample is from a cat with severe anemia and a marked leukocytosis due to marked numbers of large undifferentiated leukocytes consistent with acute lymphoid leukemia. *Source:* Courtesy of Jeremy Bessett.

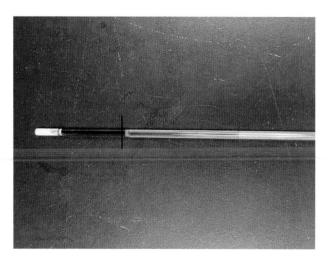

Figure 5.3 The black line indicates where the hematocrit tube should be scored. *Source:* Courtesy of Jeremy Bessett.

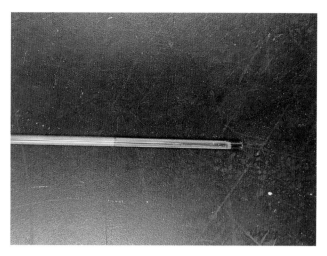

Figure 5.4 Discard the segment of the hematocrit tube containing the RBCs leaving the part of the hematocrit containing the buffy coat. Source: Courtesy of Jeremy Bessett.

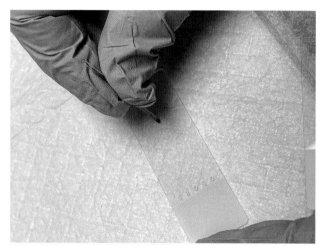

Figure 5.5 Tap or expel the buffy coat on to a slide. *Source:* Courtesy of Jeremy Bessett.

- The slides should be air-dried (not fixed) and either stained with a quick Romanowski stain or stored in a covered slide box at room temperature for evaluation later or submission for special diagnostic testing as needed.
- The buffy coat can be scanned using the 10× objective to identify large organisms, like microfilaria and large atypical cells.
- Using the 40× objective, the leukocytes can be scanned for larger intracellular organisms such as *Hepatozoon* gamonts and *Histoplasma* yeast forms.
- The 100× oil objective will need to be used to scan for smaller organisms like Rickettsial morulae and distemper inclusions.

Figure 5.6 (a) A spreader slide is placed on the buffy coat drop and it is allowed to spread. *Source:* Courtesy of Jeremy Bessett; (b) the slides are quickly pulled apart just as the buffy coat starts to spread. *Source:* Courtesy of Jeremy Bessett.

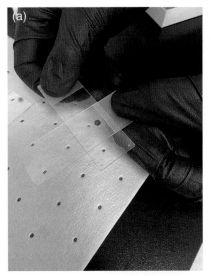
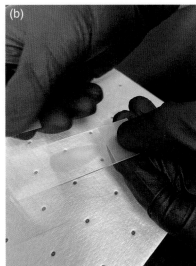

Staining the buffy coat slide

- Diff–Quik™ stain procedure (Modified Wright–Giemsa stain)
  - Check the date the stains were last changed out. Change out with fresh solutions if needed. See Procedural Tips and Troubleshooting section for recommendations on how often to change out the stain solutions.
  - Starting with solution 1 (methanol, light blue), dip the fully dried buffy coat film into the fixative solution 5–7 times (or place in solution 1 for 5–7 seconds) (see Figure 5.7).
  - Drain the slide by touching the bottom edge of the slide to the lip of the stain jar and dip the slide in solution 2 (eosinophilic stain, red/orange) 5–7 times (or place in solution 2 for 5–7 seconds) (see Figure 5.8).
  - Drain the slide by touching the bottom edge of the slide to the lip of the stain jar and dip the slide in solution 3 (basophilic stain, dark blue) 5–7 times (or place in solution 2 for 5–7 seconds) (see Figure 5.9).
  - Rinse the slide with distilled water until the water running off the slide is clear. Allow the slide to dry completely (see Figure 5.10).
  - Cap all staining containers securely when staining the slides is completed.
  - The number of times or length of time the slides are placed in each solution is not set in stone. In general, this protocol should provide good staining for buffy coat and blood films as long as the staining solutions are regularly changed. Establishing a standard protocol in your clinic laboratory will result in uniformity in the staining of slides and make evaluation easier. Note: More time may be needed in solution 3 when staining cytology slides, especially lymph node preparations.

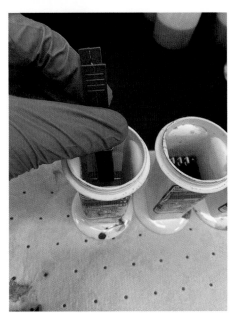

Figure 5.7 Dip the slide in the first solution 5–7 times. This solution is an alcohol fixative. *Source:* Courtesy of Jeremy Bessett.

- Procedure for Camco Quik Stain II™ (Wright–Giemsa stain). A standard Wright–Giemsa stain will provide better erythrocyte staining, especially for the identification of young polychromatic erythrocytes.
  - Check the date the stain was last changed and change out with fresh stain is needed.
  - Place the air-dried slide in the stain for 10 seconds (see Figure 5.11).
  - Without draining the stain off the slide, place the slide in the distilled water for 20 seconds (or longer if darker basophilic staining is preferred) (see Figure 5.12).

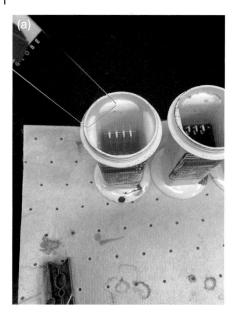

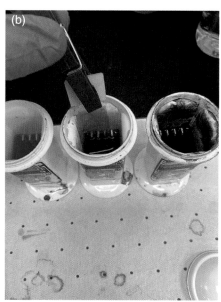

Figure 5.8 (a) Drain on the lip of the jar. *Source:* Courtesy of Jeremy Bessett; (b) dip the slide in the second solution 5–7 times. This is the eosinophilic stain that will stain erythrocytes and the granules of eosinophils. *Source:* Courtesy of Jeremy Bessett.

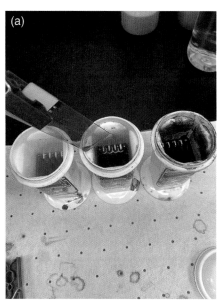

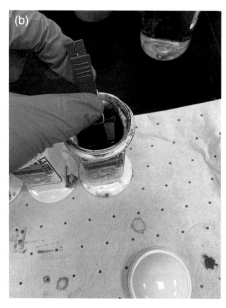

Figure 5.9 (a) Drain on the lip of the jar. *Source:* Courtesy of Jeremy Bessett; (b) dip the slide in the third solution 5–7 times. This is the basophilic stain that stains the nuclei of the leukocytes and contributes to the polychromatophilic staining of young erythrocytes. *Source:* Courtesy of Jeremy Bessett.

- Remove the slide and rinse off the remaining diluted stain with distilled water (see Figure 5.13).
- Dry the slide completely.
- Traditional Wright–Giemsa stain
  - Place an air-dried slide on a staining tray (see Figure 5.14)
  - Flood slide with fixative (alcohol solution) and leave for one minute (see Figure 5.15)
  - Tip off the fixative solution and flood the slide with the stain solution and leave for 10 minutes (see Figure 5.16)
  - Tip off the stain and slowly flood the slide with the buffer solution and gently tip the slide to mix the solutions. Leave on for five minutes (see Figure 5.17)
  - Wash off the slide with distilled water (see Figure 5.18).

There is considerable difference in the staining quality between the quick modified Romanowski (Diff–Quik) and the quick Wright–Giemsa stain. The erythrocytes in the modified stain have a red-brown appearance, which makes identification of polychromatophilic cells more difficult. The Wright–Giemsa stained erythrocytes have a brighter truer red color and polychromatophilic cells are truly bluer (see Figure 5.19).

5.5 Time Estimate to Perform Test

- Fifteen minutes including centrifugation of the sample for preparing the buffy coat slide
- Five to ten minutes to review the slide

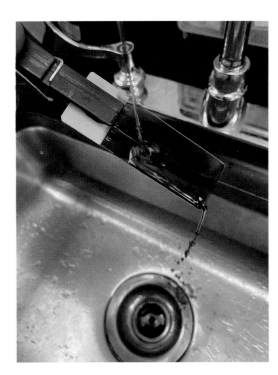

Figure 5.10 Rinse the slide briskly with distilled water to remove the stain. Poorly rinsed slides will have excessive stain precipitate that obscures some finding, especially small hemoparasites. *Source:* Courtesy of Jeremy Bessett.

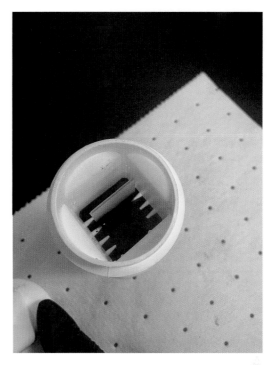

Figure 5.12 Place the slide in the distilled water for 20 seconds without draining the stain from the slide. The residual stain on the slide will mix with the distilled water to form a buffer that contributes to differential staining of the cells. The buffering of the water is best when the distilled water is at pH 6–7. A strip of pH paper can be used to test the pH of the distilled water if the stain does not differentiate appropriately. *Source:* Courtesy of Jeremy Bessett.

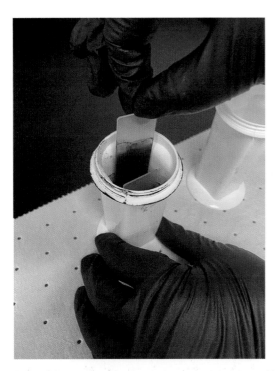

Figure 5.11 Place the slide in the stain solution for 10 seconds. This stain contains all the components (both eosinophilic and basophilic) along with the alcohol fixative to produce an appropriately stained slide. *Source:* Courtesy of Jeremy Bessett.

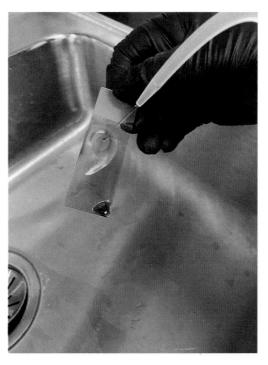

Figure 5.13 Rinse off the residual stain and allow the slide to air dry. *Source:* Courtesy of Jeremy Bessett.

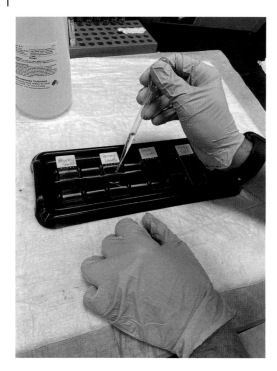

Figure 5.14 Air-dried slides are placed in a staining tray. Staining trays are relatively inexpensive and allow multiple slides to be stained quickly using this method. *Source:* Courtesy of Jeremy Bessett.

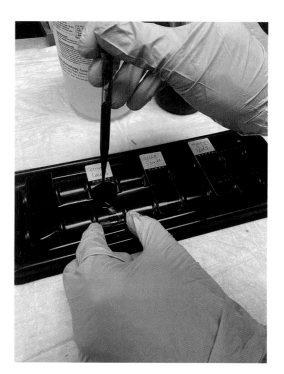

Figure 5.16 The fixative is tipped off and the slide is flooded with the stain for 10 minutes. *Source:* Courtesy of Jeremy Bessett.

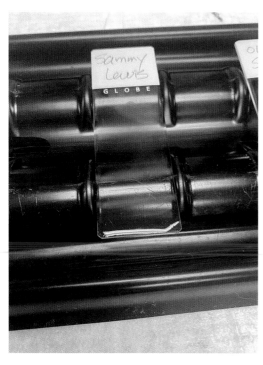

Figure 5.15 The slides are flooded with an alcohol fixative for one minute. *Source:* Courtesy of Jeremy Bessett.

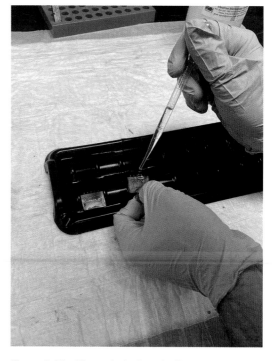

Figure 5.17 The stain is tipped off and the slide is flooded with the buffer solution and gently tilted to mix the solutions then left for five minutes. *Source:* Courtesy of Jeremy Bessett.

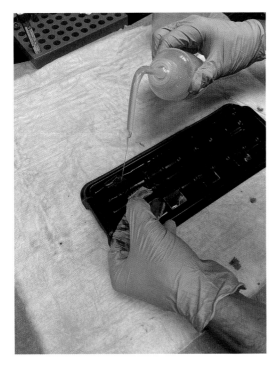

Figure 5.18 Finally, the slide is rinsed with distilled water. *Source:* Courtesy of Jeremy Bessett.

(a)

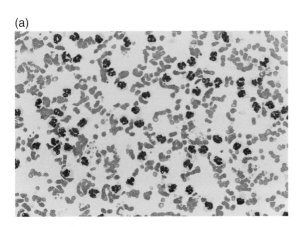

(b)

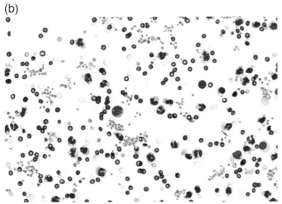

Figure 5.19 (a) Wright–Giemsa stained buffy coat; (b) Diff–Quik stain. *Source:* Courtesy of Jeremy Bessett.

5.6 Procedural Tips and Troubleshooting

- Heparinized microhematocrit tubes or samples collected in heparinized blood collection tubes are not recommended for collection of sample for buffy coat or blood film preparation. Heparin will alter the staining quality of the cells.
- It is important to remember that the buffy coat is a concentrated sample of leukocytes and platelets. As such, an occasional atypical leukocyte or reactive lymphocyte is expected on examination of the buffy coat film. These cells typically circulate in the normal animal in very low numbers. They are not commonly seen in the blood film due to their low numbers but can be seen more frequently on a buffy coat film.
- The best slide preparation method to use is the pull preparation. This will provide the largest area of monolayer for evaluation. The squash preparation can also be used but tends to have thick areas that do not lend themselves to evaluation. The squash preparation is made by placing the second glass slide on top of the slide with the sample and picking it directly up rather than pulling the slides apart.
- If the patient has significant leukopenia, it may be necessary to prepare an additional microhematocrit tube to pool the samples and provide sufficient cells for evaluation.
- Air-dried buffy coat films can be stored in a dry, room temperature environment away from dust contamination and light for several days to weeks without losing staining quality. Having a buffy coat slide prepared prior to any treatment is a good resource if the complete blood count suggests the possible presence of atypical cells or blood-borne infectious agents.
- The length of time the slides can be stored prior to submission for immunocytochemistry or PCR testing for infectious disease will depend on the specific cellular marker for immunocytochemistry and the infectious agent being investigated. Cellular proteins and DNA can degrade over time. Contact the diagnostic laboratory being used to determine if stored slides will be useful for the additional tests and how long they can be stored.

5.7 Interpreting Test Results

The buffy coat is used in the clinic to identify infectious agents [1] and to prepare a sample for submission to a reference laboratory for special diagnostic tests focused on the identification of large atypical cells that are present in low numbers on the blood film. If no atypical cells are present on the routine blood film, it is not appropriate to examine a buffy coat in search of atypical cells. It is not uncommon for immature hematopoietic cells and large lymphoid cells to be present in numbers not readily found on the blood film in a healthy patient. As a result, the buffy coat, a concentrated sample, may reveal several of these uncommon cells in patients with no hematopoietic or lymphoid disease.

Infectious agents that can be seen in higher number on a buffy coat preparation include distemper virus inclusion, morulae of Rickettsial agents, yeast such as Histoplasma capsulatum, and protozoa such as *Hepatozoon* spp.

5.8 Clinical Case Example(s)

See Part 6, cases #1, #6.

5.9 Add-On Tests That You May Need to Consider and Their Additive Value

- If organisms are seen on examination of a buffy coat, the sample should be submitted for confirmation by a veterinary clinical pathologist or for PCR for the organism suspected.

Reference

1 Mylonakis, M.E. et al. (2004). Mixed *Ehrlichia canis*, *Hepatozoon canis*, and presumptive Anaplasma phagocytophilum infection in a dog. *Veterinary Clinical Pathology* 33 (4): 249–251.

- If the blood film examination reveals atypical circulating leukocytes, submission of a buffy coat may be helpful in providing sufficient cells for immunocytochemistry or cytochemistry. In addition, a whole blood sample can be submitted for flow cytometry to identify subpopulations of atypical cells in patients suspected of leukemia.

5.10 Key Takeaways

- Buffy coat preparations allow the evaluation of a large number of leukocytes for infectious diseases that are often present in low numbers on a blood film.
- Buffy coat preparations are often requested by reference laboratories for PCR and fluorescent test for the diagnosis of canine distemper and feline leukemia virus persistent infection.
- Buffy coat preparation may be helpful in providing sufficient numbers of atypical cells in low numbers on the blood film when submitting a sample for immunocytochemical or cytochemical identification of the atypical cell origin.
- Gross evaluation of the buffy coat should be done on all centrifuged microhematocrit tubes.

6

The Blood Film

Sharon M. Dial

6.1 Procedural Definition: What Is This Test About?

The blood film is a hematological preparation in which whole blood is spread on a glass slide and stained with a Romanowsky stain to provide visual evaluation of peripheral blood cellular element morphology, number, and distribution. Historically, the blood film was an essential part of the complete blood count (CBC) and provided a differential count of the leukocytes from which absolute numbers were calculated as well as providing the opportunity for the evaluation of erythrocyte, leukocyte, and platelet morphology. With the increased availability of in-house hematology instrumentation, blood film evaluation has, regrettably, been underutilized in veterinary clinics.

6.2 Procedural Purpose: Why Should I Perform This Test?

Blood film review is now recommended for all blood samples submitted for an automated CBC by the American Society of Veterinary Clinical Pathologists (ASVCP) [1]. The blood film is considered a nonstatistical quality assurance procedure and provides an inexpensive and readily available internal quality control for the values reported using in-house hematology instruments. It also provides information not found in the automated CBC, which is essential for the evaluation of an ill patient. Identification of significant erythrocyte and leukocyte abnormal morphology or circulating hemoparasites and atypical cells cannot be done using in-house automated instruments.

While instruments can suggest the presence of a shift to immaturity in neutrophils as a component of an inflammatory leukogram, evaluation of the blood film is necessary to confirm the shift and to evaluate for changes in the neutrophils that assist in determining the degree of inflammation. While it is tempting to only evaluate a blood film when there are significant changes in erythrocyte, leukocyte, and platelet numbers, significant changes in the character of these cell populations can be present when numbers are within the reference limits.

Preparation of a blood film from a freshly collected blood sample will allow confirmation of abnormalities, such as thrombocytopenia, in samples submitted to a reference laboratory. Transport from the clinic to the laboratory and the delay in performing the automated CBC can introduce artifactual changes in morphology and cell number that can be either confirmed or refuted by a review of the blood film in the clinic. In addition, a quick review of the blood film at the clinic can provide a preview of the results that will be reported by the laboratory and allow the development of an initial treatment plan to be refined by the fully automated CBC once received. The blood film, when used in conjunction with the history and physical exam findings, will provide excellent, in the moment, information for the development of a differential diagnosis and the expedient choice of additional tests necessary for the refinement of the differential diagnosis.

6.3 Equipment

whole blood (preferably in EDTA)
glass slides
microhematocrit tubes
wooden applicator sticks
quick Romanowsky stain
distilled water
gloves

6.4 Procedural Steps: Preparing the Blood Film How Do I Perform This Test?

6.4.1 Procedure

- gather all supplies needed (see Figure 6.1)
- label slides with patient name and date
- gently mix the blood sample by either inverting it several times (five to eight inversions) or placing it on a blood tube rocker for five to eight rotations as described in Chapter 3.
- using either a micropipette, blood-filled hematocrit tube, or two wooden applicator sticks, place a small drop of blood (approximately 3 mm in diameter) on one end of a glass slide (see Figure 6.2a and b)
- hold the glass slide with the blood drop firmly in place, use a second glass slide (the "spreader" slide) to back up into the drop of blood, keeping the drop of blood behind the spreader slide in an acute angle of

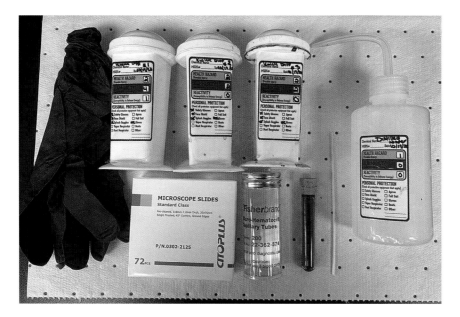

Figure 6.1 Equipment necessary for preparing a blood film include whole blood in anticoagulant, glass slides, microhematocrit tubes (or wooden applicator sticks), quick Romanowsky stain set, distilled water, and gloves. *Source:* Courtesy of Jeremy Bessett.

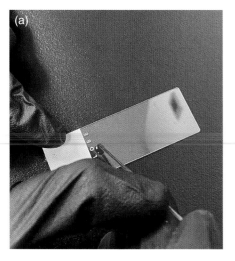 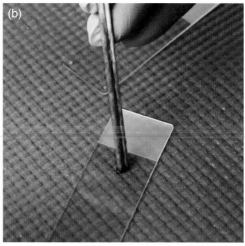

Figure 6.2 (a) A microhematocrit tube is used to place a small drop in the glass slide; (b) two wooden applicator sticks are used to place the blood on the slide. *Source:* Courtesy of Jeremy Bessett.

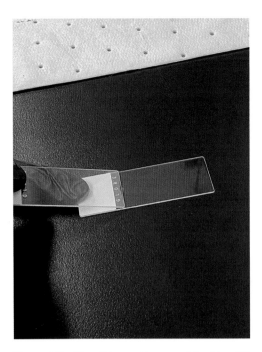

Figure 6.3 The slide used to spread the blood film should be held at a 45° angle and backed into the blood film. *Source:* Courtesy of Jeremy Bessett.

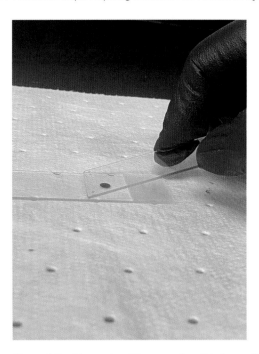

Figure 6.5 The angle of the spreader slide is smaller than 45° in this image to illustrate the angle used with blood that has a high PCV. *Source:* Courtesy of Jeremy Bessett.

- if the PCV is above the reference interval, the angle between the two slides should be less than 45° (see Figure 6.5)
- once the spreader slide has reached the drop of blood and the blood has spread out along the entire width of the spreader slide, quickly advance the spreader slide using light downward pressure and a quick fluid forward motion to the end of the horizontal slide (see Figure 6.6a and b)
- this procedure should produce a blood film that covers about 2/3 of the horizontal glass slide with a body, monolayer, and feathered edge (see Figure 6.7).

Staining the blood film: see Chapter 5, Buffy Coat.

6.4.2 Evaluating the Blood Film

Appropriate review of the blood film requires a well-defined protocol to ensure that the maximal information is obtained. Establishing a standard operating procedure for blood film review will result in consistent results regardless of who is performing the evaluation. The systematic review of the blood film should include:

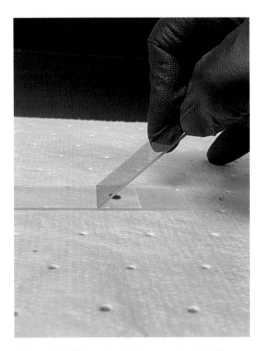

Figure 6.4 The angle of the spreader slide is greater than 45° in this image to illustrate the angle used with blood that has a low PCV. Courtesy of Jeremy Bessett. *Source:* Courtesy of Jeremy Bessett.

about 45° if the PCV is within reference interval (see Figure 6.3)
- if the PCV is below the reference interval, the angle between the two slides should be greater than 45° (see Figure 6.4)

- a gross evaluation of the blood film to note the quality of the blood film and to identify any abnormal staining like a blue tinge suggestive of high total protein or a "reverse" feathered edge suggesting significant erythrocyte agglutination

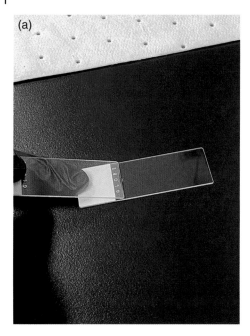 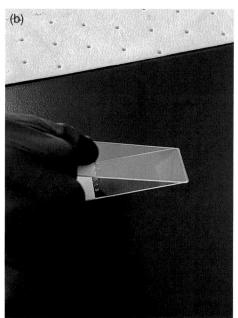

Figure 6.6 (a) Allow the blood to spread out to the edge of the spreader slide; (b) rapidly push the spreader slide in a continuous motion to the end of the slide. *Source:* Courtesy of Jeremy Bessett.

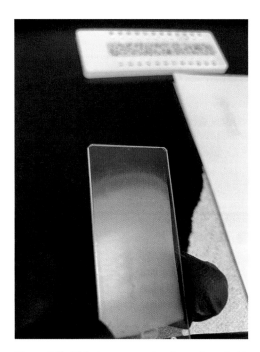

Figure 6.7 This is an example of a well-made blood film with a good-feathered edge and monolayer area. *Source:* Courtesy of Jeremy Bessett.

- using the 10× objective:
  - review of the feathered edge for platelet clumping, hemoparasites, and large, atypical cells
  - evaluate the density and distribution of leukocytes (low, appropriate, high); noting if the leukocytes are inappropriately concentrated at the feathered edge

- using the 40× objective:
  - estimate the white blood cell count; perform differential on samples with leukopenia
- using the 100× oil immersion objective:
  - evaluate platelet morphology and estimate platelet numbers
  - evaluate erythrocyte morphology with an estimate of frequency of each abnormality
- evaluate leukocyte morphology and perform a leukocyte differential count

6.4.3 Gross Examination of the Blood Film

- A properly prepared blood film should have a body, monolayer counting area, and feathered edge (see Figure 6.8). There should be no streaks, breaks, or clear droplets in the film.
- Assess the staining quality and density of the blood film. The blood film should not be too orange or too blue. If the staining quality is poor and the staining protocol has been followed, the stains should be replaced and a new slide stained.
  - Occasionally, increased blue staining of the blood film is seen with significantly high total protein. This can also be seen with altered plasma protein composition with hypergammaglobulinemia, resulting in a prominent blue hue to the stained slide (see Figure 6.9).
- If there is significant erythrocyte agglutination in the sample, the large aggregates of erythrocytes are carried

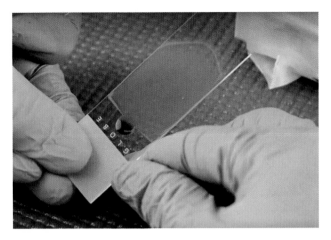

Figure 6.8 The blood film shows no streaks, breaks, or droplets and has an identifiable feathered edge and monolayer. *Source:* Courtesy of Jeremy Bessett.

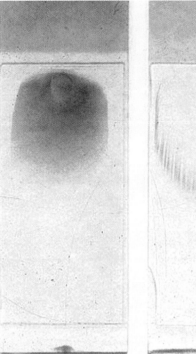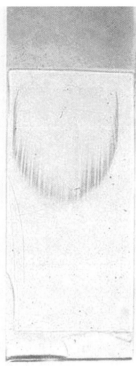

Figure 6.10 The side on the left is from a sample from a dog with a PCV in the reference interval. The slide on the right is from a dog with immune mediate hemolytic anemia and marked erythrocyte agglutination. Note the red blood cells are concentrated at the feathered edge. *Source:* Courtesy of Jeremy Bessett.

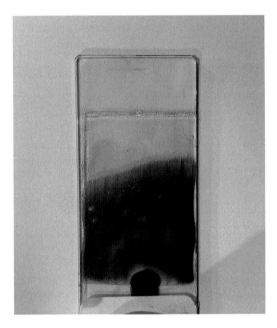

Figure 6.9 The blood film in this image is from a sample with a plasma total protein of 10.5 g/dl. *Source:* Courtesy of Jeremy Bessett.

to the feathered edge rather than being evenly distributed throughout the blood film, resulting in a "reverse" feathered edge (see Figure 6.10).

○ Slides with a "reverse" feathered edge are difficult to evaluate. The differential cell count and any estimate of cell numbers should be interpreted with care or not done. The large erythrocyte aggregates will also result in significant artifactual changes in the red cell count and indices on the automated CBC.

• If too much pressure is applied to the push slide or the blood film is made too slowly, the leukocyte distribution will be altered. A large number of leukocytes will be

carried to the feathered edge altering the leukocyte distribution and invalidating an estimate of the WBC count from the blood film (see Figure 6.11).

6.4.4 Microscopic Examination of the Blood Film

The blood film is initially reviewed using the 10x microscope objective . This degree of magnification allows an overall view of the density of leukocytes, a more precise assessment of the quality of the blood film, and evaluation of the feathered edge. After reviewing the slide with the 10x objective, most microscopists will move directly to the 100x oil emersion objective to evaluate platelet numbers and erythrocyte and leukocyte morphology, and perform a differential cell count. In doing so, the 40x objective is often overlooked as a tool in evaluation of the blood film, primarily because the use of this objective requires a coverslip to be placed on the microscope slide. Most practices do not coverslip their blood films, making it difficult to use the 40x objective, since it cannot be adequately focused without one. To utilize this objective, a temporary coverslip, using immersion oil as the mounting media, can be placed

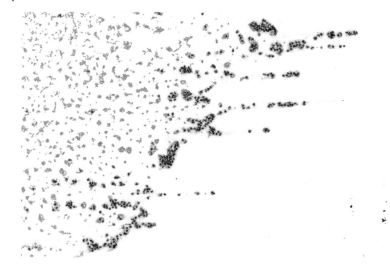

Figure 6.11 The blood film in this case was made with too much downward pressure and too slow, resulting in concentration of the leukocytes at the feathered edge. *Source:* Courtesy of Jeremy Bessett.

on the slide. The 40x objective allows the microscopist to estimate white blood cell count and perform a differential cell count quickly, especially in patients with leukopenia. Following a review of the blood film at 40x, a closer evaluation of erythrocyte and leukocyte morphology and platelet estimate can be done using the 100x oil emersion objective.

- review of the feathered edge using the 10x objective
  - The feathered edge is the thinnest area of the blood film. Platelet aggregates, larger cells, and large parasites like heartworm larvae are concentrated at the feathered edge. The feathered edge is initially evaluated using the 10x objective on the microscope. At this magnification, large platelet clumps and microfilaria are seen. With enough practice reviewing blood films, larger atypical cells can be appreciated at this power and further evaluated on the higher magnification objectives (40x and 100x oil immersion) (see Figure 6.12a–c).
  - Phagocytic cells containing the larger intracellular infectious agents that are uncommonly found in peripheral blood such as *Histoplasma capsulatum* and the schizonts of *Cytauxzoon felis* can also be found at the feathered edge [2] (see Figure 6.13a and b).
  - A very quick crude estimate of the leukocyte density can also be performed using the 10x objective. Less than 20 leukocytes/10x field is suggestive of a low leukocyte count and greater than 50 leukocytes/10x field is suggestive of a high leukocyte count (see Figure 6.14a–c).
- review of the monolayer using the 40x objective
  - Once the feathered edge of the blood film has been evaluated, a temporary coverslip can be placed on the slides as described previously. With the coverslip in place, an estimate of the WBC count can be performed.

- This estimate should provide a similar interpretation as the automated count. For instance, the WBC estimate should reveal a leukopenia, leukocytosis, or within a normal reference interval that is consistent with the automated count. It is important to remember, this is an estimate and is expected to be less accurate than the automated count, so the counts themselves can differ by several thousand WBC/µl. It should, however, be in the "ball park." If there is considerable difference between the two counts that would alter the interpretation of the leukocyte count (i.e. the automated count is significantly high and the estimate from the blood film is low), the estimate from an adequately mixed blood sample and a well-made blood film with a good leukocyte distribution is usually the best assessment of the leukocyte numbers. The sample should be re-run in the instrument and if there is still a significant difference, the sample can be submitted to a reference laboratory.
- The WBC count can be estimated by counting the total number of leukocytes in ten 40x fields in the monolayer of the blood film and then using the following formula:
  - total WBCs counted in 10 fields/$10 \times 2000 =$ estimated WBC count;
    example: if 50 leukocytes are counted in ten 40x fields, the estimated WBC count would be:
    - $50/10 \times 2000 = 10\,000$ cell/µl.
- It is important to remember that this is an estimate. How well the estimate correlates with the automated WBC count will depend on the area of the 40x objective field of view and the quality of the blood film. This formula should work for most standard 40x objectives.

(a)

(b)

(c)

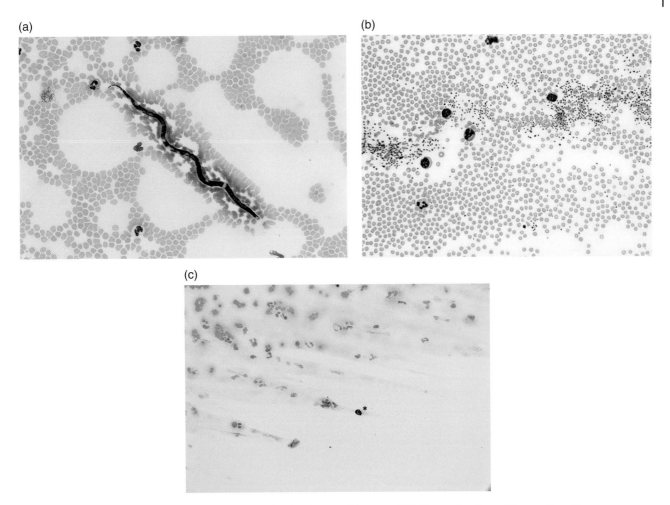

Figure 6.12 (a) *Dirofilaria immitus* microfilaria; (b) platelet clusters; (c) mast cell(*). *Source:* Courtesy of Jeremy Bessett.

(a)

(b)

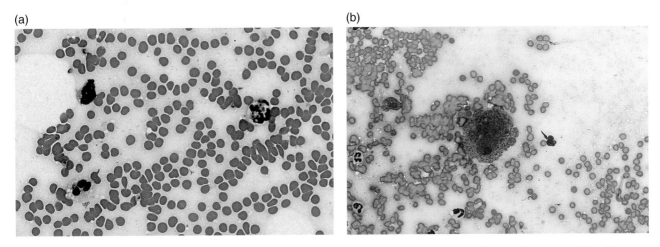

Figure 6.13 (a) Neutrophil with phagocytized *Histoplasma capsulatum* yeast forms (center right); (b) large *Cytauxzoon felis schizont* (Large cell in center). *Source:* Courtesy of Jeremy Bessett.

(a)

(b)

(c)

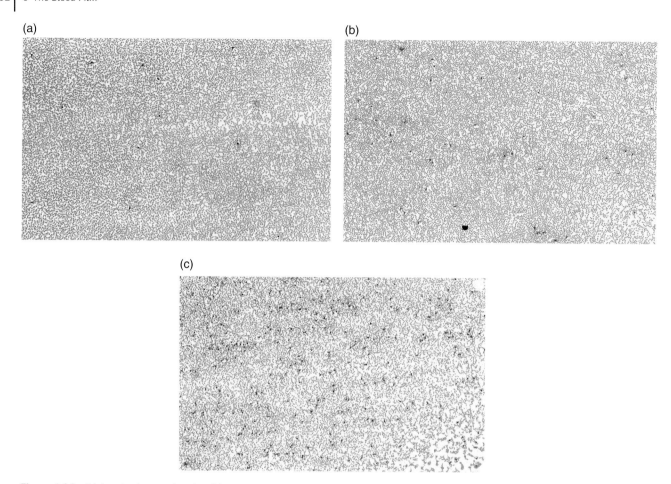

Figure 6.14 (a) Low leukocyte density; (b) appropriate leukocyte density; (c) high leukocyte density. *Source:* Courtesy of Jeremy Bessett.

○ After estimation of the WBC count, a differential leukocyte count is performed. The differential can be performed using the 40x objective much quicker than using the 100x oil immersion objective, especially in a sample with a low normal or low WBC count.

■ The procedure for the differential cell count is to categorize 100 cells into the following groups: neutrophils, lymphocytes, monocytes, eosinophils, basophils, band neutrophils, metamyelocytes, myelocytes, large undifferentiated cells, and nucleated RBCs.

■ The differential is reported as the percentage of each leukocyte type based on the number of leukocytes categorized.

■ There are several phone and tablet applications that can be used to do a manual differential cell count. However, they are inconsistently available; therefore, a stand-alone manual or electronic cell counter is recommended (see Figure 6.15a and b).

● The number of leukocytes usually counted in a manual differential is 100 cells. However, if the leukocyte count is significantly high (>30000/μl), a 200-cell differential would be needed to provide a more representative differential count. An additional 100 cells should ideally be counted in the differential for each additional 10,000 cells/μl above 30,000/μl. To calculate the final percentage when counting more than 100 cells, the number of cells in each category is divided by the total number of cells counted and multiplied by 10.

For example, in a 300-cell differential count, if 287 neutrophils are counted, the percentage of neutrophils would be: $(287/300) \times 10 = 95.6\%$

If the patient is severely leukopenic, it may be difficult to count 100 cells in the area of the monolayer. In this case, the same formula is used. If only 56 cells are found in the monolayer and 45 of them are categorized as lymphocytes, the percentage of lymphocytes in the differential would be: $(45/56) \times 10 = 83\%$.

● Review of the monolayer counting area using the 100x oil immersion objective.

Note: When evaluating blood cell morphology, it is recommended to have a good hematology atlas on hand to

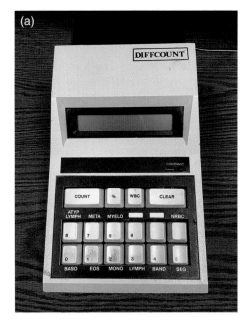
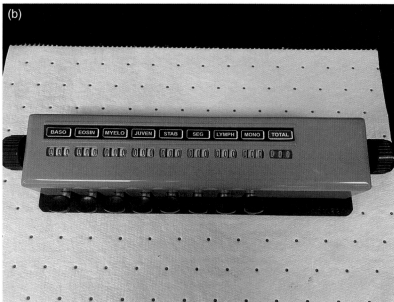

Figure 6.15 (a) The electronic cell counters not only allow counting of individual cells; they calculate the absolute numbers of the cells counted and can enumerate the number of nucleated red blood cells/100 leukocytes; (b) a manual cell counter. *Source:* Courtesy of Jeremy Bessett.

assist in the identification of blood cell morphology changes in all three cell lineages. See the suggested readings list for several available atlases for use in the clinic.

o The 100x oil immersion objective is used to closely examine the morphology of all peripheral blood formed elements and look for any hemoparasites within erythrocytes, leukocytes, and platelets.

o Evaluating platelets before focusing on erythrocytes and leukocytes is recommended because platelet morphology is often overlooked. Record the frequency of large platelets and the presence of small platelet aggregates. The presence of large platelets and small platelet aggregates can artifactually decrease automated platelet counts. In addition, since platelet aggregates are counted as one platelet in the platelet estimate from the blood film, they will negatively impact the estimated count as well.

o Erythrocyte morphology should be evaluated with a subjective estimate of frequency. Erythrocyte morphology includes changes in size (macrocytosis, microcytosis), color (polychromasia, hypochromasia), and shape (poikilocytosis).

- Consistency in reporting the frequency of erythrocyte changes is important. The literature often reports these findings as slight, mild, moderate, marked, 1+, 2+, 3+, 4+, or as a percentage of the number of cells in the field. Consider using the following guide to report red cell morphology findings based on a system developed by Weiss [3] (see Table 6.1).

Table 6.1 Standard protocol for reporting erythrocyte morphology (cells/1000× field)*.

	1+	2+	3+	4+
Anisocytosis				
Dog	7–15	16–20	21–29	>30
Cat	5–8	9–15	16–20	>20
Polychromasia				
Dog	2–7	8–14	15–29	>30
Cat	1–2	3–8	9–15	>15
Codocytes (target cells)				
Dog	3–5	6–15	16–30	>30
Hypochromasia				
Both species	1–10	11–50	51–200	>200
Poikilocytosis				
Both species	3–10	11–50	51–200	>200
Spherocytosis				
Both species	5–10	11–50	51–150	>150
Echinocytes				
Both species	5–10	11–100	101–250	>250
All other morphologies				
Both species	1–2	3–8	9–20	>20

Source: Weiss [3].

- The most common significant erythrocyte shape changes seen on blood films include burr cells, keratocytes, blister cells, Heinz bodies, eccentrocytes, spherocytes, acanthocytes, and schistocytes (see Figure 6.16a–f and h).
- Polychromasia, hypochromasia and microcytosis should be noted as well and are important in determining the underlying cause of anemia and degree of regeneration. Polychromasia can be difficult to appreciate on a quick Romanowski stain such as Diff–Quik™ since they tend to be a "muddy" blue (see Figure 6.17). Since most polychromatophilic cells are larger than normal, the size of a cell can be helpful in recognizing the staining quality of a polychromatophilic cells when using a modified Romanowski quick stain.
- Close examination for hemoparasites and other infectious agents is important in any ill patient, especially one with anemia. Common hemoparasites include *Mycoplasma hemofelis*, *C. felis*, *Babesia canis* (see Figure 6.18a–c).
- Distemper inclusion can be seen within erythrocytes in acute infection when the patient is viremic. These inclusions are best appreciated on Diff–Quik stain since they are less prominent on traditional Wright–Giemsa stains (see Figure 6.19).
  - ○ Leukocyte morphology should be evaluated with close evaluation for toxic changes in neutrophils, morphology of lymphocytes (increased basophilia, nuclear atypia, cytoplasmic granules), atypical cells (large unclassified cells, mast cells), and infectious agents.
    - Neutrophil toxic change is defined as increased cytoplasmic vacuolation, increased cytoplasmic basophilia, and the presence of Döhle bodies (in order of most to least significant). Toxic change is a cytoplasmic feature. It is important to remember that Döhle bodies are only significant in the dog. Although neutrophil toxic granulation can be seen with marked toxic change, it is rare in the dog and cat (see Figure 6.20).
    - Lymphocyte morphology should include evaluation of cell size, nuclear characteristics, cytoplasmic basophilia, and cytoplasmic granulation. Reactive lymphocytes are not uncommon in the dog and cat, especially in the young animal. They can be misidentified as neoplastic cells. Reactive lymphocytes are characterized by increased cytoplasmic basophilia, presence of a perinuclear clear zone, cytoplasmic granules, and nuclear pleomorphism (indented and lobulated nuclei) (see Figure 6.21).

They are usually present in small numbers. If there are significant numbers of these cells seen on a blood film, the sample should be referred for a pathologist's review.
- Large unclassified cells are leukocytes that are larger than a neutrophil with nuclei that have fine open chromatin with or without a nucleolus and variable amounts of cytoplasm with or without granulation. In the past, these cells were identified as "blasts" but that term is no longer used. These cells are indicative of possible myeloproliferative disease or the leukemic phase of solid tissue lymphoma. Currently, special diagnostics, such as flow cytometry, polymerase chain reaction (PCR) for antigen receptor rearrangement (PARR), immunocytochemistry, and cytochemical stains are required to confirm the lineage of these cells. Morphologic characteristics cannot reliably differentiate lymphoid cells from other lineages without evaluating phenotype (see Figure 6.22).
- Evaluation for intraleukocytic infectious agents should be done. Rickettsial organisms and *Hematozoon* sp. can be identified on a well-stained blood film (see Figure 6.23a and b).
- Distemper inclusions can also be seen in neutrophils when the patient is viremic (see Figure 6.24).

6.5 Time Estimate to Perform Test

Five to ten minutes.

6.6 Procedural Tips and Troubleshooting

- The most important aspects of preparing a uniform blood film are:
  - ○ dispensing the right amount of blood onto the slide (see Figure 6.25):
    - too large of a drop will not allow the complete incorporation of the blood drop on to the film and can produce a thick slide without an appropriate monolayer or feathered edge
    - too small a drop will not allow a large enough monolayer for evaluation
  - ○ keeping the drop of blood within the angle of the slide used to spread the blood across the horizontal glass slide. A common mistake in preparing a blood film is to try and "pull" the blood by pushing the slide up to the drop of blood instead of backing it into the drop of blood (see Figure 6.26)

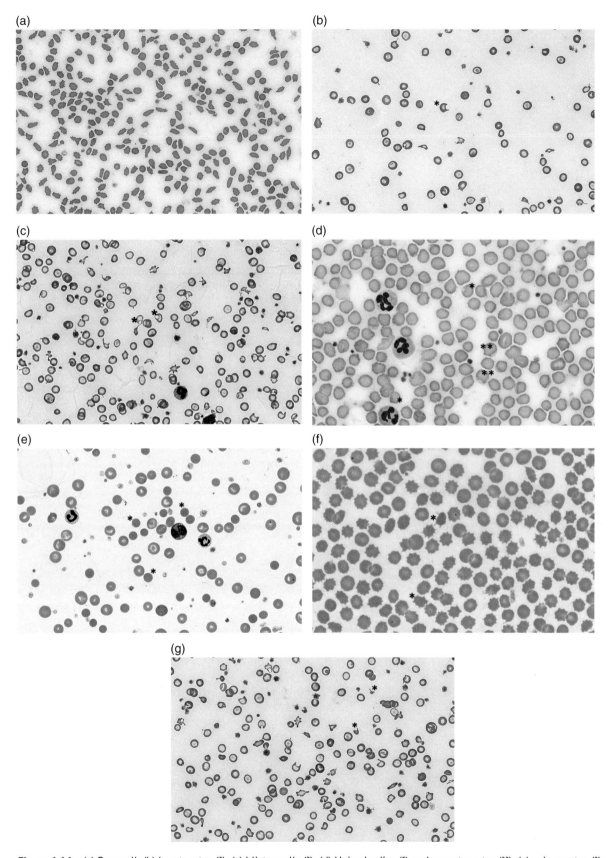

Figure 6.16 (a) Burr cell; (b) keratocytes (*); (c) blister cells (*); (d) Heinz bodies (*) and eccentrocytes (**); (e) spherocytes (*); (f) acanthocytes (*); (g) shistocytes (*). *Source:* Courtesy of Jeremy Bessett.

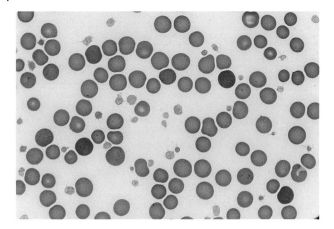

Figure 6.17 The polychromatophilic cel are not a true blue but slightly muddy in this slide stained with a modified Romanowski quick stain. *Source:* Courtesy of Jeremy Bessett.

○ using a light pressure on the spreader slide as it is quickly pushed across the horizontal slide without hesitation

○ using the correct angle of the spreader slide depending on the thickness of the blood

■ a smaller angle (<45°) between the two slides is needed for blood with a high PCV; if the angle is not small enough, a very short blood film is made

■ a larger angle (>45°) between the two slides is needed for blood with a low PCV; if the angle is not large enough, a long blood film that may run off the end of the slide is made

○ If the patient has a disease process that contributes to red cell fragility (hemolytic anemia, lipemia, iron deficiency), consider making a blood film without holding onto the spreader slide, but instead resting it on one finger to pull it back into the blood drop and push it forward. This technique is easy to perfect with

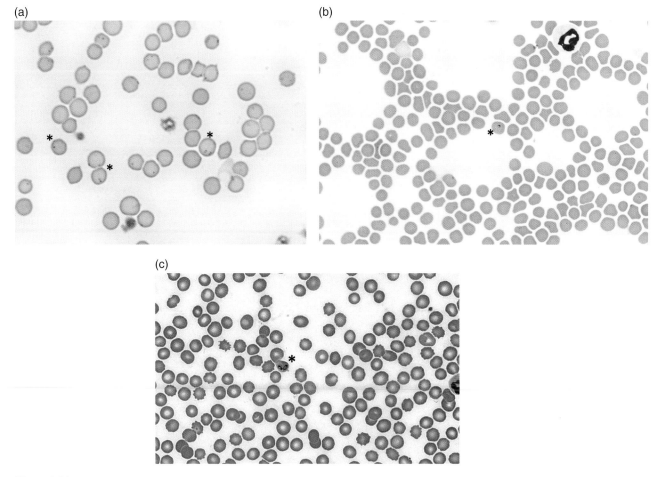

Figure 6.18 (a) *Mycoplasma hemofelis* (*); (b) *Cytauxzoon felis* (*); (c) *Babesia canis* (*).

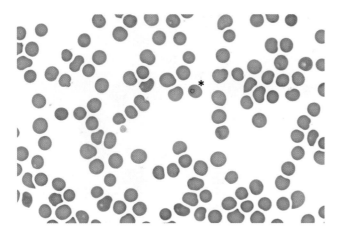

Figure 6.19 Canine distemper virus inclusion within an erythrocyte (*). *Source:* Courtesy of Jeremy Bessett.

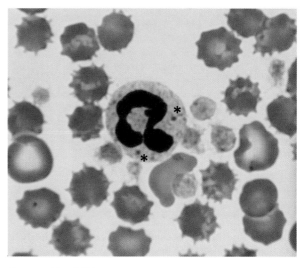

Figure 6.20 Döhle bodies in a canine neutrophil (*). *Source:* Courtesy of Jeremy Bessett.

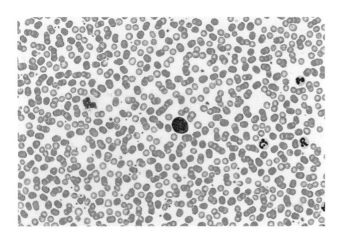

Figure 6.21 Note the large cell present in the center of the field. The cell is much larger compared to the neutrophils. This cell may or may not indicate neoplastic process. When seen on a blood film, consider submission of the sample to a reference laboratory for a pathologist review. *Source:* Courtesy of Jeremy Bessett.

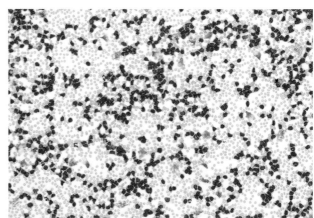

Figure 6.22 Acute myeloproliferative disease in a dog. While these cells are consistent with lymphoid origin, submitting a sample for flow cytometry would be needed to confirm the linage. *Source:* Courtesy of Jeremy Bessett.

(a)

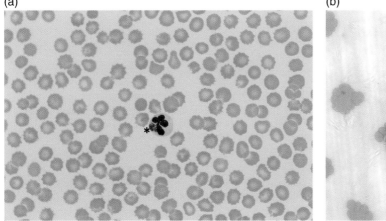

(b)

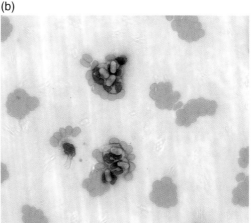

Figure 6.23 (a) A morula of *Anaplasma phagocytophilum* is present in the cytoplasm of a neutrophil (*); (b) multiple oblong lightly staining gamonts of *Hepatozoon canis* is seen in the cytoplasm of the neutrophils. *Source:* Courtesy of Jeremy Bessett.

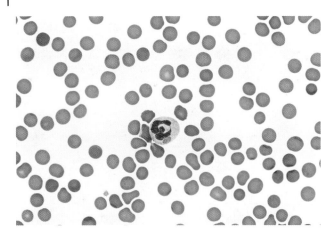

Figure 6.24 An eosinophilic canine distemper virus inclusion is present in the cytoplasm of a neutrophil. *Source:* Courtesy of Jeremy Bessett.

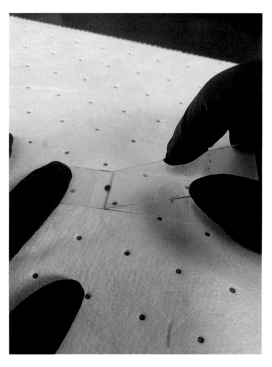

Figure 6.26 In this image, the spreader slide is in the wrong position. The drop of blood should be behind, not in front of the edge of the spreader slide. Blood cannot be spread appropriately using this configuration. *Source:* Courtesy of Jeremy Bessett.

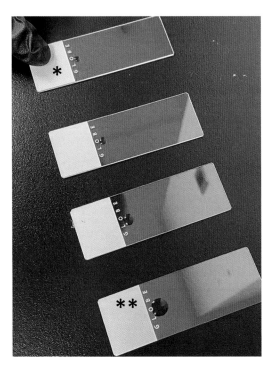

Figure 6.25 Too little blood is present on the slide at the top (*) and too much blood is present on the slide at the bottom (**). *Source:* Courtesy of Jeremy Bessett.

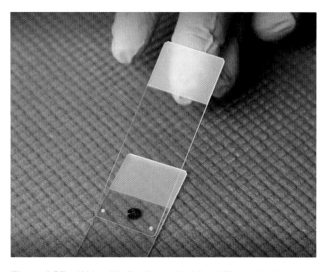

Figure 6.27 If blood is fragile or the blood film maker has a "heavy hand," a good quality blood film can be made by resting the spreader slide on a finger to pull it back to the drop of blood and push it out to make the blood film. *Source:* Courtesy of Sharon Dial.

practice. In addition to helping with fragile blood, the technique will help an individual that struggles with putting too much pressure on the spreader slide while making a blood film (see Figure 6.27)

- Defining a standard protocol for review of the blood film will ensure that all aspects of the blood film receive adequate attention
- Creating and using a standard form for recording the blood film evaluation findings encourages uniform reporting and ensures that the standard protocol is followed by each individual performing the evaluation
- monitoring of staining quality, maintenance of the stain quality by keeping the lids on the staining jars and

strictly following the appropriate staining procedure, and routine replacement of the stain solutions are essential to ensure the quality of the blood film for review.

6.7 Interpreting Test Results

The full interpretation of the blood film is beyond the scope of this text. There are numerous excellent references available to assist in the interpretation of hematological findings (see Suggested References). Having a good hematology atlas at hand when reviewing a blood film is essential. The quick blood film review will assist in determining the underlying cause of anemia by allowing evaluation of regeneration based on the degree of polychromasia, always keeping in mind that a reticulocyte count is essential to determine the full extent of the regenerative process. Review of the leukocytes will assist in differentiating physiological processes, inflammation, and myeloproliferative disease.

Close examination of red blood cell morphology will provide important information concerning causes of anemia

- increased polychromasia (≥3+ supports a regenerative bone marrow response)
  - regenerative anemias
    - blood loss
    - hemolysis
      - immune-mediated – primary or secondary
      - nonimmune-mediated – oxidative injury
    - iron deficiency
- moderate to marked numbers of spherocytes support immune-mediated hemolysis
  - occasional spherocytes can be seen with fragmentation and oxidative hemolysis
- ghost cells with hemoglobinemia and hemoglobinuria support intravascular hemolysis
  - small numbers of ghost cells can be seen as artifacts due to *in vitro* hemolysis
- Heinz bodies and eccentrocytes support oxidative injury from possible toxins
  - onions, zinc, copper, acetaminophen
- schistocytes support fragmentation anemia and suggest possible microangiopathy (disseminated intravascular coagulation) or decreased red cell deformability (iron deficiency)
- poikilocytosis with keratocytes, blister cells, and schistocytes in conjunction with hypochromasia and microcytosis support iron deficiency anemia
- burr cells suggest either liver or renal disease as an underlying process in an anemic patient

Evaluation of leukocyte distribution can support

- inflammation with or without evidence of sepsis
  - neutrophil morphology
    - toxic change
    - shift to immaturity in neutrophils
      - not all inflammatory responses result in a shift to immaturity. Lack of a shift does not rule out an inflammatory process, including infectious disease
      - compensated shift (regenerative shift) indicative of adequate bone marrow response
        - leukocytosis with neutrophilia
        - orderly shift to immaturity
          - neutrophils > bands > metamyelocytes> myelocytes
      - non-compensated shift (degenerative shift) indicative of inadequate bone marrow response
        - mild to moderate in severity
          - neutrophils within reference interval
          - orderly shift to immaturity
        - moderate to severe
          - immature forms > neutrophils
          - neutropenia with any shift to immaturity
    - marked neutropenia without a shift to immaturity
      - endotoxemia – may have a mild shift
      - immune-mediated neutropenia – may be associated with a monocytosis
      - Bone marrow suppression or injury.
- leukocytosis with atypical circulating cells suggestive of myeloproliferative disease
- Physiologic processes such as epinephrine and glucocorticoid effects
  - glucocorticoid response
    - neutrophilia
    - lymphopenia
    - ± monocytosis (dogs)
    - eosinopenia
  - Epinephrine response
    - neutrophilia
    - lymphocytosis
    - other cell types may or may not be increased
- These leukocyte patterns may be present concurrently. It is important to interpret leukocyte patterns in the context of the patient. It can be difficult to differentiate an inflammatory leukogram without a left shift from a stress leukogram. While the presence of toxic change is primarily associated with an inflammatory response and often indicative of sepsis, it can be seen in non-septic inflammation.

Examination of the blood film can reveal infectious agents such as

- *Dirofilaria immitis*
- canine distemper virus

- Rickettsial disease (*Ehrlichia, Anaplasma*)
- mycoplasmal diseases (*Mycoplasma hemofelis, Mycoplasma hemocanis*)
- *Babesia canis, Babesia gibsonii*
- *Hepatozoon* sp.
- *Cytauxzoon felis*
- circulating fungal yeast forms.

Importantly, review of the blood film will provide an excellent internal control for in-house and reference laboratory instruments. A well-made blood film done at the time of the blood drawn will provide an excellent snapshot of a patient's hematological state. In fact, in samples sent out to reference laboratories, the freshly made blood film can provide a better overview of the blood, especially in regard to platelet numbers. Depending on how long the sample is in transit, significant platelet clumping, leukocytes degeneration, and *in vitro* hemolysis can occur (especially in patients with fragile blood cells).

6.8 Clinical Case Example(s)

See Part 6, cases #1, #2, #6, #8, #15.

6.9 Add-On Tests That You May Need to Consider and Their Additive Value

- Complete blood cell count – If there are significant findings on the blood film, it is important to obtain a full CBC. Automated instruments will provide RBC indices that are necessary to evaluate anemia. In addition, the newer in-house and reference laboratory instrumentation will provide an automated reticulocyte count as well. Automated instruments usually provide a more accurate WBC count and differential. The number of cells the instrument counts for a differential is many magnitudes of order higher than the number of cells counted manually. While there are times that the instrument may have difficulty correctly categorizing leukocytes and counting RBCs and platelets, the majority of the time they provide excellent data.
- Serum chemistry profile – disease processes in many organ systems can be reflected in changes in the blood. Specifically, diseases affecting the liver, pancreas, intestinal tract, and kidney commonly are reflected in abnormalities in peripheral blood.
- Urinalysis – findings in the urinalysis can assist in supporting *in vivo* hemolysis, suggest significant inflammation providing a source for a focus of sepsis or blood loss.
- Infectious disease PCR or titers – PCR can be used to confirm the presence of infectious agents if the clinical presentation is suggestive of infectious disease, but no organisms are found. In addition, PCR can be used to confirm the presence of an organism if they are present in low numbers or their morphology is not typical.

6.10 Key Takeaways

- Review of a freshly made blood film is an excellent quick evaluation of the peripheral blood and can add significant information to the values obtained with regard to the automated CBC.
- It is recommended to make and keep a blood film to review if the results of the automated CBC is not consistent with the clinical findings in the patient.
- Significant changes can occur in the blood sample if there is a significant delay in performing the automated CBC, leukocytes may degenerate and platelets clumping is common. Having a freshly made blood film may preclude having to redraw a sample.
- The estimate of the platelet count from the blood film can be a better representation of platelet mass than an automated platelet count, especially in samples that are sent to reference laboratories that may be in transit for significant amount of time.

References

1 Flatland, B., Freeman, K.P., Vap, L.M. et al. (2013 Dec). ASVCP guidelines: quality assurance for point-of-care testing in veterinary medicine. *Veterinary Clinical Pathology* 42 (4): 405–423.

2 Sleznikow, C.R., Granick, J.L., Cohn, L.A. et al. (2022 Jan). Evaluation of various sample sources for the cytologic diagnosis of *Cytauxzoon felis*. *Journal of Veterinary Internal Medicine* 36 (1): 126–132.

3 Weiss, D.J. (1984). Uniform evaluation and Semiquantitative reporting of hematologic data in veterinary laboratories. *Veterinary Clinical Pathology* 13 (2): 27–31.

Suggested Bench-Side Reference

Reagan, W.J.I., Rovira, A.R., and Denicola, D.B. (2019). *Veterinary Hematology: Atlas of Common Domestic and Non-domestic Species*, 3e. Hoboken: Wiley Blackwell.

Harvey, J.W. (2012). *Veterinary Hematology a Diagnostic Guide and Color Atlas*. St. Louis, Mo: Elsevier/Saunders.

7

Blood Glucose
Sharon M. Dial

7.1 Procedural Definition: What Is This Test About?

Whole blood glucose can be a very useful window into a patient's metabolic state. Numerous diseases are associated with changes in whole blood glucose concentration. Determination of whole blood glucose is used both diagnostically and in monitoring the response to therapy. Handheld glucometers allow a rapid patient-side determination of whole blood glucose concentration and are especially useful when evaluating a patient with history and clinical findings suggestive of diabetes mellitus, Cushing's disease, liver disease, sepsis, or neurologic disease involving either seizures or changes in mentation.

7.2 Procedural Purpose: Why Should I Perform This Test?

Glucose is the primary source of energy for cellular metabolism and one of the few clinical chemistry tests that can be considered a true STAT test, especially in a patient with seizures or altered mentation. With the onset of reliable in-house handheld glucometers, this test can be easily performed on a small amount of whole blood for both diagnosis and monitoring of patients with altered metabolic needs.

Whole blood glucose concentration can be altered by many pathophysiological mechanisms including increased or decreased metabolic consumption, decreased or increased production, and decreased glycogen stores. Many disorders of glucose metabolism are the result of changes in hormone activity. The primary hormones involved in glucose metabolism are insulin (decreases blood glucose), glucagon (increases blood glucose). Diabetes mellitus is common in both dogs and cats and depends on the identification of persistent hyperglycemia with glucosuria. In

addition, high circulating concentrations of glucocorticoids, catecholamines, and growth hormone can oppose the activity of insulin (insulin antagonists) increasing blood glucose concentration in stressed or excited patients. Decreased circulating glucocorticoids can result in hypoglycemia by increasing peripheral insulin sensitivity and inhibiting gluconeogenesis.

Since the liver is a primary site for storage of glucose in the form of glycogen and production of glucose by gluconeogenesis or glycogenolysis, loss of greater than 75% of liver mass can result in hypoglycemia. Starvation-induced hypoglycemia is rare in the adult dog and requires severe depletion of glycogen stores and protein as a source of amino acids for gluconeogenesis. In contrast, young animals, especially toy breeds, have a higher frequency of hypoglycemia associated with starvation or hyporexia. This is due to their limited glycogen storage and reduced capacity for gluconeogenesis. One of the most common abnormalities seen in starvation is decreased urea nitrogen rather than hypoglycemia. See Chapter 8 for evaluation of whole blood urea nitrogen using in-house test strips.

Sepsis, due to the production of inflammatory cytokines that are insulin antagonists, is also associated with alterations in blood glucose concentration. Both hyperglycemia and hypoglycemia can be seen with sepsis depending on the time frame of the disease. Acute sepsis is often associated with increased circulating corticosteroids and catecholamines resulting in hyperglycemia. As the septic process proceeds, depletion of hepatic glycogen stores, decreased hepatocyte gluconeogenesis, and decreased insulin clearance by the liver result in the development of hypoglycemia. As with all clinical pathology data, blood glucose should be interpreted within the context of the patient and other laboratory data.

Whole blood glucose is required when evaluating any patient with clinical history or physical exam findings suggestive of diabetes mellitus, such as polyuria, polydipsia, weight loss (especially in the face of a good appetite), hyporexia, chronic inflammatory, or infectious disease, such as chronic urinary tract infections, and cataracts. Both in clinic and at home monitoring of whole blood glucose is essential when following a patient with diabetes mellitus [1]. Since stress and excitement can alter blood glucose concentration, teaching a client how to use a handheld glucometer to perform glucose monitoring in a less stressful environment for the patient is not uncommon. Given adequate guidance and training, most owners can perform a glucose curve at home when needed to assist in evaluating a patient's insulin needs. As with all tests, it is important to assure that the owner understands and uses a standard protocol and maintains proper recording of the results.

Glucose is the primary source of energy for maintenance of neuronal activity. The brain requires a constant source of glucose to maintain normal function and mentation. Any patient with altered mentation, ataxia, weakness, convulsions, or seizures should have a blood glucose concentration determination done. It is important to remember that a rapid drop in blood glucose concentration will result in acute clinical signs at a higher blood glucose concentration than is seen when there is a gradual decrease. It is difficult to predict clinical signs based on a single blood glucose value, clinical history, and other physical findings are important factors in the interpretation of blood glucose.

Urine glucose evaluation is important in evaluating the underlying cause of hyperglycemia. Stress or excitement induced hyperglycemia may or may not be associated with glucosuria. The hyperglycemia of stress and excitement are transient and usually not sufficiently high to exceed the renal tubular glucose reabsorption threshold except in the cat. When hyperglycemia and glucosuria are present concurrently along with the appropriate history and physical exam findings, a diagnosis of diabetes mellitus is warranted. Hyperadrenocorticism can result in or exacerbate diabetes mellitus due to insulin antagonism and should be considered in a patient that appears refractory to appropriate insulin therapy (insulin resistant). Glucosuria without hyperglycemia can occur when there is proximal renal tubular injury or a hereditary defect in renal tubular transport mechanisms (Fanconi's syndrome).

Currently, there are several handheld glucometers available for use in veterinary medicine with some variation in accuracy. In one study, the AlphaTrak 2® and OneTouch were shown to have the best performance [2]. Hematocrit may have an effect on glucose values. In this study, comparing a human glucometer and a glucometer for use in veterinary medicine (AlphaTrak2®), the veterinary glucometer had the best performance in samples with a hematocrit that is within reference interval or higher [3]. While there is an expectation that the glucose concentration from a glucometer should correlate with the glucose concentration obtains from a reference laboratory, they will not be the same. The concentrations should, however, result in the same clinical interpretation of hypoglycemic, euglycemic, or hyperglycemic based on each instrument's reference intervals. In most studies comparing glucometers to other instruments used in reference laboratories, when there is a difference in interpretation, it is usually because the glucose concentration obtained from the glucometer is lower, resulting in the interpretation of hypoglycemia versus euglycemia or euglycemia versus hyperglycemia [2].

7.3 Equipment

- Handheld in-house glucometer for use in veterinary patients
- Reagent strips within the expiration date
- Recommended whole blood sample type (see instrument manual for list of appropriate sample types)
- Syringe or lancet for collection of a fresh venous blood sample
- Whole blood in a blood collection tube containing approved anticoagulant (see instruction manual for appropriate anticoagulants)
- Standard operating procedure or instrument manual

7.4 Procedural Steps: How Do I Perform This Test?

This procedure is for using whole blood collected in ethylenediaminetetraacetic acid (EDTA) and describes the general steps for glucometers. Each glucometer will have a specific protocol in the instruction manual, which should be closely adhered to when performing a glucose determination.

7.5 A Note on Quality Control

Most instruments supply a control product. A control test can be done before performing the test on a patient sample to ensure that the instrument is working properly or for troubleshooting the instrument. See the instrument manual for proper use of the control product recommended by the manufacturer.

- The procedure for performing the control test is the same as that for the patient's sample. However, there are additional aspects regarding expiration dates to keep in mind.
  - Like the test strips, the control product will have an expiration date. In most cases, the expiration date for

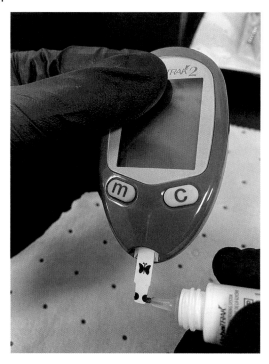

Figure 7.1 Place a small droplet of control product close to the sample port of the test strip and allow capillary action to draw the sample into the test strip. *Source:* Courtesy of Jeremy Bessett.

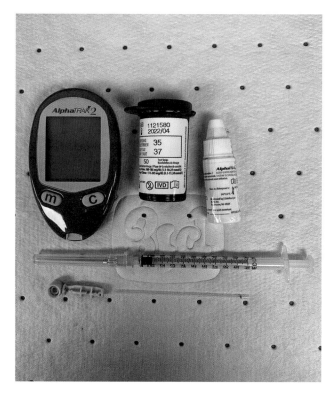

Figure 7.2 Equipment needed to perform this test include a glucometer, reagent strips in their vial, control product, and a syringe or lancet to obtain a small blood sample (note: blood from a blood collection tube containing ethylenediaminetetraacetic acid or heparin can also be used). *Source:* Courtesy of Jeremy Bessett.

storing the unopened control product is fixed. Once the product is opened, it may have an expiration date based on the date it is opened.

o For example, the fixed expiration date for a control product is 4/12/2022 but the product cannot be used after three months of being opened. If the product was opened on 3/13/2022, it will expire on 4/12/2022. If it is opened on 12/2/2021, it will expire on 3/2/2022. To be sure that these dates are monitored, each vial of control product should have the date it is opened written on the vial.

o The control products usually come in small dropper bottles. Prior to introducing the product, wipe the tip with tissue and discard the first two drops. Introduce the control product into the test strip using the dropper bottle (see Figure 7.1).

7.6 Procedure for Patient Samples

- Assemble all equipment and have the standard operating procedure or instrument manual available to assist if any error messages are displayed when performing the test (see Figure 7.2).
- Gently mix the whole blood collection tube containing approved anticoagulant type (for most glucometers

either EDTA or heparin anticoagulant can be used). See Chapter 3 for appropriate methods to mix whole blood in a collection tube.

- Check the expiration data on the test strip vial and remove a test strip from the vial being careful not to touch the sample port (see Figure 7.3).
- Insert the test strip into the glucometer. (Do not try to load the test strip with blood before it is placed in the instrument; see Figure 7.4).
- The test trip will activate the instrument and a screen will indicate that the system is ready for the sample to be loaded. Most instruments will require that a code from the test strip vial be entered to ensure the correct reading will be displayed. Each vial/lot of test strips require their own algorithm to determine the glucose value and the code instructs the instrument which algorithm to use. In addition, the code is specific for the species and determines the reference interval that is used to indicate if the value is high or low. See instrument manual for directions on entering the code. Some have preloaded codes the user scrolls through to find the code for the vial. Others may have a way to enter the code via keypad strokes (see Figure 7.5).

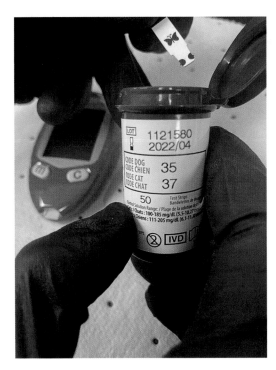

Figure 7.3 Note the expiration date (April 2022), the lot number (1121580), and the code for dog (35) and cat (37). Each of these numbers are important for running the samples and obtaining an accurate result. *Source:* Courtesy of Jeremy Bessett.

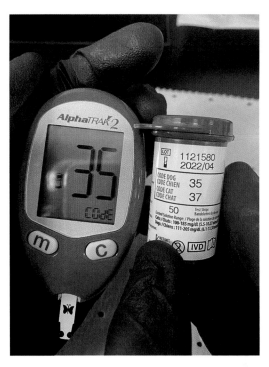

Figure 7.5 Follow the instruction manual on how to enter the code for the test strip being used, enter the code indicated on the test strip vial. In this case, the sample is from a dog and the code entered would be 35. If the sample were from a cat, the code to be entered would be 37. *Source:* Courtesy of Jeremy Bessett.

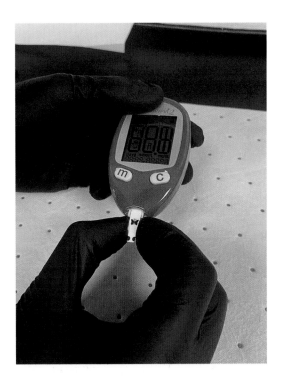

Figure 7.4 Inserting the test strip will activate the screen. Remember to not touch the sample port when inserting the test strip. *Source:* Courtesy of Jeremy Bessett.

- The instrument will indicate when to add the sample to the sample port of the test strip (see instrument manual for appropriate indicator). Capillary action will pull the blood into the sample end of the test strip.
- Using a 1 ml syringe or the end of a microhematocrit tube filled with well-mixed blood from the blood collection tube or freshly collected from the patient, bring a droplet of blood to the blood sample end of the test strip and allow the sample to be drawn into the test strip (see Figures 7.6 and 7.7).
- The instrument will indicate that the sample has been properly introduced (see instrument manual for the method used to indicate a properly applied sample).
  - In most instruments, the instrument will not provide a result if the sample is too small, the sample was applied too soon or too late (meters will often turn off if the sample is not applied within a specific window), the test strip is defective, or the instrument is no longer functioning properly. (Consult the instrument manual for appropriate action to troubleshoot these errors.)
- If no errors are reported by the instrument, a glucose concentration will show in the instrument display (see Figure 7.8). Record the value obtained.

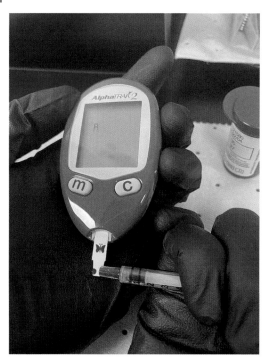

Figure 7.6 A 1 ml syringe is used to introduce the sample onto the sample port. *Source:* Courtesy of Jeremy Bessett.

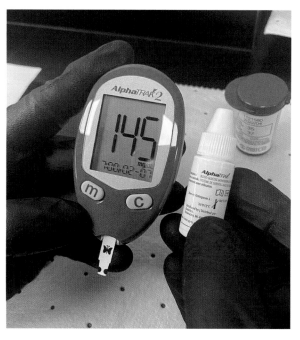

Figure 7.8 The instrument display will show the reading for the sample or control product. In this case, the high-level control product was tested and the reading is 145 mg/dl. *Source:* Courtesy of Jeremy Bessett.

- The manual for the instrument should have good documentation for all error messages that may appear during the procedure and troubleshooting recommendations. In addition, most instrument manufacturers will have a customer service department that can assist if the problem persists following the appropriate recommended actions in the manual.

7.7 Time Estimate to Perform Test

Five to ten minutes.

7.8 Procedural Tips and Troubleshooting

All individuals using a glucometer should be well trained on how to use the instrument, including how to troubleshoot error messages before performing the test on a patient sample. Access to the instruction manual or an in-house standard operating procedure specific for the instrument should be readily available when performing the test.

Since this is an in-house instrument, an appropriate quality control log should be used to document appropriate controls have been run as indicated in the standard operating procedure (see Figure 7.9). The log should at minimum record when the control product is used, the control product lot number, control product expiration date, the test strip lot number and expiration date, and the value determined, any

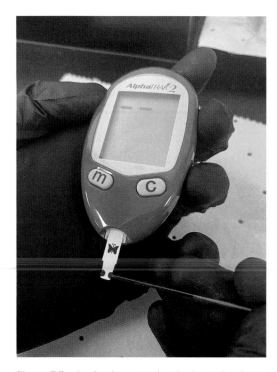

Figure 7.7 A microhematocrit tube is used to introduce the sample onto the sample port. *Source:* Courtesy of Jeremy Bessett.

Glucometer Quality Control Record								
Date	Test Strip Lot#	Test Strip Expiration Date	Control Solution Range used	Control Solution Lot#	Control Solution Expiration Date	Glucometer Reading	Notes (error messages, troubleshooting actions taken)	Operator Initials

Figure 7.9 Excel sheets are commonly used for creating and maintaining procedure logs. The blank form can be printed for manual entry or the log can be maintained electronically. *Source:* Courtesy of Jeremy Bessett.

error messages and the troubleshooting procedure done to obtain a valid control value prior to performing a patient sample, and the initials of the individual performing the test. The American Society for Veterinary Clinical Pathology has published an excellent guideline to assist in developing an appropriate quality assurance program within a veterinary clinic that uses in-house instruments [4].

7.9 Interpreting Test Results

Changes in whole blood glucose are commonly seen in veterinary medicine. The most common change in glucose is due to physiological changes in response to excitement or stress. Both increased circulating epinephrine and glucocorticoid hormones will result in a mild to moderate increase in the dog. In the cat, hyperglycemia associated with stress or excitement can be moderate to marked and often exceeds the renal threshold, resulting in glucosuria. Hyperglycemia can also be seen in postprandial samples.

Diseases associated with hyperglycemia include:

- diabetes mellitus
  - Lack of insulin – dog
  - Insulin resistance – cat

- hyperadrenocorticism (Cushing's disease) – increased circulating endogenous glucocorticoids
  - Iatrogenic hyperadrenocorticism – increased circulating exogenous glucocorticoids.
- hepatic lipidosis in the cat
- acromegaly
- pheochromocytoma – increased circulating catecholamines.

Diseases associated with hypoglycemia include:

- neoplasia – beta-cell tumors, paraneoplastic production of insulin-like growth factor
- sepsis
- insulin overdose in diabetic patients
- juvenile hypoglycemia in puppies
- end-stage liver disease
- prolonged starvation.

Decreased blood glucose can be an artifact associated with prolonged time from collection of a sample and centrifugation to collect the plasma or serum. This is not commonly seen when using a glucometer to determine whole blood glucose since the test is generally performed imediately after collection of the sample.

7.10   Clinical Case Example(s)

See Part 6, cases #3, #5, #7, and #8.

7.11   Add-On Tests That you May Need to Consider and Their Additive Values

A CBC may support hyperglycemia secondary to stress, excitement, or hypoglycemia associated with sepsis.

A full chemistry profile will allow evaluation of liver and electrolytes to support liver or endocrine disease as a cause of changes in glucose concentration.

Urinalysis will allow the confirmation of glucosuria to support a clinical diagnosis of diabetes mellitus.

Serum fructosamine is recommended to assist in differentiating transient hyperglycemia of stress or excitement from persistent hyperglycemia associated with diabetes mellitus in the cat.

Adrenocorticotropic hormone stimulation or low dose dexamethasone suppression tests will assist in identifying underlying adrenocortical abnormalities that may be the cause of changes in glucose concentration (hyperadrenocorticism and hypoadrenocorticism can both result in altered glucose concentration).

7.12   Key Takeaways

- Hyperglycemia is a common clinical chemistry finding and can be caused by several mechanisms.
- Any patient with convulsions, seizures, or altered mentation should be evaluated for both hypoglycemia and marked hyperglycemia (hyperosmolar syndrome).
- An appropriate quality control protocol is important in maintaining the accuracy and value of a blood glucose determination using a glucometer.
- Veterinary glucometers provide adequate accuracy for in-house determinations of blood glucose concentrations in the dog and cat.

References

1 Wiedmeyer, C.E. and DeClue, A.E. (2011). Glucose monitoring in diabetic dogs and cats: adapting new technology for home and hospital care. *Clinics in Laboratory Medicine* 31 (1): 41–50.

2 Cohen, T.A., Nelson, R.W., Kass, P.H. et al. (2009). Evaluation of six portable blood glucose meters for measuring blood glucose concentration in dogs. *Journal of the American Veterinary Medical Association* 235 (3): 276–280.

3 Paul, A.E.H., Shiel, R.E., Juvet, F. et al. (2011). Effect of hematocrit on accuracy of two point-of-care glucometers for use in dogs. *American Journal of Veterinary Research* 72 (9): 1204–1208.

4 Flatland, B., Fry, M.M., LeBlanc, C.J., & Rohrbach, B.W. 2013. ASVCP guidelines: quality assurance for point-of-care testing in veterinary medicine. *Veterinary Clinical Pathology* 42(4), pp. 405–423.

8

Blood Urea Nitrogen

Sharon M. Dial

8.1 Procedural Definition: What Is This Test About?

The Azostix™ urea nitrogen reagent pad is a semiquantitative measurement of the urea nitrogen concentration in whole blood. The color change is the result of the action of the enzyme urease on urea in the blood. The urease acts on urea to release ammonium ions. The release of ammonium results in a pH change, resulting in the color change to increasingly darker green based on the reaction of the ammonium with the pH indicator in the reagent pad (bromothymol blue).

Urea is the waste product of protein catabolism. It is produced in the liver and excreted by the kidney. It can increase in the blood with decreased excretion due to a decrease in glomerular filtration rate (GFR). Increased protein intake can also increase the concentration of blood urea nitrogen (BUN). Since blood has a high protein content, hemorrhage into the gastrointestinal tract results in an increase in protein intake and can also cause an increase in BUN. The Azostix reagent pad does not replace the more accurate methodology used in clinical chemistry instrumentation. Nor can it be used alone to assess renal function. It does provide a good screening test for changes in BUN that indicate either decreased GFR or gastrointestinal hemorrhage.

8.2 Procedural Purpose: Why Should I Perform This Test?

Urea nitrogen is one of the two analytes used to assess glomerular filtration rate. Urea is produced in the liver as a result of protein catabolism and is both filtered and passively reabsorbed by the kidney. Creatinine is filtered with minimal secretion or reabsorption. Azotemia, the presence of an increase in one or both of these analytes in the blood

due to decreased excretion by the kidney, can be caused by prerenal, renal, or postrenal disease. Urea is freely filtered by the kidney but can diffuse back into the blood as the urine filtrate moves through the nephron. The amount of urea reabsorbed depends on how quickly urine filtrate flows through the nephron. Creatinine is freely filtered by the kidney with minimal reabsorption or secretion making it a better indicator of total GFR.

The reagent pad urea nitrogen is a quick screening test for any patient with a history of polydipsia/polyuria, dehydration, or clinical evidence of uremia. The test is not a stand-alone test for renal function. If increased concentration is found using the reagent pad test, the BUN concentration should always be interpreted in the context of clinical findings and urinalysis. A complete blood count, chemistry profile, and urinalysis are recommended as follow-up.

Causes of increased BUN:

- any cause of decreased GFR (prerenal, renal, and postrenal)
- increased protein intake (high protein feed, gastrointestinal hemorrhage)
- increased protein catabolism unrelated to dietary intake (less common).

There are a few important caveats with regard to the interpretation of increased BUN concentration without an increase in creatinine concentration. Gastrointestinal hemorrhage will result in increased BUN with normal creatinine. This is due to the high protein content of blood making gastrointestinal hemorrhage a "high protein meal" as it is digested and the blood proteins are absorbed in the intestinal tract. The liver produces urea as a waste product of protein catabolism.

Decreased liver function occurs either by loss of hepatic mass (chronic liver disease) or shunting of blood past the liver (congenital or acquired portosystemic shunts). Patients with decreased liver function may have a significantly decreased BUN as a result of decreased hepatic production. In these patients, decreased GFR can result in a BUN concentration within the reference interval and increased creatinine.

Causes of decreased BUN:

- low protein diet
- decreased production by the liver
- increased renal excretion
  ○ increased urine filtrate flow through the nephron
    ▪ osmotic diuresis
    ▪ increased GFR.

Clinical indications for performing a reagent pad BUN include:

- clinical findings suggestive of renal disease
  ○ polydipsia/polyuria
  ○ weight loss
  ○ anorexia or hyporexia
  ○ vomiting
  ○ ammonia smell of breath
- clinical findings indicative of dehydration
  ○ pale tacky mucous membranes
  ○ tachycardia
  ○ decreased skin turgor
  ○ thin or thready pulses
  ○ sunken eyes.

8.3 Equipment

The following equipment are used to perform this test:

- whole blood in tube with anticoagulant
- Azostix® reagent strips
- pipette
- distilled water in a wash bottle
- minute timer
- gloves.

8.4 Procedural Steps: How Do I Perform this Test?

- Gather all equipment needed (see Figure 8.1).
- Gently mix the blood sample on a rocker or manually as described in Chapter 3.
- Remove one reagent strip from the container and place it print side up on a level surface.
- Set timer for 60 seconds.

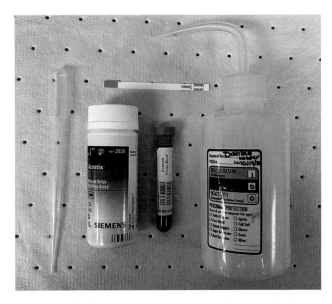

Figure 8.1 Equipment needed to perform this test includes: Azostix reagent strips (within expiration date), whole blood with anticoagulant, a pipette, distilled water in a wash bottle, and gloves. *Source:* Courtesy of Jeremy Bessett.

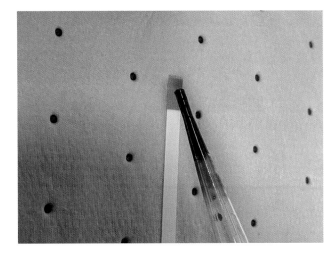

Figure 8.2 Use a pipette to place a large drop of blood on the reagent pad. Do not dip the reagent pad into the blood tube. *Source:* Courtesy of Jeremy Bessett.

- Using a disposable pipette, place a large drop of blood that covers the entire reagent pad at the end of the reagent strip (see Figure 8.2).
- Start timer as soon as the reagent pad is fully covered (see Figure 8.3).

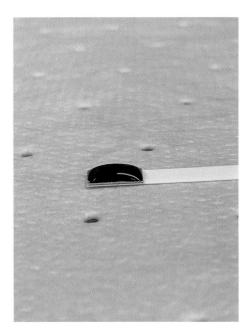

Figure 8.3 Completely cover the reagent pad as shown in this image. Incomplete coverage of the pad will negatively impact the final reading. *Source:* Courtesy of Jeremy Bessett.

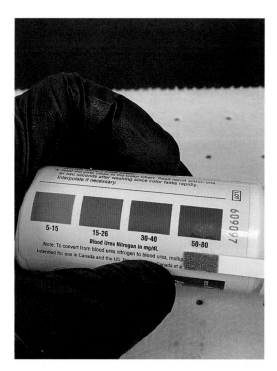

Figure 8.5 Holding the reagent strip to the color chart, determine which color most closely matches the reagent pad. In this sample, the recorded value would be 50–80 mg/dl. *Source:* Courtesy of Jeremy Bessett.

- After 60 seconds, quickly wash the blood off the reagent pad with a strong stream of water from the wash bottle for about 1–2 seconds (see Figure 8.4).
- Compare the color of the reagent pad to the color chart on the reagent container and record the reading from the chart that best matches the color in the reagent pad (see Figures 8.5 and 8.6).

8.5 Time Estimate to Perform Test

Five minutes.

8.6 Procedural Tips and Troubleshooting

The timing of the sample from application of the blood to the pad and washing must be consistent to provide a valid test.

Quick and complete washing of the reagent strip is necessary for accurate results.

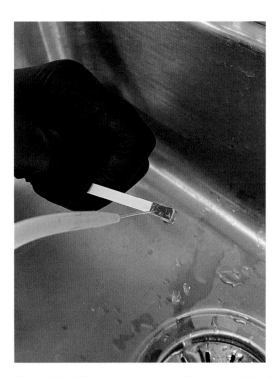

Figure 8.4 Using a steady stream of water, wash the blood from the reagent pad for about one to two seconds. *Source:* Courtesy of Jeremy Bessett.

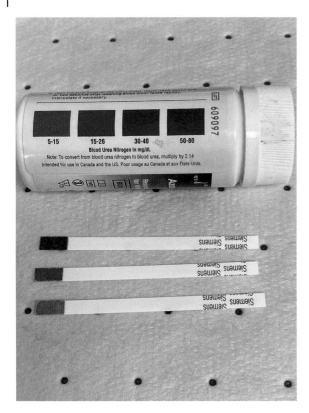

Figure 8.6 In this image, three samples are shown with three different BUN results. Top: 50–80 mg/dl, Middle: 30–40 mg/dl, Bottom: 5–15 mg/dl. *Source:* Courtesy of Jeremy Bessett.

The primary cause of poor interobserver consistency is the interpretation of the color range when compared with the color chart. The difference between the two midrange values is subtle. If there is any question in reading the color change by an observer, it is appropriate to get an additional observer to read the strip.

8.7 Interpreting Test Results

An increased BUN concentration must be interpreted in the context of the patient's clinical findings and urinalysis.

In the dehydrated patient with increased BUN concentration, a urine specific gravity is necessary to determine if the increase is due to prerenal factors alone or if either primary renal disease or renal function due to nonrenal disease is present.

- If the urine specific gravity is greater than 1.030 in the dog or 1.035 in the cat, the increased BUN is due to pre-renal causes of decreased GFR. In dehydration, the increase in plasma osmolality and, if severe enough, the decreased blood volume/pressure will result in increased secretion of antidiuretic hormone. Antidiuretic hormone results in increased permeability to water in the collecting ducts of the kidney, water is conserved by increasing

the movement of water from the lumen of the collecting duct back into the extracellular fluid compartments, and the urine becomes concentrated.

- If the urine specific gravity is in the isosthenuric range (1.008–1.012) or the range of inadequate concentration (1.012–1.035 in the dog; 1.015–1.040 in the cat), the patient's kidney is not adequately conserving water. This may be due to primary renal disease with loss at 75% of renal mass or a nonrenal disease process that inhibits the kidney's ability to concentrate urine.
  - Nonrenal diseases that impair renal concentrating ability include:
    - diabetes mellitus
    - hypoadrenocorticism (Addison's disease)
    - hyperadrenaocorticism (Cushing's disease)
    - endotoxemia – sepsis
    - hypercalcemia
      - hypercalcemia of malignancy
      - primary hyperparathyroidism
      - vitamin D toxicity.

Note: Hypercalcemia can also result in direct injury to the kidney as a result of metastatic calcification.

Increased BUN in an ill patient with mild to no clinical evidence of dehydration may or may not indicate a decrease in GFR.

- Increased BUN with concentrated urine specific gravity indicates appropriate renal function. Consider:
  - gastrointestinal blood loss or increased protein catabolism
    - fever
    - excessive exogenous or endogenous corticosteroids
  - high protein diet
  - other causes of prerenal azotemia
    - cardiac disease with decreased cardiac output
    - hypovolemia due to hemorrhagic or distributive shock.

If the BUN concentration is less than 26 mg/dl in a dehydrated polyuric patient, consider evaluating for diseases that can result in alteration of the renal medullary osmotic gradient or secondary nephrogenic diabetes mellitus.

8.8 Clinical Case Example(s)

See Part 6, cases #3, #8, #10, and #14.

8.9 Add-On Tests That You May Need to Consider and Their Additive Value

A concurrent urinalysis is essential when interpreting an increased BUN. Specifically, urine specific gravity, glucose, and protein will assist in determining the underlying cause of increased BUN.

A full chemistry profile and CBC are warranted whenever an ill patient has increased BUN. Since creatinine is a better indicator of GFR, serum creatinine concentration is necessary to support decreased GFR as a cause of the increased BUN. Assessment for underlying disease processes that can affect renal function in the normal kidney can be supported by evaluation of analytes related to liver disease, endocrine disease, and electrolyte balance.

8.10 Key Takeaways

- BUN is not a stand-alone test. To fully determine the reason for an increased BUN, additional testing should be done.

- A full chemistry profile and urinalysis should be performed on patients with an increased BUN by reagent strip.
- BUN can be increased due to a decreased GFR or gastrointestinal bleeding. Additional test and consideration of clinical findings are necessary to determine which of these mechanisms is most likely in the patient.
- BUN cannot be interpreted without a urine specific gravity.

9

Whole Blood Lactate
Sharon M. Dial

9.1 Procedural Definition: What Is This Test About?

Increased whole blood lactate concentration measured by a lactate meter reflects a switch from aerobic to anaerobic metabolism and is often seen in diseases associated with tissue hypoxia due to hypoperfusion or hypoxemia, diseases that are associated with decreased oxygen utilization and renal disease associated with decreased glomerular filtration rate (GFR) with decreased clearance of lactic acid produced during normal metabolic activity. In addition, hyperlactatemia can be seen when there is an increase in oxygen utilization. A small amount of lactate is produced in the healthy animal because of anaerobic respiration. If oxygen is not available or cannot be used by the tissues, the pyruvate produced by glycolysis results in the production of lactic acid rather than being fully oxidized in the mitochondria to produce adenosine triphosphate. Increased anaerobic metabolism in the hypoxic environment results in less energy production per glucose molecule and produces excess lactic acid, resulting in decreased tissue and blood pH (acidemia).

Several studies have evaluated and compared the use of the handheld lactate meter for use in the dog and cat [1, 2].

9.2 Procedural Purpose: Why Should I Perform This Test?

The measurement of whole blood lactate is used primarily as a prognostic indicator in the critically ill patient. Diseases that result in significant hyperlactatemia include:

- diseases associated with decreased availability of oxygen
  - decreased tissue perfusion
    - cardiac insufficiency
    - distributive shock – sepsis
    - hypovolemia
      - dehydration
      - hemorrhage
  - decreased blood oxygen-carrying capacity
    - anemia
    - methemoglobinemia
    - carbon monoxide toxicity
  - decreased blood oxygenation
    - pneumonia
- diseases associated with increased oxygen utilization
  - seizures
  - excessive exercise or exercise without adequate training
- disease associated with decreased oxygen utilization
  - sepsis without distributive shock.

Measurement of whole blood lactate is indicated in any patient with clinical evidence of alterations in oxygen utilization including:

- pale, hyperemic, or cyanotic mucous membranes
- significant tachyarrhythmia/dyspnea
- fever
- seizures
- thready pulse
- marked dehydration
- collapse
- peritoneal fluid accumulation with clinical signs suggestive of sepsis.

An additional use of the measurement of lactate is evaluation of body cavity fluid lactate in comparison with whole blood lactate. Lactate concentration in body cavity fluids can increase in association with sepsis or neoplasia. There is insufficient consensus in the literature concerning the specificity of fluid lactate concentration in the identification of sepsis. However, comparing the fluid lactate concentration to peripheral blood lactate concentration appears to be much more specific and warrants culture if bacterial agents are not identified in the cytologic preparations of the fluid [3]. A differential lactate concentration of greater than 2 mmol/l between the fluid and peripheral blood is strongly indicative of sepsis. Lactate concentration also increases in neoplastic effusions. Both neoplastic cells and microbial organisms can increase lactate due to their metabolic use of glucose within the fluid.

9.3 Equipment

The following equipment is used in performing this test:

- lactate meter
- lactate reagent strips
- syringe and needle
- microhematocrit tubes
- control product (recommended).

9.4 Procedural Steps: How Do I Perform This Test?

This procedure is for testing when using freshly collected capillary whole blood and describes the general steps involved in the lactate meter. Each lactate meter will have a specific protocol in the instruction manual, which should be closely adhered to when performing a lactate determination test.

9.5 A Note on Quality Control

Most instruments supply a control product. A control test can be done before using a patient sample to ensure that the instrument is working properly or for troubleshooting the instrument. See the instrument manual for proper use of the control product recommended by the manufacturer.

- The procedure for performing the control test is the same as that for the patient's sample. However, there are additional aspects regarding expiration dates to keep in mind.
  - Like the test strips, the control product will have an expiration date. In most cases, the expiration date for storing the unopened control product is fixed. Once the product is opened, it may have an expiration date based on the date it is opened.
  - For example, the fixed expiration date for a control product is 4/12/2022 but the product cannot be used after three months of being opened. If the product was opened on 3/13/2022, it will expire on 4/12/2022. If it is opened on 12/2/2021, it will expire on 3/2/2022. To be sure that these dates are monitored, each vial of control product should have the date it is opened written on the vial.
  - Control products usually come in small dropper bottles. Prior to introducing the product, wipe the tip with tissue and discard the first two drops. Introduce the control product into the test strip using the dropper bottle. This is the same protocol for using the control product as described in Chapter 7 for use of the glucometer.

9.6 Procedure for Patient Samples

Assemble all equipment and have the standard operating procedure or instrument manual available to assist in any error messages that may be displayed when performing the test (see Figure 9.1).

- Collect a small amount of fresh blood in a 1 ml syringe or a hematocrit tube without coagulant.
- Check the expiration date on the test strip vial and remove the test strip from the vial being careful not to touch the sample port (see Figure 9.2). Some test strips may come in a foil pack instead of a vial.
- The test trip will activate the instrument and a screen will indicate that the system is ready for the sample to be loaded (see Figure 9.3). Some instruments may require that a code from the test strip vial be entered to ensure the correct reading will be displayed. Each vial/lot of test strips require their own algorithm to determine the lactate value and the code instructs the instrument which

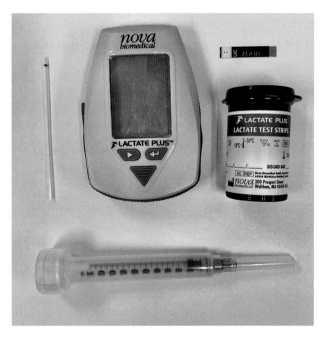

Figure 9.1 Equipment needed to perform this test includes a lactate meter, reagent strips in their vial, control product (not shown), a syringe or lancet and microhematocrit tube to obtain a small blood sample. *Source:* Courtesy of Jeremy Bessett.

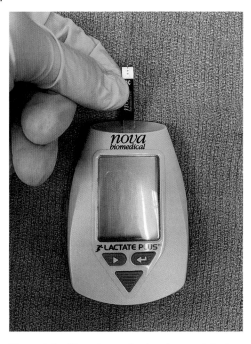

Figure 9.2 Note the expiration date and the lot number. Insert the test strip into the lactate meter. *Source:* Courtesy of Jeremy Bessett. (Do not try to load the test strip with blood before it is placed in the instrument.)

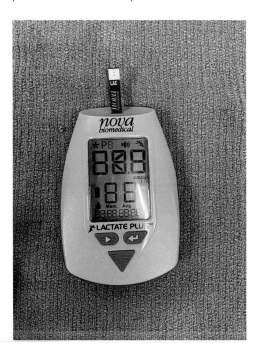

Figure 9.3 Inserting the test strip will activate the screen. *Source:* Courtesy of Jeremy Bessett.

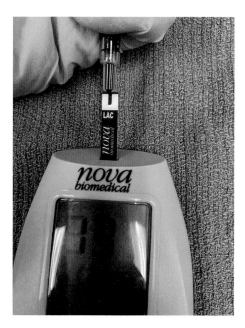

Figure 9.4 A 1 ml syringe is used to introduce the sample onto the sample port. *Source:* Courtesy of Jeremy Bessett.

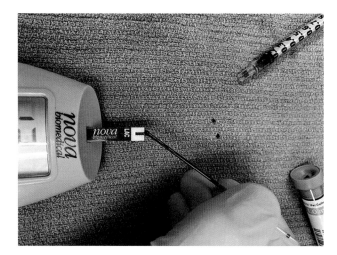

Figure 9.5 A microhematocrit tube is used to introduce the sample onto the sample port. *Source:* Courtesy of Jeremy Bessett.

algorithm to use. See instrument manual for directions on entering any code needed. Some have preloaded codes the user scrolls through to find the code for the vial. Others may have a way to enter the code via keypad strokes.

- The instrument will indicate when to add the sample to the sample port of the test strip (see instrument manual for appropriate indicator). Capillary action will pull the blood into the sample end of the test strip.
- Using a 1 ml syringe or the end of a microhematocrit tube filled with well-mixed blood from the blood collection tube or freshly collected from the patient, bring a droplet of blood to the blood sample end of the test strip and allow the sample to be drawn into the test strip (see Figures 9.4 and 9.5).

Lactate Meter Quality Control Record								
Date	Test Strip Lot#	Test Strip Expiration Date	Control Solution Range used	Control Solution Lot#	Control Solution Expiration Date	Lactate meter Reading	Notes (error messages, troubleshooting actions taken)	Operator Initials

Figure 9.6 Excel sheets commonly are used for creating and maintaining procedure logs. The blank form can be printed for manual entry or the log can be maintained electronically. *Source:* Courtesy of Jeremy Bessett.

- The instrument will indicate that the sample has been properly introduced (see instrument manual for the method used to indicate a properly applied sample).
  - In most instruments, the instrument will not provide a result if the sample is too small or if the sample is applied too soon or too late (meters will often turn off if the sample is not applied within a specific window), the test strip is defective, or the instrument is no longer functioning properly. (Consult the instrument manual for appropriate action to troubleshoot these errors).
- If no errors are reported by the instrument, a lactate concentration will show in the instrument display. Record the value obtained.
- The manual for the instrument should have good documentation for all error messages that may appear during the procedure and troubleshooting recommendations. In addition, most instrument manufacturers will have a customer service department that can assist if the problem persists following the appropriate recommended actions in the manual.

Since this is an in-house instrument, an appropriate quality control log to document appropriate controls have been run as indicated in the standard operating procedure (see Figure 9.6). The log should at minimum record when the control product is used, the control product lot number, control product expiration date, the test strip lot number and the test strip expiration date, and the value determined, any error messages and the troubleshooting procedure done to obtain a valid control value prior to performing a patient sample, and the individual performing the test. The American Society for Veterinary Clinical Pathology has published an excellent guideline to assist in developing an appropriate quality assurance program within a veterinary clinic that uses in-house instruments [4].

9.7 Time Estimate to Perform Test

Five minutes.

9.8 Procedural Tips and Troubleshooting

Always check the expiration date on the reagent strips and control product before using.

A control test should be performed:

- at least once per week
- before performing each patient sample, if the meter is used less than once per week
- each time a new lot of reagent strip is used
- if the results are inconsistent with the patient's clinical presentation.

As with any in-house instrument, maintaining a quality control log is essential to produce trustable test results.

9.9 Interpreting Test Results

The available lactate meters do not usually provide a reference interval for whole blood lactate. In general, lactate concentration should be less than 2.5 mmol/l. If lactate is commonly used as an in-clinic test, the clinic can create a reference interval for their patient population [4].

Increased lactate concentration in whole blood is indicative of increased anaerobic metabolism and is seen in several disease processes:

- cardiac disease resulting in decreased tissue perfusion
- respiratory disease resulting in decreased hemoglobin oxygenation
- anemia
- shock
  - cardiogenic
  - distributive
  - hypovolemic
    - dehydration
    - hemorrhage
- seizures
- renal disease with retained metabolic acids due to decreased GFR
- sepsis without evidence of distributive shock

- toxicity with inhibition of oxygen utilization
  - carbon monoxide
  - strychnine
  - acetaminophen.

A single point lactate concentration can assist in providing evidence of the underlying disease process. Serial determinations of whole blood lactate are often used to provide prognostic information. Persistent hyperlactatemia in the face of appropriate therapy for the underlying disease process has a negative prognosis [3].

Increased lactate concentration can be seen in peritoneal fluid with sepsis or neoplasia. A lactate concentration differential of greater than 2 mmol/l between peritoneal fluid and whole blood strongly supports sepsis. The use of lactate concentration in pericardial or pleural fluid is not recommended.

9.10   Clinical Case Example(s)

See Part 6, cases #3 and #9.

9.11   Add-On Tests That You May Need to Consider and Their Additive Value

- An arterial blood gas profile will provide additional support for underlying diseases associated with hyperlactatemia including those affecting respiratory/cardiac and metabolic systems.
- Chemistry profile will assist in the evaluation of organ function to identify evidence of alterations in liver, renal, gastrointestinal, and endocrine functions that may be contributing to the increased production or retention of lactic acid.
- A CBC will assist in identifying inflammatory changes related to sepsis.
- Thoracic and abdominal imaging will assist in identifying disease processes within these body cavities that are contributing to hyperlactatemia.
- If abdominal fluid is found on physical examination or imaging, a fluid analysis is recommended to identify the underlying mechanism of the fluid accumulation. Culture of the fluid is recommended if it is found to be inflammatory with or without identifiable infectious agents.

9.12   Key Takeaways

- A single determination of decreased blood lactate concentration supports the presence of a disease process that promotes anaerobic metabolism or retention of metabolic acids.
- A single determination of blood lactate concentration should only be used as a prognostic indicator in the context of the individual patient. Significant hyperlactatemia does not equate to a poor prognosis in all cases.
- Serial determination of blood lactate concentration is of more prognostic value than a single determination. Persistent hyperlactatemia in the face of appropriate therapy predicts a negative prognosis.
- The lactate concentration differential of greater than 2.0 mmol/l between peritoneal fluid and whole blood is strongly supportive of sepsis.

References

1 Acierno, M.J. and Mitchell, M.A. (2007). Evaluation of four point-of-care meters for rapid determination of blood lactate concentrations in dogs. *Journal of the American Veterinary Medical Association* 230 (9): 1315–1318. https://doi.org/10.2460/javma.230.9.1315. PMID: 17472555.

2 Hughes, D., Rozanski, E.R., Shofer, F.S. et al. (1999). Effect of sampling site, repeated sampling, pH, and PCO$_2$ on plasma lactate concentration in healthy dogs. *American Journal of Veterinary Research* 60 (4): 521–524. PMID: 10211699.

3 Pang, D.S. and Boysen, S. (2007). Lactate in veterinary critical care: pathophysiology and management. *Journal of the American Animal Hospital Association* 43 (5): 270–279.

4 Flatland, B., Fry, M.M., LeBlanc, C.J., and Rohrbach, B.W. (2013). ASVCP guidelines: quality assurance for point-of-care testing in veterinary medicine. *Veterinary Clinical Pathology* 42 (4): 405–423.

10

Saline Agglutination Test
Sharon M. Dial

10.1 Procedural Definition: What Is This Test About?

True immune-mediated erythrocyte agglutination can be seen in primary and secondary immune-mediated hemolytic anemia. When aggregation of erythrocytes is seen macroscopically in the blood collection tube or microscopically on examination of the blood film, it is important to determine if the aggregation is antibody mediated or nonspecific adherence. The saline agglutination test is used to determine whether erythrocyte agglutination is due to antibody-specific cross-linkage or nonspecific adherence due to high protein or altered proteins in the plasma. The principle of the test is to dilute the blood sample and observe whether or not the erythrocytes disperse into individual cells or if they remain aggregated.

10.2 Procedural Purpose: Why Should I Perform This Test?

Immune-mediated hemolytic anemia is not uncommon in the dog but less common in the cat. In some forms of immune-mediated hemolytic anemia, antibody-dependent agglutination of the erythrocytes is seen. In patients that present with a regenerative anemia and gross or microscopic evidence of erythrocyte agglutination, it is essential to confirm that the agglutination is antibody mediated. High plasma protein or increased concentration of inflammatory proteins with higher affinity for the erythrocyte surface can result in nonspecific erythrocytes aggregation. The saline agglutination test is an inexpensive screening test that can assist in differentiating these two mechanisms of erythrocyte aggregation or agglutination.

Immune-mediated anemia in the dog and cat can be a primary or secondary disease. Primary immune-mediated disease is diagnosed by confirming antibody-mediated removal or destruction of erythrocytes, ruling out secondary disease as a cause of the immune-mediated erythrocyte destruction and ruling out nonimmune causes of the agglutination.

The saline agglutination test has a long history of use in veterinary medicine. However, it is somewhat controversial. The protocol for the test has not been standardized.

10.3 Equipment

Equipment used for this test include:

- whole blood in blood collection tube with anticoagulant
- glass slides
- pipette
- saline (0.9% NaCl)
- coverslips
- gloves
- Optional: clean conical centrifuge tube.

10.4 Procedural Steps: How Do I Perform This Test?

Gather all the necessary supplies for the test (see Figure 10.1).

10.4.1 Quick slide method

- Gently mix the whole blood sample as described in Chapter 3.

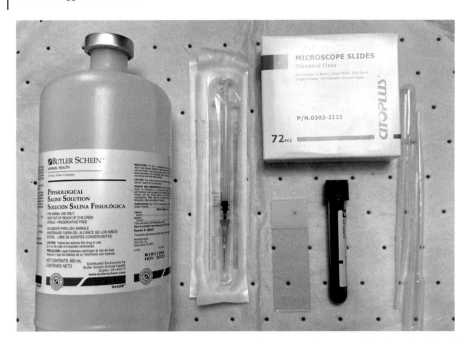

Figure 10.1 Supplies necessary for a saline agglutination test include whole blood with anticoagulant, glass slides, pipette, 0.9% saline, coverslips, and gloves. *Source:* Courtesy of Jeremy Bessett.

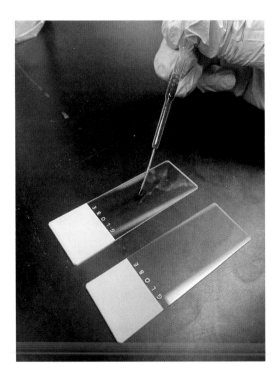

Figure 10.2 Using a small pipette place a drop of blood onto a glass slide. *Source:* Courtesy of Jeremy Bessett.

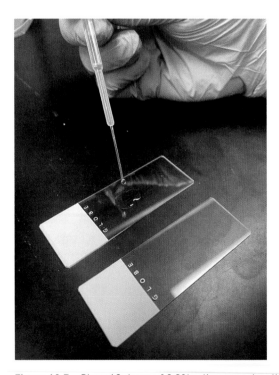

Figure 10.3 Place 10 drops of 0.9% saline onto the slide. At least 10 drops should be used. To keep from flooding the slide, a small caliber micropipette is used. *Source:* Courtesy of Jeremy Bessett.

- Using a pipette, place one drop of blood onto a glass slide (see Figure 10.2).
- Using a pipette, place 10 drops of 0.9% saline onto the glass slide (see Figure 10.3).

- Gently rotate the slide to mix the saline with the whole blood (see Figure 10.4).
- Place a coverslip on the glass slide for examination under the microscope (see Figure 10.5).

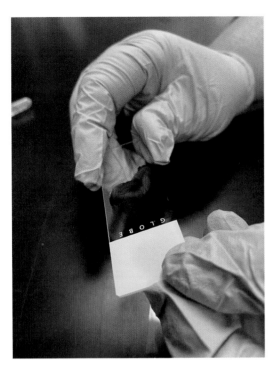

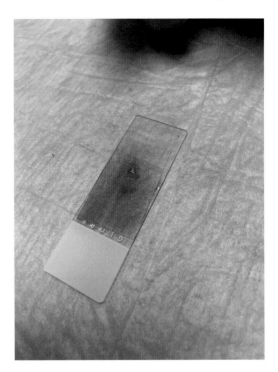

Figure 10.4 Gently rotate the slide to be sure the sample is adequately mixed. Adequate mixing is necessary to ensure the saline can dilute any nonspecific proteins adhered to the erythrocytes. *Source:* Courtesy of Jeremy Bessett.

Figure 10.5 A coverslip is placed on the slide to provide an even layer and distribution of the erythrocytes for evaluation. *Source:* Courtesy of Jeremy Bessett.

(a)

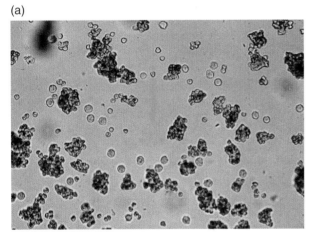

(b)

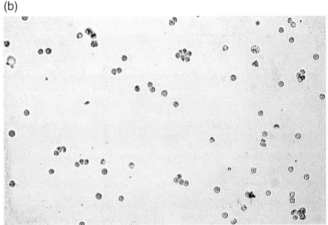

Figure 10.6 (a) Erythrocytes have remained in large aggregates indicating a positive test; (b) erythrocytes have dispersed into individual cells or doublets. *Source:* Courtesy of Sharon M. Dial.

- View the preparation using the 10× objective to determine if the erythrocyte aggregates have dispersed (see Figure 10.6a and b).

10.5 Time Estimate to Perform Test

Five minutes.

10.6 Procedural Tips and Troubleshooting

The most common error in performing this test is not using sufficient saline to dilute the blood or not mixing the sample sufficiently to allow the erythrocytes to disperse if there is nonspecific aggregation. A more stringent test would be to place 5 drops of blood in a small centrifuge tube with

3 ml of saline, mix well, and view at 10×. In most cases, diluting at least 1 : 10 blood to saline should allow adequate dilution of any proteins causing nonspecific agglutination. The slide agglutination test as described above is a good screening test. The more stringent test can be reserved for those samples when agglutination remains after a 1 : 10 dilution is reviewed.

10.7   Interpreting Test Results

A positive saline agglutination test is indicative of antibody-mediated erythrocyte agglutination and supports the diagnosis of immune-mediated disease. A negative saline agglutination test does not rule out immune-mediated anemia in a patient with a regenerative anemia with icterus or hemoglobinemia. Close examination of the blood film for other indicators of immune removal of erythrocytes is necessary. The presence of significant numbers of spherocytes is strong evidence of immune-mediated hemolysis regardless of the results of the saline agglutination test.

The direct Coombs test can be performed at a reference laboratory to support the diagnosis of immune-mediated anemia in patients with a negative saline agglutination test suspected of having immune-mediated anemia. The direct Coombs test detects the presence of antibody on erythrocytes using reagents with species-specific antibodies directed at the different isotypes of antibodies. Most laboratories use a polyvalent reagent that can detect all isotypes plus complement. Since the end-point of the Coombs test is agglutination, it is often recommended that a positive saline agglutination test precludes submission of a sample for a direct Coombs test.

The presence of true agglutination is indicative of antibody-mediated agglutination and, in the anemic animal, supports an immune-mediated mechanism for the anemia. However, it is important to remember that immune-mediated anemia can be primary (autoimmune) or secondary to infectious diseases or neoplasia. Prior to instituting aggressive immune-suppressive therapeutics, a full screening for infectious agents, and underlying neoplasia is essential. *Babesia* spp., in the dog, and *Mycoplasma hemofelis*, in the cat, are two infectious agents that are associated with secondary immune-mediated agglutination. The 2019 ACVIM consensus statement on the diagnosis of immune-mediated hemolytic anemia in dogs and cats is an excellent reference for the underlying mechanisms of both primary and secondary immune-mediated hemolytic anemia and the diagnostic tests, including the saline agglutination test, used for the diagnosis of this disease [1].

The suggested protocol for the saline agglutination test is less stringent than proposed in this chapter. Regardless of the procedure used, consistency is essential.

10.8   Clinical Case Example(s)

See Part 6, case #2.

10.9   Add-On Tests That You May Need to Consider and Their Additive Value

A blood film evaluation is an essential companion test for the saline agglutination test. The findings of spherocytes or ghost cells on review of the blood film provide evidence that the agglutination is related to immune-mediated mechanisms. Close examination for hemoparasites may identify an underlying cause for secondary immune-mediated hemolytic anemia. In addition, identification of an inflammatory leukogram would support the possibility of nonspecific agglutination due to increased inflammatory proteins.

Evaluation of plasma color and a urinalysis may reveal hemoglobinemia/hemoglobinuria or icterus/hyperbilirubinemia/bilirubinuria and support the diagnosis of immune-mediated hemolytic anemia.

A complete chemistry profile will further evaluate for secondary organ dysfunction as comorbidities in patients with suspected immune-mediated hemolytic anemia are not uncommon. This is especially true in the anemic patient with icterus. Not all icteric patients with anemia have prehepatic icterus. Primary liver disease and sepsis can be associated with both secondary immune-mediated mechanisms of anemia and nonimmune mechanisms of anemia.

10.10   Key Takeaways

- Sufficient dilution of the blood sample is necessary to reduce erythrocyte aggregation due to increased plasma proteins. A 1 : 1 or even a 1 : 4 ratio of blood to saline may result in a false positive result.
- A positive saline agglutination test in the anemic animal should be supported by additional findings associated with immune-mediated erythrocyte destruction, such as spherocytes, ghost cells, hemoglobinemia/hemoglobinuria, and icterus/hyperbilirubinemia/bilirubinuria.

- The saline agglutination test is not a stand-alone test for immune-mediated disease. There is no "gold standard" or pathognomonic test for immune-mediated hemolytic anemia. The diagnosis of this disease requires a constellation of history, physical exam findings, and supportive diagnostic tests.

Reference

1 Garden, O.A., Kidd, L., Mexas, A.M. et al. (2019). ACVIM consensus statement on the diagnosis of immune-mediated hemolytic anemia in dogs and cats. *Journal of Veterinary Internal Medicine* 33 (2): 313–334.

11

Activated Clotting Time
Sharon M. Dial

11.1 Procedural Definition: ("What Is This Test About?")

The activated clotting time (ACT) is a measurement of the activity of the intrinsic and common coagulation pathways. It measures the time from activation of the pathways by introduction of blood into a tube containing clot activator to the formation of fibrin strands that cause the blood to thicken when tilted.

11.2 Procedural Purpose: Why Should I Perform This Test?

Patients that present with evidence of bleeding without previous trauma or prolonged bleeding with trauma should be evaluated for abnormalities in hemostasis. The ACT is especially useful to evaluate patients with evidence of a coagulation factor deficiency, either inherited or acquired. Clinical signs associated with coagulopathies include:

- bruising (ecchymosis)
- hematoma formation
- body cavity hemorrhage
- rebleeding (bleeding that occurs after initial clotting)
- excessive bleeding during surgery.

In these patients, a quick assessment of clotting ability is warranted.

The ACT test is a measure of the activity of the coagulation factors in the intrinsic pathway (Factors XII, XI, IX, and VIII) and the common pathway (Factors X, II, XIII, and V). It is much less sensitive than the activated partial thromboplastin time (APTT) and may not be prolonged

unless there is a marked decrease in coagulation factor activity. Common coagulation abnormalities that can result in the prolongation of the ACT test include:

- Factor VIII deficiency (Hemophilia A)
- disseminated intravascular coagulation (DIC)
- Rodenticide poisoning (vitamin K antagonists).

Significant thrombocytopenia will result in a prolongation of the ACT test. A platelet count is advised before performing this test. If the platelet count is <10000/µl, the ACT time will be affected.

11.3 Equipment

Equipment used for this test include:

- ACT vacutainer blood collection tubes
- serum vacutainer blood collection tubes
- syringes (3 or 5 ml)
- vacutainer needles and sleeve
- butterfly catheter
- heating block or water bath
- stopwatch or watch with a second hand
- gloves

11.4 Procedural Steps: How Do I Perform This Test?

- Gather equipment and supplies for performing the test (see Figure 11.1).
- Turn on the heating block and heat to 37°C.
- Place the ACT blood collection tube in one of the heating blocks or water baths and preheat the tube at 37°C for

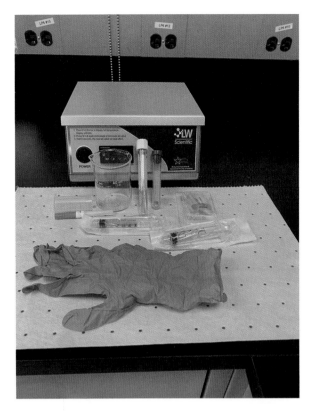

Figure 11.1 Equipment and slides needed to perform the activated clotting time (ACT) test include blood drawing supplies (syringes, vacutainer needles and sleeve, butterfly catheter) blood collection tubes (ACT vacutainer tubes, serum vacutainer tubes), a tube heating block or waterbath, stopwatch or watch with a second hand, and gloves. *Source:* Courtesy of Jeremy Bessett.

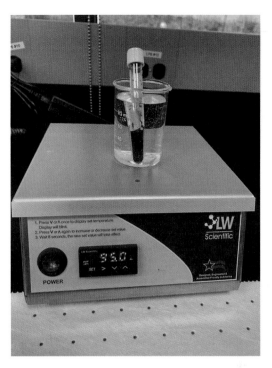

Figure 11.2 If a tube heating block is not available, a beaker of water can be placed on a heating plate and heated to 37°C to use as a water bath. *Source:* Courtesy of Jeremy Bessett.

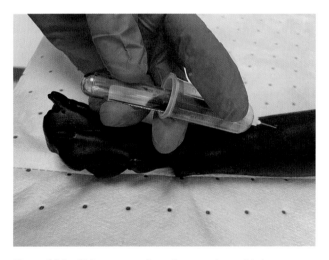

Figure 11.3 Using a vacutainer sleeve and a multi-draw vacutainer needle, draw 2 ml of blood into a serum blood collection tube first and discard or save for other diagnostic testing. This clears the needle of any substances like tissue factor that can initiate coagulation prior to placing the blood in the activated clotting time tube. *Source:* Courtesy of Jeremy Bessett.

5–10 minutes. **This is an essential step.** The tubes must be at 37°C when used to allow consistent results.

Note: If a tube heating block is not available, a water bath can be used. A simple water bath can be created using a beaker of water, thermometer, and an adjustable hot plate with a low setting that can hold steady at 37°C (see Figure 11.2). If neither of these are available, warming the tube in the axilla can suffice.

- Draw 2 ml of fresh whole blood into a serum vacutainer from a clean venipuncture using a vacutainer needle and sleeve or from a butterfly catheter (22 or 21 gauge is recommended for using either method).
- When obtaining the sample from a direct venipuncture, the use of a vacutainer needle and sleeve is recommended. Place the needle in a peripheral vein (usually the cephalic vein), draw 1–2 ml into a serum tube (no anticoagulant), discard or save for other testing (see Figure 11.3), then draw directly into the ACT tube until filled (sample size is 2 ml) (see Figure 11.4).
- When obtaining the sample using a butterfly catheter, draw 1–2 ml into a syringe, discard this initial blood sample (see Figure 11.5), and using a new syringe, draw 2 ml to dispense into the ACT tube (see Figure 11.6).

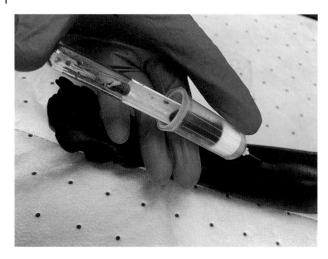

Figure 11.4   Change to the activated clotting time tube and allow the tube to fill completely by vacuum. *Source:* Courtesy of Jeremy Bessett.

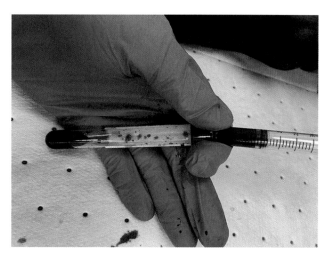

Figure 11.6   Once the line and needle of the catheter has been cleared, change syringes and draw 2 ml of blood to dispense into the activated clotting time tube. It is essential that exactly 2 ml is dispensed. Overfilling or underfilling the tube will adversely affect the results of the test. *Source:* Courtesy of Jeremy Bessett.

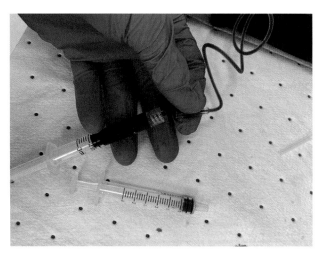

Figure 11.5   When drawing the blood using a butterfly catheter, follow the same principle as when using a vacutainer sleeve. Draw 2 ml of blood to discard or save for other tests. *Source:* Courtesy of Jeremy Bessett.

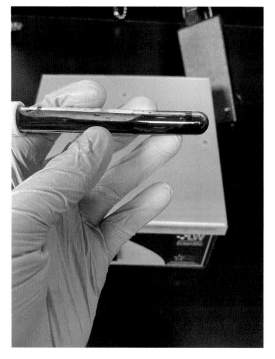

Figure 11.7   The tube should be gently tilted just off of horizontal to observe for thickening of the blood. Do not wait until a visible clot is formed. *Source:* Courtesy of Jeremy Bessett.

- Start a stopwatch timer as soon as blood is placed into the ACT tube. The tube is mixed gently five times and placed into the 37°C heating block or water bath.
- The tube is taken out of the heating block at 50 seconds and every 5 seconds after and gently tilted to determine if a change in viscosity (thickening) or clumping has occurred (Figure 11.7). Do not wait until a firm visible clot is seen.
- Record the length of time from start to identification of initial clotting.

11.5   Time Estimate To Perform Test

Twenty minutes (including time taken for blood collection).

11.6   Procedural Tips and Troubleshooting

Adequate warming of the ACT tube is essential for performing this test. If the tubes are not adequately warmed, the ACT may be artificially prolonged.

To ensure consistent and valid results for the ACT test, the timer should be started as soon as the blood is added to the ACT tube and the test must be monitored and checked at 50 seconds and every five seconds after that. This test is not a "walk away" test and requires the full attention of the operator.

The reference intervals for each type of ACT tube are specific for that manufacturer and are not interchangeable. Reference values can vary as much as 30 seconds between different ACT tube manufacturers. If the source for the ACT tube changes, new reference intervals should be included in the standard operating procedure. If the tube being used does not have a published reference interval, consider testing a blood sample collected from a healthy dog or cat with the patient's sample as a comparison.

The ACT test should not be done without knowing the platelet count. Platelet counts less than 10 000/µl will prolong the time.

11.7   Interpreting Test Results

A prolonged ACT test indicates a significant and severe coagulopathy. In clinical practice, rodenticide poisoning and DIC are common disease processes that result in severe coagulopathy due to decreased coagulation factor activity.

A complete coagulation profile should be done if patients show clinical evidence of a coagulopathy and have a prolonged ACT test. A complete profile that includes fibrinogen, fibrin(ogen) degradation products or d-dimers will assist in differentiating rodenticide toxicity, clotting factor deficiencies, and DIC.

The interpretation of the ACT test and a coagulation profile should be done in the context of the patient's history and clinical exam findings. There can be significant overlap in the results of coagulation testing between patients with consumptive coagulopathy (DIC) and rodenticide toxicity. Occasionally, patients with rodenticide toxicity will have evidence of fibrin and fibrinogen degradation (increased fibrin(ogen) degradation) products and d-dimer formation. Patients with consumptive coagulopathy usually have significant underlying inflammatory disease and are often considerably more ill compared with patients with rodenticide toxicity. They present with more comorbidities that predispose them to widespread systemic activation of coagulation.

11.8   Clinical Case Example(s)

See Part 6, case #3 and #9.

11.9   Add-On Tests That You May Need to Consider and Their Additive Value

A complete coagulation profile (prothrombin time [PT], activated partial thromboplastin time [APTT], total clotting time (TCT), fibrin(ogen) degradation products (FDPs), d-dimer, fibrinogen) should be performed whenever a patient has a prolonged ACT test.

A complete blood count and chemistry profile will be essential for identifying underlying inflammatory or infectious disease processes as well and significant organ dysfunction that may result in a consumptive coagulopathy.

Diagnostic imaging is recommended to assist in localizing possible inflammatory or neoplastic diseases that may result in coagulopathy.

11.10   Key Takeaways

- The ACT test is a screening test that can be used to screen patients with clinical findings indicative of a coagulopathy and should be followed up with a full coagulation profile when prolonged.
- The ACT test is less sensitive than the APTT and may be within reference interval in patients with significant factor deficiency. A significant coagulopathy is not ruled out with an ACT test within the reference interval.

Part 3

Quick Assessment Tests (QATS) Involving Urine

12

Assessing Urine's Physical Properties
Ryane E. Englar

12.1 Procedural Definition: What Is This Test About?

Urinalysis is a diagnostic test that involves both macroscopic and microscopic examination of the patient's sample. Urine samples are routinely obtained via cystocentesis, the preferred method of urine collection for urinalysis and urine culture. Alternate methods of urine collection include urethral catheterization, "free catch" of voided urine, or aspiration of samples off floors and tabletops, the primary disadvantage of the latter being sample contamination. Ideally, six milliliters of urine are obtained by the method of choice to allow for adequate sample size while minimizing trauma to the urinary bladder and urethra during collection.

Urinalysis begins with a macroscopic assessment of the sample. The sample is inspected to characterize its physical properties. This chapter will concentrate on the following properties of urine:

- volume
- color
- clarity
- odor.

A subsequent chapter (see Chapter 13) will cover the remaining physical property of urine, so-called urine specific gravity (USG).

12.2 Procedural Purpose: Why Should I Perform This Test?

The evaluation of urine is a critical diagnostic tool that is used in the detection and management of a wide range of medical conditions from local involvement of the urinary tract (e.g. urinary tract infection, UTI) to systemic disease (e.g. diabetes mellitus).

Urinalysis is an essential part of the diagnostic workup for patients that present with aberrant micturition histories, including, but not limited to:

- dysuria – difficult or painful urination
- hematuria – bloody urine
- oliguria – reduced urine production
- pollakiuria – increased frequency of urination
- polyuria – excessive urine volume or output
- stranguria – straining during urination
- periuria – urinary "accidents" or house soiling
- unusual or otherwise distinct urine odor.

Urinalysis is also an essential part of monitoring disease progression and/or patient response to case management of urinary tract disease.

Because of its utility as a diagnostic tool, urine is often referred to by clinicians as "liquid gold."

Urinalysis involves multiple steps:

1) assessment of urine's physical features: volume, color, clarity, and odor
2) measurement of urine specific gravity (USG)
3) chemical examination of urine constituents
4) microscopic examination of urine sediment.

As diagnostic machinery advances to the point that laboratory equipment can perform steps three and four on their own, it may be tempting to gloss over urine's physical features. This is not a new phenomenon. When Laennec invented the stethoscope in 1816, this diagnostic tool in many ways replaced what had previously been used to assess cardiovascular health: the patient's subjective impressions and physician's observations. However, clinicians gather unique and essential clues about disease processes through observation.

Low-Cost Veterinary Clinical Diagnostics, First Edition. Ryane E. Englar and Sharon M. Dial.
© 2023 John Wiley & Sons, Inc. Published 2023 by John Wiley & Sons, Inc.

Gross observations about urine include both visual and olfactory determinations about the sample's volume, color, clarity, and odor.

12.2.1 Sample Volume

Urine production ranges from 20 to 40 ml/kg/day in the average canine or feline patient. This equates to roughly 1–2 ml/kg/h [1]. This amount is contingent upon hydration status and the kidney's ability to concentrate.

Note that oliguria may be pathologic, as from feline lower urinary tract disease (FLUTD) or compensatory, as in a patient's appropriate response to dehydration.

Likewise, polyuria may be physiologic, as from overconsumption of water because of psychogenic polydipsia, or pathologic, as from diabetes insipidus.

Sample volume must be interpreted along with sample color and concentration, as measured through USG, to obtain a more complete clinical picture.

12.2.2 Sample Color

Urine color is a useful feature because it can be indicative of hydration status or a variety of diseased states. For example, urine that is dark yellow may suggest marked bilirubinuria whereas urine that is discolored red may suggest macroscopic hematuria.

A more comprehensive list of urine colors and their associations will be provided under the subheader, interpretation of test results.

12.2.3 Sample Clarity

Clarity is sometimes referred to as transparency. The opposite of clear urine is turbid urine. Turbidity or cloudiness may suggest increased number of cells, crystals, casts, or organisms.

A more comprehensive list will be provided under the subheader, interpretation of test results.

12.2.4 Sample Odor

Urine odor may be linked to intermediate or end-products of metabolism. For instance, patients with ketoacidosis may develop urine that smells like acetone.

A more comprehensive list will be provided under the subheader, interpretation of test results.

In isolation, observations are cheap, readily available, and easy-to-identify diagnostic clues. They prompt pattern recognition. For instance, observing hematuria generates a list of the most common differential diagnoses: UTI, urolithiasis, urinary bladder or urethral neoplasia, and thrombocytopenia.

Observations tell us where to look next within our patient and which steps we should take *now* to rule out differentials.

Observations must therefore be paired with chemical examination of the urine and microscopic examination of the sediment to provide a complete portrait of the patient. This more thorough snapshot of patient health is necessary to diagnose with accuracy.

12.3 Equipment

Examination of urine's volume, color, clarity, and odor requires the least "supplies." You need only:

- exam gloves for handling biofluids
- a fresh sample of urine within a clean, clear collection container
- a clear conical centrifuge tube or alternate means of measuring urine volume (see Figure 12.1)
- your eyes to see
- your nose to smell
- a white background against which to assess urine color
- graph paper or text on a white background against which to assess turbidity.

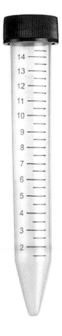

Figure 12.1 A 15 ml sterile polypropylene conical centrifuge tube with printed graduations to enable measurement of urine volume. *Source:* Courtesy of Ryane Englar, DVM, DABVP (Canine and Feline Practice).

12.4 Procedural Steps

1) Collect urine sample:
   √ Cystocentesis
   Advantages:
   o Ideal for urine culture *if handled and transferred sterilely* because the sample is not contaminated by the lower urinary tract
   o Minimal risk for iatrogenic UTI
   o Well-tolerated by most cats and dogs with minimal restraint and without sedation
   Disadvantages:
   o Client cannot collect sample at home
   o Requires technical skill to palpate and isolate the urinary bladder
   o Challenging to perform blind cystocentesis if urinary bladder is small
   o Ultrasound-guided cystocentesis is preferred, but requires equipment that not all veterinary practices have access to
   o Common to see iatrogenic microscopic hematuria (<50 red blood cells [RBCs]/ high-powered field [HPF])
   o Laceration of the urinary bladder is rare, but possible, particularly if the patient flails while the procedure is being performed
   o It is possible to inadvertently aspirate the intestinal tract and/or major abdominal vessels
   o Potential for seeding neoplastic cells throughout the abdomen if there is a mass within the urinary bladder
   o Potential for inducing uncontrolled hemorrhage if the patient has an underlying coagulopathy
   o Potential for urinary bladder rupture if the organ is extremely distended, as from urinary tract obstruction (UTO). Note that in some cases, we intentionally perform therapeutic cystocentesis in cats with UTO to reduce intravesicular pressure.
   √ "Free catch" (e.g. voided; tabletop see Figure 12.2)
   Advantages:
   o Noninvasive
   o Client can collect sample at home
   o Does not require restraint
   o Does not cause iatrogenic hematuria, which can result from cystocentesis or urethral catheterization
   o Easily obtainable from both male and female dogs
   o Can be obtained from cats by providing a box that contains non-absorbable litter, such as commercially available hydrophobic sand, or even aquarium gravel.
   Disadvantages:
   o Not ideal in cases that require urine culture due to potential for contamination with leukocytes,

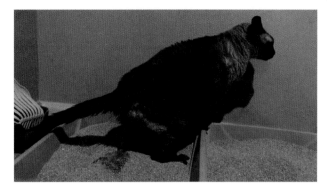

Figure 12.2 Cat voiding in litter box. Note that if the cat were tolerant, the cat's owner could slide a sterile urine collection container under the stream of urine to collect a midstream sample. This technique is typically more common in canine patients than feline patients because cats tend to eliminate in the absence of spectators. *Source:* Courtesy of Ryane Englar, DVM, DABVP (Canine and Feline Practice).

   epithelial cells, bacteria, or other debris from the distal urinary tract, skin, and/or fur
   o Contamination may also be due to the collection container itself if a sterile, single-use container is *not* used.
   √ Manual urinary bladder expression
   Advantages:
   o Easily performed in patients who are under general anesthesia (e.g. immediately prior to ovariohysterectomy or orchiectomy)
   o Part of routine care for patients with urine retention, as from decreased detrusor contractility; these patients require manual expression of the urinary bladder.
   Disadvantages:
   o Too much force can cause iatrogenic hematuria and proteinuria, +/− urinary bladder rupture
   o Not ideal in cases that require urine culture due to potential for contamination with leukocytes, epithelial cells, bacteria or other debris from the distal urinary tract, skin and/or fur
   o Inappropriate in patients who have just undergone cystotomy.
   √ Urethral catheterization
   Advantages:
   o Relatively easy to perform in male dogs
   Disadvantages:
   o Client cannot collect sample at home
   o Challenging to place urethral catheters in female dogs and female cats
   o Requires sedation and/or anesthesia for female dogs, female cats and male cats

o Catheter-induced trauma may contaminate the sample with iatrogenic hematuria and transitional epithelial cells; iatrogenic proteinuria is common

o Increased risk of iatrogenic UTI secondary to the procedure, particularly in female dogs

o Not advised to place urethral catheters in male cats unless they are presenting with UTO, in which case urethral catheterization constitutes essential therapy. Placing a urethral catheter in an otherwise healthy male cat for the sole purpose of collecting urine is not advised because there is a risk of iatrogenic UTO by irritating the lining of the anatomically narrow urethra.

2) Place urine sample in a clean, sterile, leak-proof container with a closed lid or top, labeled with the following details:
   - animal identification (e.g. name and case number)
   - owner identification: (e.g. client last name)
   - date and time of sample collection
   - how sample was obtained.

3) Analyze the urine sample within 30 minutes of collection to maximize accuracy of the results [2].

   Prolonged storage may potentiate bacterial overgrowth as well as secondary artifacts such as decreased glucose and changes in pH [2].

   If analysis must be delayed beyond the 30-minutes mark, then refrigeration of the sample is essential to slow bacterial proliferation and degeneration of both cells and casts [3].

   Refrigerated samples should not be analyzed beyond 24 hours after collection.

   Delayed analysis may result in changes that influence observations.

   For instance, hemoglobin, as from the breakdown of erythrocytes, imparts a red color to the urine. Prolonged exposure of urine to the elements will oxidize hemoglobin. The iron that is contained within hemoglobin (Hb) will transition from the ferrous [Fe+2] to ferric [Fe+3] state, forming methemoglobin (MetHb). MetHb is unable to bind oxygen and will therefore convey a brownish color to the urine instead of reddish (see Figures 12.3a and b). An observer may interpret this brown color as true methemoglobinuria secondary to toxicosis, as from acetaminophen, onion, or garlic toxicosis, when in fact, the color has resulted from delayed analysis.

4) If the urine sample has been refrigerated, allow it to come to room temperature before analyzing further.

5) Mix the urine sample well by inverting the sealed container.

(a) 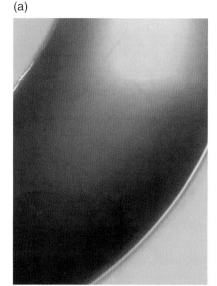 (b)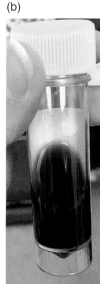

Figure 12.3 (a) An example of feline hemoglobinuria. *Source:* Courtesy of Dr. Whitney Rouse; (b) an example of feline methemoglobinuria. *Source:* Courtesy of Ryane E. Englar, DVM, DABVP (Canine and Feline Practice).

Particles that contribute to turbidity may settle out if the sample is left to stand. Turbidity is a measure of sample cloudiness (the opposite of clarity) and is a subjective measurement.

6) Transfer 0.5–1.0 ml of the sample to a sterile urine collection tube if urine culture is indicated.
   - Select a clean (empty; unused; sterile) red-top vacutainer tube.
   - Label this vacutainer tube as containing urine to differentiate from serum.
   - Swab the top of the unused (clean; empty) red-top vacutainer tube with alcohol.
   - If the urine sample was collected via cystocentesis and is still contained within the syringe, remove the used needle from the syringe safely and place a new needle on the syringe.
   - Insert the clean needle (with syringe attached) into the top of the red-top vacutainer tube.
   - The vacuum in the red-top vacutainer tube will begin to draw urine into the tube.
   - You need less than 1.0 ml of urine to perform a urine culture. After this volume has been drawn into the tube, you can pull the needle and syringe out of the tube.
   - Remove the used needle from the syringe safely.
   - Uncap a new urine collection tube.
   - Fill this new collection tube with the remainder of your urine sample.

7) Measure the volume of the remaining sample by pouring the urine into a conical centrifuge tube with printed graduations or any alternate measuring tool, as in a graduated cylinder. Record this volume.

Note that if the volume measured exceeds 10 ml, then it is acceptable to record this value as ">10 ml."

8) Identify and record the color of the urine sample using the appropriate descriptor:
   a) colorless (meaning transparent, like water)
   b) pale yellow
   c) yellow
   d) yellow amber
   e) yellow green
   f) deep yellow
   g) yellow orange
   h) orange
   i) peach
   j) pink
   k) pink-brown
   l) red
   m) red-brown or rust
   n) brown
   o) black
   p) blue-green
   q) milky white
   r) "other."

Refer to the subsection below, "Interpreting Test Results," to consider what each color may indicate.

9) Evaluate the sample for clarity or turbidity and record the appropriate descriptor:
   a) clear
   b) slightly cloudy
   c) cloudy
   d) turbid
   e) flocculent.

Refer to the subsection below, "Interpreting Test Results," to consider what each category of turbidity may indicate.

10) Smell the urine and record any unusual features.

Waft air over the open sample toward your nose to take in the aroma without inhaling urine droplets.

Wearing a mask during this phase of urinalysis will minimize risk of inhalation. Certain infectious diseases are transmitted through the urine, including, but not limited to, leptospirosis.

Refer to the subsection below, "Interpreting Test Results," to consider what specific scents may indicate.

12.5 Time Estimate to Perform Test

Five minutes.

12.6 Procedural Tips and Troubleshooting

12.6.1 Urine Collection

- Choose a method of urine collection that takes into consideration the presenting complaint and the patient's current medical condition. For example:
  ○ patients with known or suspected coagulopathies should not undergo cystocentesis [4]
  ○ patients that are being reassessed for hematuria may not benefit from cystocentesis because the procedure itself is likely to cause microscopic hematuria [3]. You cannot discern whether hematuria in the sample is preexisting or iatrogenic, therefore, the approach to urine collection does not support your diagnostic aim.
- In the case of "free catch" samples, collect urine in a sterile container that is free of contaminants such as food, detergent, or other residues.
- If clients do not have access to sterile, single-use urine collection cups, then they are likely to collect samples in plastic or glass containers that previously held food. It is understandable why clients reach for these; however, these makeshift containers risk contamination of the urine. The author has had urine submitted to her in pickle, jam, and jelly jars, many of which were not cleaned prior to filling. This impeded accurate observations about that sample's physical properties because the urine was discolored and cloudy, but not because of its own constituents.
- It is good practice to provide clients with medical-grade (sterile) urine collection cups. This practice maximizes macroscopic assessment of urine's physical properties and facilitates microscopic assessment as well.
- Once the sample has been collected, make sure that the lid of the container is tightly closed. This prevents evaporation of water if the urine is exposed to the air for a prolonged period [4].

12.6.2 Urine Color

- Even when a sample is contained within a clear vial, it can be challenging to discern the sample's color. Holding the collection tube against a white background provides the contrast that is needed to accurately assess sample color [3].
- Macroscopic hematuria may be caused by an overzealous manual expression of the urinary bladder in rabbits.

12.6.3 Urine Turbidity

- If obtaining a urine sample by "free catch," try to avoid the first part of the urine stream and collect a midstream

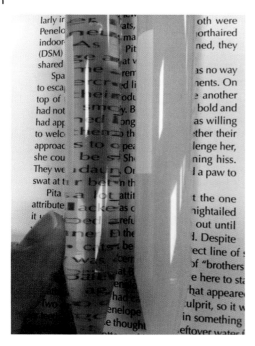

Figure 12.4 Using text against a white background to differentiate turbidity of urine samples. The sample on the left is clear; you can read with ease the words on the far side of the sample. The sample on the right is cloudy; you cannot see through the urine at all. *Source:* Courtesy of Ryane Englar, DVM, DABVP (Canine and Feline Practice).

sample instead to reduce the potential for contamination with exudate from the distal urethra, genital tract, and external skin. Such exudate may cause the sample to appear cloudy or even gritty.

- Even when a sample is contained within a clear vial, it can be challenging to discern the sample's turbidity. Subtle distinctions between clear and slightly cloudy, or between slightly cloudy and cloudy, may be challenging to detect without holding the sample against graphing paper or text on a white background (see Figure 12.4) [3]. How easy the text is to read through the urine sample can help you to distinguish which category of turbidity to classify it as.

12.7 Interpreting Test Results

12.7.1 Sample Color

Dogs and cats typically produce yellow- to light amber-colored urine. This normal pigmentation results from the

presence of metabolic byproducts urochrome and urobilin [3, 5]. Urochrome is a sulfur-containing yellow pigment that forms when the colorless metabolite urochromogen is oxidized [3, 5]. Urobilin is a byproduct of the degradation of hemoglobin [5].

Certain physiologic states, such as fever, and nutritional planes, such as starvation, can increase excretion of urochrome, impacting urine color. Hydration status also influences urine color. Dilute urine is paler than normal whereas concentrated urine takes on a darker yellow or yellow-orange appearance.

Abnormal urine color results from endogenous or exogenous pigments.

Because it is readily apparent, abnormal urine color is a common presenting complaint among companion animal owners, who may report concurrent inappropriate elimination behaviors. For example, clients often seek veterinary advice when cats urinate outside of litterboxes and the resultant puddle leaves an unusual stain behind. Furthermore, clients in geographical regions that experience wintry weather may report discoloration of white snow with abnormal shades of urine.

Urine color is easily identified by observant owners, particularly if patients exhibit concurrent dysuria, stranguria, oliguria, and/or pollakiuria. These clinical signs prompt clients to seek veterinary medical attention for presumptive urinary tract disease. Clinicians also need to prepare clients that certain prescribed drugs have been linked to transient discoloration of the urine and that such changes are to be expected so as not to incite panic.

Because urine discoloration is such a visible characteristic and because pigmenturia can be associated with so many diseased states, it is critical that clinicians familiarize themselves with the many shades of urine [2, 5–9] (see Table 12.1).

Note that normal urine color varies among species. For instance, dietary pigments often cause urine from horses and cattle to appear darker yellow.

Rabbit urine is also unique in that it ranges in color from white to yellow-white to light brown. Consumption of hay and vegetables and some metabolized antibiotics by rabbits may even cause a transient orange-red urine secondary to porphyrinuria. This may be mistaken as hematuria when in fact it is not truly pathological.

The intensity of urine color is partly dependent upon the sample volume and partly dependent upon the sample's concentration.

Table 12.1 The many shades of urine in cats and dogs and what each may be indicative of when identified during the macroscopic component of urinalysis.

Color of urine	Possible explanation(s) for color	Accompanying photograph
Colorless to pale yellow	Dilute urine, as from polyuria	Figure 12.5
	Colorless to pale yellow urine may be normal for the patient if the diet is significantly low in protein or high in sodium chloride	
	Colorless to pale yellow urine may result from: [10] • overhydration (as from psychogenic polydipsia) • compromised renal concentration of the urine (as from diabetes insipidus) • osmotic diuresis (as from glucosuria in patients with diabetes mellitus)	
	Colorless to pale yellow urine is expected if: [10] • the patient is receiving glucocorticoid therapy • the patient has a known endogenous glucocorticoid excess, as from hyperadrenocorticism • the patient is receiving diuretics • the patient is in renal failure • the patient has appreciable hypercalcemia	
	Colorless to pale yellow urine is *not* appropriate in a patient that is dehydrated; hence it is important to consider urine color in light of urine specific gravity	
Yellow to light amber	Normal color for canine/feline urine due to: • urochromes • urobilin	Figure 12.6
Yellow-green or yellow-brown	Bile pigments: • bilirubin • biliverdin (in birds and reptiles) causes a greenish tint	Figure 12.7
Deep yellow or yellow-orange	• highly concentrated urine • bilirubin (bilirubinuria) • excessive urobilin (as from fever or starvation)	Figure 12.8
Deep amber	• highly concentrated urine • increased bile pigments	
Peach, pink, red-pink, pink-brown, orange	Hematuria, hemoglobin, myoglobin, porphyrinuria, treatment with clofazimine or rifampin/rifampicin	Figures 12.9–12.11
Red, rust, brown	• blood (hematuria) • hemoglobin (hemoglobinuria) • bilirubin (bilirubinuria) • beetroot ingestion; beetroot contains betacyanin, in particular betanin, which may impart a bright red color to the urine • myoglobin (myoglobinuria)	Figures 12.12 and 12.13
Dark brown or black	• methemoglobin • melanin	Figures 12.14 and 12.15
Green, blue-green, blue	• methylene blue • oxidation of bilirubin to biliverdin (old urine sample) • UTI involving *Pseudomonas aeruginosa*	None
Milky white	• pyuria (with or without concurrent UTI[3]) • lipiduria (may be seen in healthy patients; frequently develops in cats with hepatic lipidosis[3]) • crystalluria • spermaturia	Figure 12.16

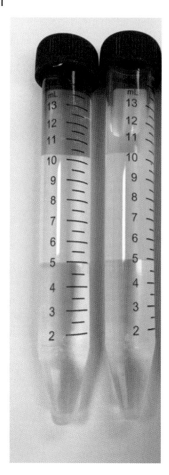

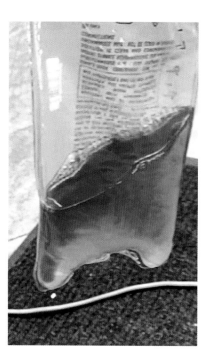

Figure 12.7 Yellow-green urine. Courtesy of Dr. Danelle Capobianco.

Figure 12.5 Two urine samples in canine patients. The sample on the left is colorless; the sample on the right is pale yellow. *Source:* Courtesy of Ryane Englar, DVM, DABVP (Canine and Feline Practice).

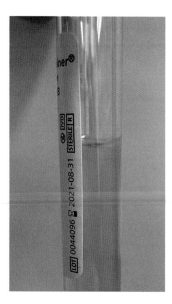

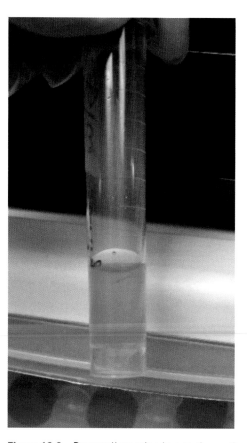

Figure 12.6 The expected color (straw yellow) in a canine patient. *Source:* Courtesy of Ryane Englar, DVM, DABVP (Canine and Feline Practice).

Figure 12.8 Deep yellow urine in a canine patient. *Source:* Courtesy of Ryane Englar, DVM, DABVP (Canine and Feline Practice).

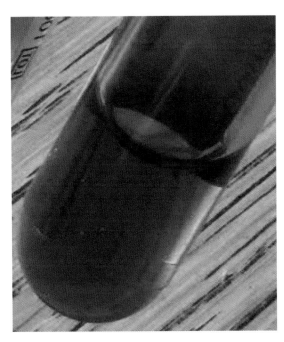

Figure 12.9 Orange-colored urine in a patient that had been prescribed rifampicin. *Source:* Courtesy of Ryane Englar, DVM, DABVP (Canine and Feline Practice).

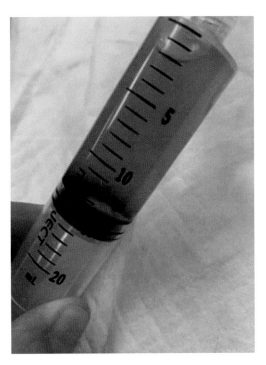

Figure 12.11 Pink-colored urine in a feline patient with UTO. *Source:* Courtesy of Dr. Danelle Capobianco.

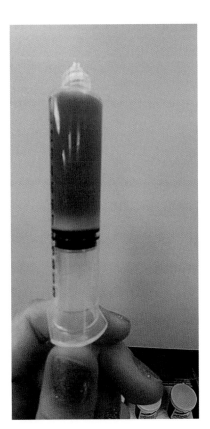

Figure 12.10 Peach-colored urine in a feline patient with UTO. *Source:* Courtesy of Dr. Lori Kruse.

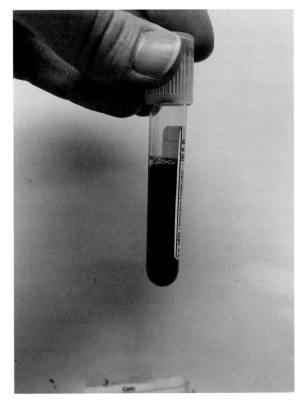

Figure 12.12 Red urine in a feline patient with UTO. *Source:* Courtesy of Jackie Kucskar, DVM.

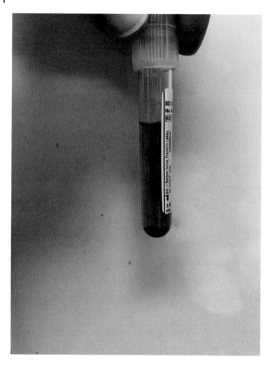

Figure 12.13 Rust-brown colored urine in a canine patient with urolithiasis. This urine sample is old, hence the change in color from red to rust-brown. *Source:* Courtesy of Jackie Kucskar, DVM.

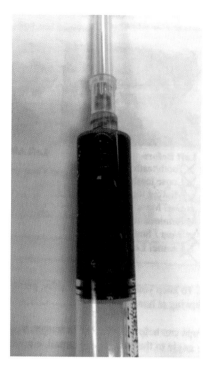

Figure 12.15 Brown-black urine in a veterinary patient. *Source:* Courtesy of Ryane E. Englar, DVM, DABVP (Canine and Feline Practice).

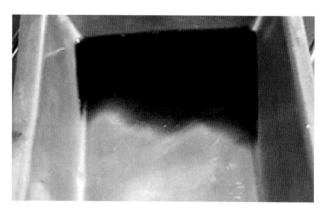

Figure 12.14 Brown urine in a cat that ingested acetaminophen. *Source:* Courtesy of Ryane E. Englar, DVM, DABVP (Canine and Feline Practice).

12.7.2 Sample Turbidity

Normal canine and feline urine is typically clear to slightly cloudy (see Figure 12.17).

Turbid urine is opaque.

Urine cloudiness, so-called turbidity, results from one or more of the following (see Figure 12.18):

- bacteriuria
- casts
- crystalluria

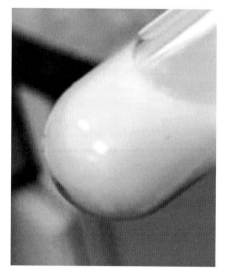

Figure 12.16 Milky white urine due to pronounced pyuria. *Source:* Courtesy of Ryane Englar, DVM, DABVP (Canine and Feline Practice).

- epithelial cells
- fecal contamination of the urine
- increased cellular content (e.g. erythrocytes and/or leukocytes)
- lipiduria
- mucus
- pyuria
- semen.

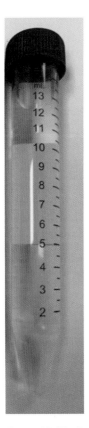

Figure 12.17 Example of clear urine in a canine patient.

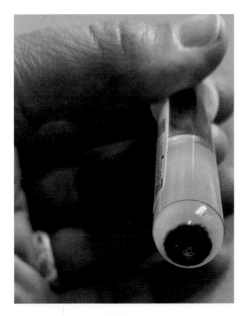

Figure 12.18 Example of cloudy urine in a feline patient with urinary tract obstruction, post-centrifugation. Note the sizable pellet that consists of cells and crystals; however, the supernatant remains cloudy. Although the authors have not yet guided you through the process of centrifugation to evaluate the urine sediment, this is a good example of turbid urine. *Source:* Courtesy of Jackie Kucskar, DVM.

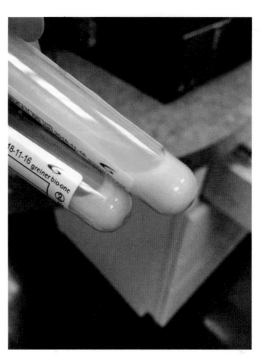

Figure 12.19 Example of turbid urine in a canine patient. Urine culture disclosed beta hemolytic *Streptococcus*. *Source:* Courtesy of Ryane E. Englar, DVM, DABVP (Canine and Feline Practice).

Turbid urine is opaque. It is an abnormal feature in dogs and cats (see Figures 12.19 and 12.20).

Turbid urine is normal in horses and rabbits (see Figure 12.21).

The turbidity that is associated with equine urine is due to high concentrations of mucus and calcium carbonate crystals, which are considered normal in this species.

Calciuria is responsible for the turbidity of a rabbit's urine.

Flocculent urine contains macroscopic particulate matter. These pieces of floating debris may indicate an abundance of cellular material, fat, and/or mucus.

12.7.3 Sample Odor

Normal urine typically has a subtle smell of ammonia; however, this aroma will strengthen as urine becomes increasingly concentrated. For this reason, the first voided morning sample can smell quite strong.

Odor is infrequently documented; however, it constitutes observable data that is easily gathered and may provide a diagnostic clue (see Table 12.2).

12.8 Clinical Case Example(s)

- A young adult male cat is presented for wellness examination. The cat was adopted as a stray. The cat has no visible or palpable scrotal testicles, so the client assumes that the

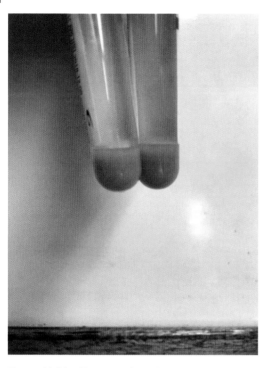

Figure 12.20 Example of turbid urine in a dog with a prostatic abscess. *Source:* Courtesy of Ryane E. Englar, DVM, DABVP (Canine and Feline Practice).

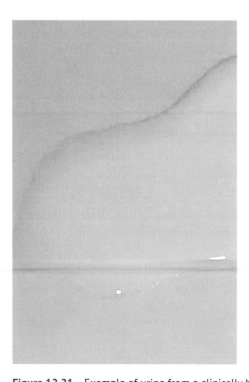

Figure 12.21 Example of urine from a clinically healthy rabbit. Note that this degree of turbidity is considered normal. *Source:* Courtesy of Ryane Englar, DVM, DABVP (Canine and Feline Practice).

Table 12.2 Scents that may be associated with urine and what they may indicate.

Odor of urine	Possible explanation(s) for odor
Fruity smell +/− undertones of nail polish remover	Ketonuria
Pungent	Intact male (especially cats and goats)
Putrid	Bacteriuria and/or protein degradation within an old sample, especially one that was not stored properly (e.g. not refrigerated)
Strong ammonia or the smell of stale sweat	Certain types of UTI-causing bacteria that metabolize urea via the enzyme urease
Sweet	Glucosuria

cat was owned at one point and neutered. During history-taking, the client's only complaint is that the cat's urine smells "strong." This odor is detracting from the client's bond with the cat and has made the client reconsider whether the cat should retain its indoor-only lifestyle. The client's comment about the pungency of the urine – "he smells like a tomcat!" – makes you wonder if the cat is bilaterally cryptorchid, so you conduct a thorough physical examination. When you manually extrude the penis from the prepuce, you find penile spines. This exam finding suggests that the cat has circulating levels of testosterone. This is confirmed via a paired blood test in which baseline serum testosterone is compared with that which results from the administration of gonadotropin-releasing hormone. Both testicles are located within the abdomen during exploratory laparotomy and are surgically excised. Testosterone levels decline significantly within 24–48 hours post-castration, and tomcat odor vanishes within a week. The relationship between client and cat is salvaged, and the cat can remain within the household as an indoor-only companion.

- A three-year-old spayed female domestic shorthaired (DSH) cat presents for evaluation of house soiling. The client is frustrated because they came home from work late last night to find that the cat had urinated in the bathtub. Both litter boxes were clean so the client cannot explain the acute change in elimination behavior. The urine also looks "odd." The client took a photograph with their smartphone and brought it in to show you: (see Figure 12.22).
- You examine the photograph that the client provides and note that the urine appears bloody. Given the signalment of the patient, you are concerned about idiopathic (sterile) cystitis as a differential diagnosis. Because stress is thought to play a primary role in the development of idiopathic cystitis, you take a patient history to establish what, if anything, has changed at home. Your client discloses

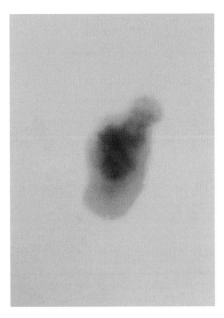

Figure 12.22 Example of feline house soiling. *Source:* Courtesy of Ryane Englar, DVM, DABVP (Canine and Feline Practice).

that the patient had been the "only child" in the home until five days ago. At that time, the client's partner moved into the one-bedroom apartment along with their two Jack Russell terriers. According to the client, introductions between the pets did not go well and the cat spends most of its time hiding beneath the bookcase. These historical details pique your interest and prompt you to proceed with urinalysis. Subsequent evaluation of the urine sediment rules out UTI; however, pyuria and both macroscopic and microscopic hematuria are supportive of the presumptive diagnosis, feline idiopathic cystitis. You prescribe pain management to support the cat through this episode, and you discuss environmental modification with the client as a means of stress reduction. The cat responds well to a combination of anxiolytics and analgesics. House soiling ceases once synthetic feline facial pheromone has been provided in the form of plug-in diffusers within the home. The cat was also given escape routes from the dogs in the form of vertical space (e.g. cat trees).

12.9 Add-On Tests That You May Need to Consider and Their Additive Value

Gross observation of the urine is merely the first step of urinalysis. Following gross observation, you should proceed with three additional steps:

- measurement of USG (see Chapter 13)
- chemical examination of the urine's constituents (see Chapter 14)

- microscopic examination of the urine sediment (see Chapter 15).

A word of caution: discolored urine is likely to alter results of the urine dipstick analysis (see Chapter 14) because this diagnostic test relies upon semiquantitative reagent strips. These test strips are colorimetric. In particular, the accuracy of the results for the following dipstick tests may be impacted by pigmenturia: [2]

- pH
- proteins
- glucose (particularly in the presence of marked bilirubinuria)
- ketones.

When urine is discolored red, rust, or brown, you cannot differentiate between hemoglobinuria (secondary to hemoglobinemia), bilirubinuria (secondary to hyperbilirubinemia), and myoglobinuria (secondary to myoglobinemia). In this case, examine the patient's plasma: [5]

- Pink plasma is suggestive of hemoglobin. Hemoglobinemia and accompanying hemoglobinuria are due to intravascular hemolysis.
- Yellow plasma is suggestive of bilirubin; hyperbilirubinemia and accompanying bilirubinuria may be due to liver disease, posthepatic obstruction, or hemolysis.
- Clear plasma is suggestive of myoglobin; myoglobinuria may result from muscle damage. If this is true, then you would expect to also see an elevation in the patient's serum creatine kinase.

Urinalysis is often paired with bloodwork to screen for occult disease in healthy patients or to further characterize overt clinical illness. Many values within a chemistry panel are influenced by the patient's ability to produce urine and/or concentrate it. Interpretation of these values in the context of the patient's urinalysis results helps guide the diagnosis. For example, bloodwork may disclose azotemia; however, urine facilitates the determination of etiology. A patient with concentrated urine and elevations in blood urea nitrogen (BUN) and creatinine is likely to have prerenal azotemia, as from dehydration.

12.10 Key Takeaways

- Urinalysis is incomplete unless observable and olfactory features of patient samples are examined. These include urine volume, urine color, urine clarity (turbidity), and urine odor.
- Observable and olfactory features alone are not pathognomonic for disease; however, they provide clues that guide the diagnostic plan. For instance, red

discoloration of the urine should prompt the clinician to consider urolithiasis as a differential diagnosis, indicating the need for diagnostic imaging as part of the patient workup.

- To maximize accuracy, urine samples should be analyzed within 30 minutes of collection. *in vitro* changes can and will occur in unpreserved urine that is stored at room temperature. These include the oxidation of hemoglobin to MetHb causing a change in color from urine that may have once been red to urine that is now rust-colored or brown.

- Urine color is easily determined when samples are examined through a clear container against a white background; urine turbidity is more easily discerned when samples are examined through a clear container against a white background that contains text.

- Urine samples should be well-mixed prior to analysis because particles that contribute to turbidity may settle out if the sample is left to stand.

- Urine turbidity can be artificially induced by refrigeration, which may cause crystals to precipitate that were not present at room temperature. Refrigerated samples should be returned to room temperature before analysis to lessen this artifact; however, doing so may not eliminate it.

12.11 Clinical Pearls

- Do not run a urinalysis without taking patient history. History-taking remains one of the most important tools in diagnostic medicine and it is cheap! Approximately two-thirds of diagnoses in human healthcare can be made based upon the patient's history alone [11]. The patient history-taking is likely to play a greater role in veterinary medicine because details about our patient's health must be relayed to us by observant clients. The clients have the answers we need, but it is up to us to actively solicit their perspective.

- Ask the client to describe what they are seeing and when it started. Ask about:
  - elimination behavior and location
    - Litter boxes: how many, where are they, and how often are they cleaned?
    - Is the patient house soiling? If so, where?
      - If a cat is peeing in a sink or tub, they are trying to tell you something.
    - What, if anything, has changed at home?
    - Have there been any additions or subtractions within the home in terms of other people and animals?
  - changes in thirst

  - changes in urine volume
  - changes in urine stream
    - If the owner says that the urine stream is different, listen.
  - changes in voiding frequency
    - The patient may ask to go outdoors more often.
    - The patient may urinate in multiple spots in the yard rather than emptying their whole bladder the first time.
  - changes in comfort of voiding
    - Is the patient visibly uncomfortable when voiding?
      - A cat that goes in and out of the litter box is trying to tell you something.
    - Is the patient vocalizing during urination?
      - A cat that is crying in the litter box is trying to tell you something.
  - inability to hold their bladder all night, whereas they were capable of doing so in the past
  - changes in urgency to void
  - changes in urinary continence
    - Is the patient aware that they are urinating?
    - Is the patient urinating when it is asleep?
  - changes in hygiene
    - Is the male dog licking his penis excessively?
      - Is there a change in penile discharge (color or amount)?
    - Is the fe(male)/cat or female dog licking at their perineum excessively?
      - Is there vulvar discharge?
        - If so, what is the color and consistency?
        - What is the patient's sexual status?
          - Is the patient in heat?
          - When were they in heat last?
  - changes in urine color
  - changes in urine odor
  - If the owner says the urine smells, listen to them.
  - Is this a new problem or it is recurrent?
- Examine the whole patient.
  - Assess the prepuce and the penis.
    - penile trauma and balanoposthitis both cause dysuria
    - male dogs with transmissible venereal tumor (TVT) may have a mass at the base of the penis; this may contribute to hematuria.
  - Examine the vulva.
    - Perivulvar dermatitis often causes painful urination.
    - Abnormal vulvar conformation (e.g. hypoplastic or recessed vulva) predisposes patients to UTIs.
  - Palpate the urinary bladder. Doing so may redirect your thoughts on the urine.
  - Assess the patient's mucous membranes. Patients are likely to be pale if hematuria is severe enough to incite

anemia [12]. They may also have a prolonged capillary refill time (CRT) [12].

   o Assess the patient for any evidence of disorders involving hemostasis, including petechial or ecchymotic hemorrhages [12].

   o Perform a rectal examination in male dogs to assess the prostate in dogs with hematuria [12].

- Contaminated urine is better than no urine at all. If the client sucked it up off the kitchen floor with a turkey baster, test it anyway.

- Any amount of urine is still worth testing. One drop is still one drop more than you had.

- Do not get hung up if the urine is 35 minutes old and the author said it should be tested within 30 minutes. Ask clients when the urine was collected and if they refrigerated it overnight, test it anyway.

- If the client brings in a "free catch" sample that appears bloody, ask if the urine consistently looked bloody or if the blood-tinge appeared at the beginning or end of the stream.

   o When the urine stream initially appears bloody, then it is likely that the patient has a lower urogenital tract issue [12].

   o When the urine stream is clear initially, but becomes bloody at the end of urination, then it is more likely that a focal lesion exists within the urinary bladder, as in a polyp or urolith. Blood associated with this location is voided last as opposed to blood associated with a lesion in the distal urethra, which is voided first [12].

- If your patient pees on clothing, rug, etc. and the urine has dried up, ask the client if it feels sandy. Grittiness could be indicative of crystalluria or urolithiasis.

   o Ask the client what color the urine stain is.

   o Ask the client if the stain smells unusual and, if so, in what way.

- Abnormal urine color indicates pathology; however, it is nonspecific. In addition, pathology may exist in the presence of urine that is normal in color. Therefore, urine color is just one of many clues. It is not intended to be used as a stand-alone diagnostic test.

- If urine color is abnormal, ask questions about:
     o diet
     o medication
     o collection techniques

- Urine color may align with concentration (e.g. pale urine is often dilute; dark urine is often concentrated); however, it is never appropriate to skip USG assessment.

- If urine is discolored such that you are not sure if the patient has true hematuria or hemoglobinuria, centrifuge the sample. If erythrocytes are intact, they will settle out into the bottom of a sample, leaving the supernatant clear.

References

1 Sirois, M. (2020). *Laboratory Procedures for Veterinary Technicians*, 7e. St. Louis, Missouri: Elsevier.

2 Grauer, G.F. and Pohlman, L.M. (2016). *Canine and Feline Urinalysis: From Collection to Interpretation*. Zaragoza, Spain: Grupo Asís Biomedia, S.L.

3 Reppas, G. and Foster, S.F. (2016). Practical urinalysis in the cat: 1: urine macroscopic examination 'tips and traps'. *Journal of Feline Medicine and Surgery* 18 (3): 190–202.

4 Polzin, D.J. and Osborne, C.A. (2012). Urinalysis in acutely and critically ill dogs and cats. In: *Advanced Monitoring and Procedures for Small Animal Emergency and Critical Care* (ed. J.M. Burkitt Creedon and H. Davis), 409–420. Chichester, West Sussex: Wiley-Blackwell.

5 Callens, A.J. and Bartges, J.W. (2015). Urinalysis. *The Veterinary Clinics of North America. Small Animal Practice* 45 (4): 621–637.

6 Englar, R.E. (2019). Grossly abnormal urine. In: *Common Clinical Presentations in Dogs and Cats* (ed. R.E. Englar), 821–830. Hoboken, NJ: Wiley-Blackwell.

7 Bellwood, B. and Andrasik-Catton, M. (2014). *Veterinary Technician's Handbook of Laboratory Procedures*. Oxford: Wiley-Blackwell.

8 Skeldon, N. and Ristić, J. (2016). Urinalysis. In: *BSAVA Manual of Canine and Feline Clinical Pathology* (ed. E. Villiers and J. Ristić), 183–218. Quedgeley, Gloucester, United Kingdom: BSAVA.

9 Chew, D.J., DiBartola, S.P., and Schenck, P.A. (2011). Urinalysis. In: *Canine and Feline Nephrology and Urology*, 2e (ed. D.J. Chew, S.P. DiBartola, P.A. Schenck and D.J. Chew), 1–31. St. Louis, Mo: Elsevier/Saunders.

10 Englar, R.E. (2019). Polyuria and polydipsia. In: *Common Clinical Presentations in Dogs and Cats* (ed. R.E. Englar), 799–809. Hoboken, NJ: Wiley-Blackwell.

11 Lichstein, P.R. (1990). The medical interview. In: *Clinical Methods: The History, Physical, and Laboratory Examinations* (ed. H.K. Walker, W.D. Hall and J.W. Hurst). Boston: Butterworths.

12 Forrester, S.D. (2004). Diagnostic approach to hematuria in dogs and cats. *The Veterinary Clinics of North America. Small Animal Practice* 34 (4): 849–866.

13

Urine Specific Gravity
Ryane E. Englar

13.1 Procedural Definition: What Is This Test About?

Urine specific gravity (USG) is measured during routine urinalysis as a test of how well the kidneys can modify urine concentration by adjusting its solute content [1]. When we measure the specific gravity (SG) of a solution, we are determining that solution's density [2]. Density is a measure of the mass of an object relative to the space that it occupies [2]. When we consider density of a solution, then what we are really investigating is the mass of solute per volume of solution. Urine is a mixture of solutes. Therefore, urine's density is a measure of the mass of all solutes within a given volume of solution. To interpret this, we compare the density of urine to the density of an equal volume of distilled water [3]. This ratio is essentially what defines USG [1–3].

Fresh water has a SG of 1.000 at 4° Celsius at sea level [2].

Substances that are less dense than water will float. These include gasoline, automotive oil, kerosene, jet fuel, lard oil, and corn oil. These substances have a SG less than 1.000.

Substances that are denser than water will sink. These include milk, 5% sodium chloride, and propylene glycol. These substances have a SG greater than 1.000.

Urine is always denser than water because it is excreted by the kidneys and based upon the physiologic process by which urine is produced, the kidneys are incapable of excreting pure water.

Urine always consists of water plus solutes of varying densities. In addition to water, urine contains:

- electrolytes
  - calcium
  - chloride
  - magnesium
  - sodium
  - potassium
- hormones

- nitrogenous substances
  - creatinine
  - urea
- organic acids
  - uric acid
- other organic compounds
- vitamins.

Therefore, USG will always exceed 1.000.

How much of each solute is contained within a given volume of urine determines the degree to which USG exceeds 1.000. For example, adding one of the following substances to 100 ml of urine will increase USG by 0.001 [2]:

- 0.147 g of sodium chloride (NaCl)
- 0.27 g of glucose
- 0.4 g of albumin.

What determines how much solute is excreted by the kidneys depends upon the patient's hydration status and renal function. The kidneys must be able to sense and respond appropriately to the tonicity of the patient's plasma. Response depends upon renal tubular function, which determines the degree to which urine will be diluted within the loop of Henle or the degree to which urine will be concentrated within the distal tubules.

In addition to renal function, how much urine is produced and how concentrated that urine will be depends upon several factors: [4, 5]

- factors external to the patient
  - ambient temperature
  - humidity
- factors related to the patient
  - activity level
  - diet
    - moisture content
    - sodium content
  - thirst and water consumption.

In health, urination, and thirst are interrelated. Assuming adequate renal function, a dehydrated patient will both maximally concentrate urine to conserve water and be driven to drink [5].

Urine formation requires a balancing act by the kidneys [5]. If the body has too little water, then the kidneys step in to conserve water and urine output will decline [5]. On the other hand, if the body is experiencing water overload, then the kidneys will eliminate the excess as urine [5].

In this way, the kidneys work in concert with the rest of the body to achieve water balance. Water balance is made possible by the following factors working in concert: [4–12]

- antidiuretic hormone (ADH) or vasopressin
- tubular function
- medullary hypertonicity.

ADH is produced by the hypothalamus [4, 6]. ADH is secreted when plasma tonicity increases [4, 6, 11]. ADH conserves water by reabsorbing it from the distal tubules and collecting ducts of the nephrons through aquaporin channels [4, 6, 13]. This action reduces urine output and results in concentrated urine [4, 6].

Urine cannot be adequately concentrated unless at least one-third of nephrons are operational [6]. Renal medullary hypertonicity is also required for water to be passively reabsorbed in the distal tubule and collecting duct [6]. This concentration gradient is established and maintained by the movement of sodium, chloride, and urea out of the nephrons and into the medullary interstitial space [14].

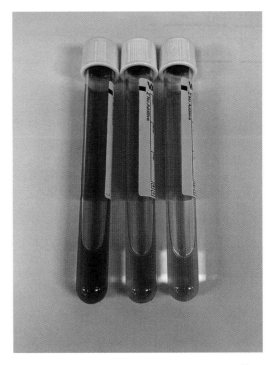

Figure 13.1 Three different samples of urine with varying degrees of concentration. The sample on the far left is hypersthenuric. The sample on the far right is hyposthenuric. The sample in the middle is isosthenuric. We cannot determine this without measuring USG. However, the color of the urine on the far left suggests that the sample is highly concentrated as opposed to the sample on the far right, which appears to be very dilute. *Source:* Courtesy of Jeremy Bessett, Inaugural Class of 2023, University of Arizona College of Veterinary Medicine.

13.2 Procedural Purpose: Why Should I Perform this Test?

Measuring USG is an easy, cheap, and convenient way to gain information about a patient's hydration status and their renal tubular function. As clinicians, we want to know how well the kidneys are regulating water balance and excreting waste. USG is our attempt to describe urine concentration (see Figure 13.1).

The gold standard approach to estimating urine concentration is to measure urine osmolality. Osmolality describes the number of particles in a solution irrespective of particle size or weight, a feature that makes it more accurate [15]. For example, USG overestimates urine solute concentration if many high molecular weight molecules (e.g., albumin, synthetic colloids, iohexol) are present in the urine whereas urine osmolality does not [15, 16].

Despite its accuracy, osmolality is not easily measured in clinical practice as compared with USG. Because USG can be performed in-house with ease, it has become a standard part of routine urinalysis.

USG and osmolality are linearly correlated; thus, it is appropriate to extrapolate urine concentration from USG [15]. Four canine studies have reported excellent correlations between USGs determined by refractometry and urine osmolality measurements [17].

USG provides baseline data as well as an opportunity for repeat measurements, which are essential when monitoring patients with known or suspected alterations in fluid volume status, renal dysfunction, and other metabolic conditions, including, but not limited to, diabetes insipidus.

13.3 Equipment

The preferred method of in-house measurement of USG requires refractometry [1, 2, 18]. Traditionally, refractometers are handheld tools that indirectly measure USG by detecting how solutes in solution refract light as compared with light refraction in air [1]. This so-called refractive index (RI) depends upon the sample's temperature and concentration [1]. Because cells, casts, and most crystals do not refract light, they do not influence the RI of urine; however, electrolytes, protein, glucose, urea, and creatinine do [1]. So, too, do particles that are suspended in solution; therefore, samples that are turbid should be centrifuged first such that only the supernatant is used to measure USG [1].

Traditional handheld refractometers contain the following components:

- adjustable eyepiece to focus the image
- measuring prism
- optical measuring surface
- illuminator flap or cover
- bimetallic strip (hidden from external view)
- calibration screw to adjust the position of the bimetallic strip, which allows the refractometer to be calibrated prior to measuring the USG of a patient sample
- scales
  - USG, urine gravity (UG), or specific gravity (SG) scale
  - serum protein (SP) scale in g/dl (g/100 ml) to measure total protein in a serum or plasma sample (see Chapter 4)
  - +/− RI scale (nD or ND) to measure the concentration of many other solutions.

Note that there are many types of handheld refractometers. Veterinary-specific models have historically been promoted over those with human-based USG scales out of concern that the latter led to spuriously high results, particularly for highly concentrated feline samples [1]. Because of this, conversion tables were created to adjust feline USG values when human health-care refractometers were used to perform veterinary urinalysis. Feline USG can be calculated as follows [1, 19]:

$$\left[\left(\text{Human refractometer USG reading}\right)\times0.846\right]+0.154$$

Veterinary-specific refractometers are commercially available and most incorporate different USG scales for canine and feline patients. However, it is unclear whether feline-specific scales are truly necessary [20, 21]. The accuracy of some feline-specific refractometers has been called into question [20, 21]. It is important to consider that refractometers are likely to vary in terms of their results; therefore, using the same type of refractometer in clinical practice is important when making comparisons between patient samples. If, for instance, your patient has USG measured every month, then it would be important to use the same tool each time to evaluate patient data for trends.

Regardless of whether it is manufactured for human health care or veterinary medicine, the in-clinic refractometer should be temperature-compensated. This feature adjusts for temperatures up to 100° Fahrenheit, which affects the density of urine [1]. If the clinic only has access to nontemperature-compensated refractometers, then

samples should be read at or near 20° Celsius, which is roughly room temperature or 68° Fahrenheit [22].

In addition to access to a refractometer, you will need the following to measure USG in-house:

- exam gloves for handling biofluids
- a fresh sample of urine within a clean collection container
- a clean, plastic pipette or alternative means by which to apply urine to the optical measuring surface, which overlies the prism
- adequate lighting overhead to facilitate reading the refractometer's scale
- a means to calibrate the refractometer daily
  - distilled water (USG 1.000)
  - alternatively, 5% NaCl solution in distilled water (USG 1.022)
- distilled water to clean the surface of the refractometer where the sample is applied
- specifically designed optic cleaning wipes (e.g. Kimwipes) that will not scratch the optical measuring surface.

13.4 Procedural Steps

Digital refractometers are now commercially available. These are easier to read and eliminate the subjectivity of interpretation. However, most clinics continue to use traditional handheld models to measure USG. The following instructions assume that you will be using a traditional refractometer.

1) Gather supplies (see Figure 13.2).
2) Check to be certain that the refractometer is calibrated prior to use.
   a) Lift the illuminator flap or stage cover (see Figures 13.3 and 13.4).
   b) Inspect the optical measuring surface ("the stage") to ensure that it is clean and dry.
   c) Using a clean pipette, apply a drop of distilled water (USG 1.000) to the stage (see Figures 13.5 and 13.6).
   d) Close the stage cover.
   e) Hold the eyepiece of the refractometer up to your eye as if the refractometer were a telescope (see Figure 13.7).
   f) Point the end opposite the eyepiece toward a light source.
   g) Now look through the eyepiece to visualize the USG scale.
      i) Twist the eyepiece as necessary to sharpen the image.
      ii) To obtain a sharper image, you may need to apply gentle downward pressure onto the dorsal

surface of the stage cover with your fingers from the hand that is not holding the refractometer.

h) Look for the shadow line where the illuminated and dark areas meet.

i) Read where the shadow line crosses the UG or SG scale on the refractometer. The UG or SG scale should read 1.000 (see Figure 13.8).

   i) If the reading is indeed 1.000, then your refractometer is calibrated appropriately, and you are ready to dive into measuring your sample's USG.

   ii) If the reading is more than 50% of a single graduation above 1.000, then your refractometer is not calibrated appropriately, and you are not ready to dive into measuring your sample's USG.

3) Let us assume that your refractometer is not appropriately calibrated.
Skip to Step #4 if your UG or SG scale did in fact read 1.000.
To calibrate your refractometer:
- Keep the distilled water on the stage.

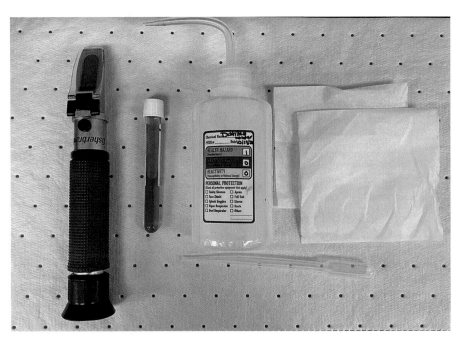

Figure 13.2 Supplies for USG by Refractometry. *Source:* Courtesy of Jeremy Bessett, Inaugural Class of 2023, University of Arizona College of Veterinary Medicine.

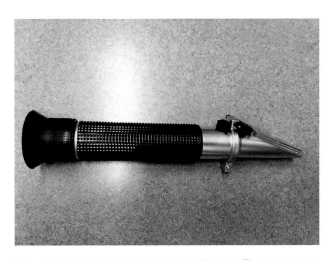

Figure 13.3 Refractometer prior to calibration. The stage cover is closed. Ryane E. Englar (Author).

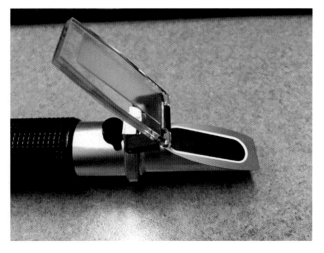

Figure 13.4 Refractometer ready for calibration. The stage cover has been lifted. *Source:* Ryane E. Englar (Author).

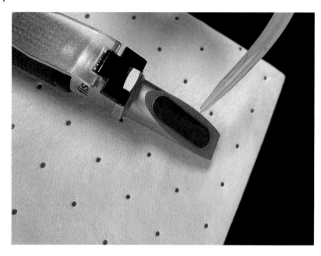

Figure 13.5 Applying a drop of distilled water to the stage for the purpose of calibration. *Source:* Courtesy of Jeremy Bessett, Inaugural Class of 2023, University of Arizona College of Veterinary Medicine.

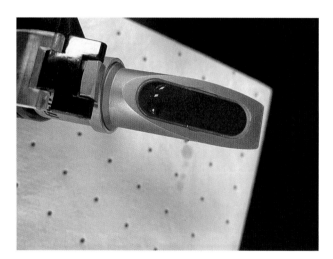

Figure 13.6 Distilled water has been placed on the stage for the purpose of calibration. *Source:* Courtesy of Jeremy Bessett, Inaugural Class of 2023, University of Arizona College of Veterinary Medicine.

- There may be a cap over the calibration screw. If so, remove the cap.
- Insert the small screwdriver that came with your refractometer into the calibration screw that sits at the back of or behind the stage (see Figure 13.9).
- Twist the screw as you are looking through the eyepiece.
- You should see the shadow line move up or down, depending upon the way in which you turn the screw.
- Adjust the shadow line until it rests at 1.000 on the UG or SG scale.
- Congratulations, your refractometer is calibrated!

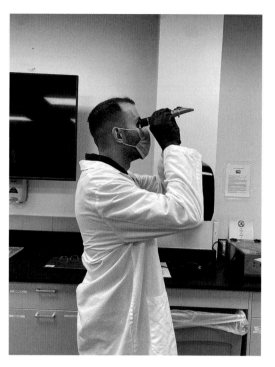

Figure 13.7 The correct positioning of the examiner's eye relative to the refractometer to obtain a reading.
Source: Courtesy of Jeremy Bessett, Inaugural Class of 2023, University of Arizona College of Veterinary Medicine.

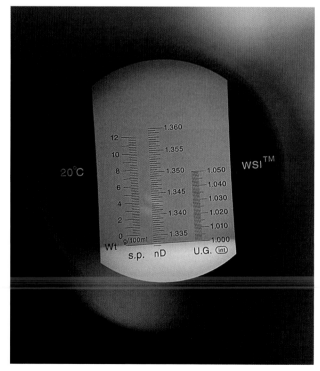

Figure 13.8 The correct reading for a properly calibrated refractometer. *Source:* Courtesy of Jeremy Bessett, Inaugural Class of 2023, University of Arizona College of Veterinary Medicine.

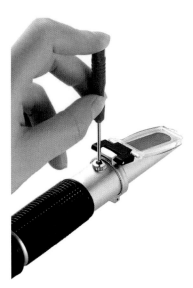

Figure 13.9 Inserting the refractometer's screwdriver into the calibration screw to calibrate the refractometer. *Source:* Ryane E.Englar (Author).

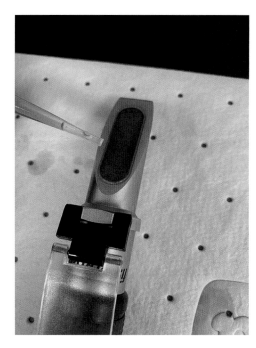

Figure 13.11 Preparing to load the patient's sample onto the stage of the refractometer. *Source:* Courtesy of Jeremy Bessett, Inaugural Class of 2023, University of Arizona College of Veterinary Medicine.

- Dry off the stage using specifically designed optic cleaning wipes (e.g., Kimwipes) that will not scratch the optical measuring surface (see Figure 13.10).
- Now you are ready to read your sample's USG.
4) Lift the illuminator flap or stage cover.
5) Inspect the optical measuring surface ("the stage") to ensure that it is clean and dry.
6) Use a clean transfer pipette to apply 2–3 drops of your patient's urine sample to the stage without touching the optical measuring surface (see Figures 13.11–13.13).
7) Close the illuminator flap or stage cover.

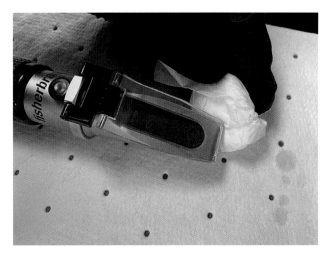

Figure 13.10 Drying the stage of the refractometer following calibration in preparation for loading the patient's sample. *Source:* Courtesy of Jeremy Bessett, Inaugural Class of 2023, University of Arizona College of Veterinary Medicine.

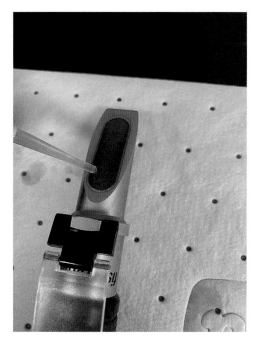

Figure 13.12 Loading the stage of the refractometer with the patient's sample. *Source:* Courtesy of Jeremy Bessett, Inaugural Class of 2023, University of Arizona College of Veterinary Medicine.

8) The urine will spread out across the stage (see Figure 13.14).
9) Pick up the refractometer.

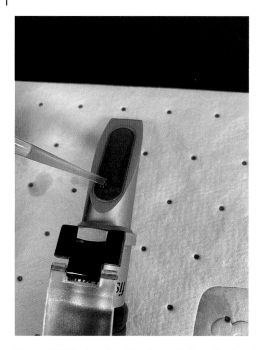

Figure 13.13 Loading the stage of the refractometer with the patient's sample. *Source:* Courtesy of Jeremy Bessett, Inaugural Class of 2023, University of Arizona College of Veterinary Medicine.

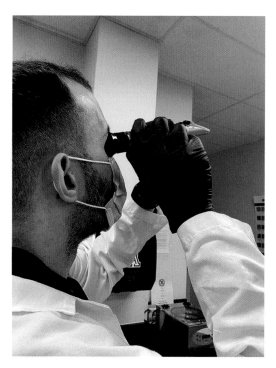

Figure 13.15 Close-up of the correct positioning of the examiner's eye relative to the refractometer to obtain a reading. *Source:* Courtesy of Jeremy Bessett, Inaugural Class of 2023, University of Arizona College of Veterinary Medicine.

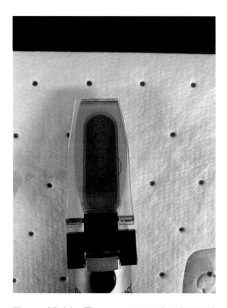

Figure 13.14 The stage cover has been closed, causing the patient sample to spread across the stage. *Source:* Courtesy of Jeremy Bessett, Inaugural Class of 2023, University of Arizona College of Veterinary Medicine.

10) Hold the eyepiece of the refractometer up to your eye as if the refractometer were a telescope (see Figure 13.15).
11) Point the end opposite the eyepiece toward a light source.
12) Now look through the eyepiece to visualize the USG scale.

   a) Twist the eyepiece as necessary to sharpen the image.
   b) To obtain a sharper image, you may need to apply gentle downward pressure onto the dorsal surface of the stage cover with your fingers from the hand that is not holding the refractometer.
13) Look for the shadow line where the illuminated and dark areas meet.
14) Read where the shadow line crosses the UG or SG scale on the refractometer. This is the USG of your patient's urine (see Figures 13.16–13.19).
15) Document the USG in the patient's medical record.
16) Lift the illuminator flap or stage cover.
17) Soak up the urine sample from the stage using a specifically designed optic cleaning wipe (e.g., Kimwipes) so as not to scratch the optical measuring surface.
18) Clean off the stage using an alcohol swab.
   Note that some clinics only clean off the stage using distilled water. That is an appropriate substitute for ensuring that the next sample will not be contaminated by the previous sample that was read; however, it is important to note that distilled water is not a disinfectant.
19) Wait until the alcohol (or distilled water) has completely evaporated before storing the device or using it again.

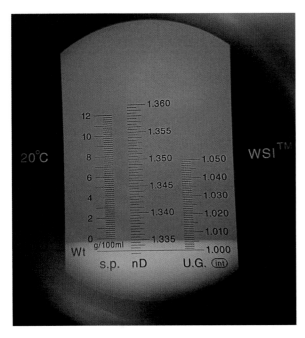

Figure 13.16 Urine specific gravity reading for hyposthenuric urine. *Source:* Courtesy of Jeremy Bessett, Inaugural Class of 2023, University of Arizona College of Veterinary Medicine.

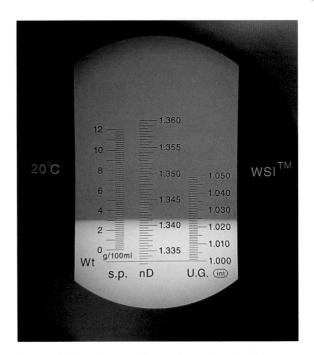

Figure 13.18 Urine specific gravity reading for midrange concentrated urine. *Source:* Courtesy of Jeremy Bessett, Inaugural Class of 2023, University of Arizona College of Veterinary Medicine.

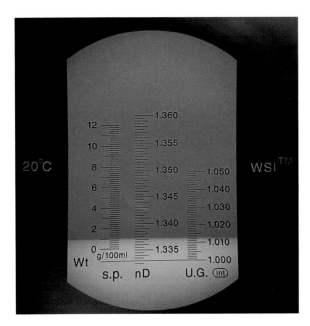

Figure 13.17 Urine specific gravity reading for isosthenuric urine. *Source:* Courtesy of Jeremy Bessett, Inaugural Class of 2023, University of Arizona College of Veterinary Medicine.

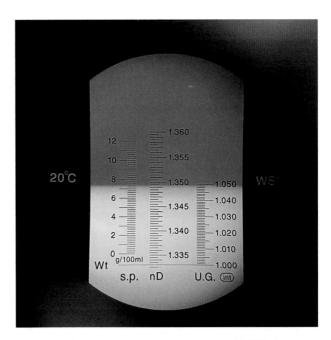

Figure 13.19 Urine specific gravity reading of 1.050, the highest measurement possible on this refractometer's scale. *Source:* Courtesy of Jeremy Bessett, Inaugural Class of 2023, University of Arizona College of Veterinary Medicine.

13.5 Time Estimate to Perform Test

Less than five minutes.

13.6 Procedural Tips and Troubleshooting

13.6.1 Tips

- Calibrate your refractometer daily.
- Collect a first morning sample of urine and measure its USG. This is likely to reflect the maximal concentrating ability of the patient because this urine will have the highest solute concentration [23].
- Recognize that USG varies throughout the day [23]. Contributing factors are appetite, thirst, and activity.
- Measure USG prior to the administration of any treatments (e.g. fluid therapy, diuretics, corticosteroids) that have the potential to alter USG [23].

  This baseline measurement becomes an important data point against which you can compare serial measurements of USG to assess how the patient is responding to treatment.
- Use a veterinary-specific refractometer.

  These typically have scales that measure USG up to 1.060 as compared with human health-care refractometers, which tend to measure USG up to 1.035 [23].
- If your patient's sample exceeds the UG or SG scale, do not simply report it as greater than "x." [23]
  - o Mix an equal volume of distilled water and urine.
  - o Determine the USG of the mixture.
  - o Multiply the numbers to the right of the decimal point by 2.
  - o The product is the patient's actual USG.
- If your patient's USG is lower than anticipated, repeat the test on serial samples of urine, collected on different days. Abnormal renal function is likely if values are consistently low.
- Consider the patient's USG in the context of their hydration status.
  - o A dehydrated patient should have concentrated urine.
  - o If a dehydrated patient does not have concentrated urine, then renal function is likely compromised.

13.6.2 Difficulties Reading the UG or SG Scale

Is the scale blurry or is the shadow line distinct?

- Did you inspect the stage prior to use? A scratched surface may impede your ability to see the shadow line on the UG or SG scale.
- Was the stage cleaned prior to use? Dried urine caked onto the stage may also impede your ability to see the shadow line on the UG or SG scale.

- Did you remember to sharpen the image by twisting the eyepiece as necessary to sharpen the image?
- Did you remember to sharpen the image by applying gentle downward pressure to the stage cover with your fingers from the hand that is not holding the refractometer?
- You might have inadvertently loaded air bubbles onto the stage, or you may not have completely covered the stage with urine. Consider adding more droplets of urine to the stage or better yet, start over.
- Is your patient's urine sample turbid? Recall that suspended particles interfere with light transmission. This will make the shadow line hard to read. Centrifuge the urine and use the resulting supernatant to measure your patient's USG.

13.6.3 Unusual Results

Are you reading the correct scale?

- The UG or SG scale should begin with 1.000; the scale should advance in graduated increments (e.g. 1.005, 1.010, 1.015, 1.020, 1.025, 1.030, 1.035, 1.040, 1.045, 1.050...)
- If you are getting a reading that ranges from 0 to 12, then you are likely reading the SP scale instead of the UG or SG scale. Double-check that you are reading the correct scale.

13.7 Interpreting Test Results

USG must be interpreted considering the following factors:

- Time of day when sample was taken (e.g. first morning sample vs evening sample)
  - o USG is highest for the first urine of the morning [23, 24].
  - o USG is generally lower in the evening as compared with the morning [24].
- Sample temperature
  - o Cold temperatures increase USG; therefore, refrigerated samples should be warmed to room temperature before measuring USG.
- Sample turbidity
  - o Turbidity increases USG; therefore, turbid samples should be centrifuged first such that only the supernatant is used to measure USG.

Additional factors that increase USG include: [1, 22]

- glucosuria
- hemoglobinuria
- lipiduria

- proteinuria
- radiographic contrast media, such as iohexol, that has been excreted in the urine.

Factors that decrease USG include: [1]

- ○ prescribed medications
  - corticosteroids
  - diuretics
  - fluid therapy
- ○ prescribed diets [5]
  - high sodium
  - low protein
- ○ moist (as opposed to dry) food, particularly in female cats [25].

What constitutes normal versus abnormal USG varies between species. The values for USG that Cornell University College of Veterinary Medicine references are as follows: Adapted from [26]

Species	Possible range for USG	Usual range for USG
Canine	1.001–1.065	1.015–1.045
Feline	1.001–1.085	1.035–1.060
Large animals	1.001–1.050	1.015–1.030

Other ranges have been reported in the literature; however, the author appreciates the utility of this approach. The possible range has been provided along with what is more typically seen in clinical practice.

Based upon their USG, patients can then be classified as either hyposthenuric, isosthenuric, or hypersthenuric.

Patients that exhibit hyposthenuria (USG < 1.008 in companion animals; <1.008–1.010 in horses) have dilute urine [26, 27]. The nephrons' proximal convoluted tubules and loops of Henle are functional; however, there is an issue at the level of the connecting tubules that prevents them from being able to concentrate urine [26]. This may be because the patient lacks ADH, as in cases of central diabetes insipidus, or because the renal tubules themselves are nonresponsive to ADH, as in cases of nephrogenic diabetes insipidus [26]. Note that there are additional causes of hyposthenuria, including, but not limited to, urinary tract infections (UTIs) [1].

Patients that exhibit isosthenuria (USG 1.008–1.012 in companion animals; USG 1.010–1.014 in horses) produce urine that is unchanged by the kidneys [1, 27]. When this occurs in cats that are dehydrated and/or azotemic, this may be an early sign of renal dysfunction [1].

Patients that exhibit hypersthenuria (USG > 1.012 in companion animals) produce concentrated urine [1].

For instance, when they are dehydrated or azotemic, cats should concentrate to a USG of, at minimum, 1.040 [1].

Patients that have low USG may have a history of polyuria and polydipsia (PU/PD).

Urine output varies day-to-day, between patients and within the same patient; however, urine production averages 20–40 ml/kg/day in dogs and cats [5, 14]. This equates to roughly 1–2 ml/kg/h [5, 14].

To compensate for this loss of water as urine, dogs consume 50–60 ml/kg/day of water [5, 14]. This volume has not been quantified for cats.

Water consumption increases in the normal patient if dietary moisture is low, if ambient temperature is high, or if activity level is high [5, 14]. Although this is an example of a normal fluctuation in a healthy patient, it is important to recognize that changes in urine output may also be pathological. Urine output may be greater or less than expected [4].

Polyuria occurs when urine is overproduced [4, 12, 14]. Urine production exceeds 45 ml/kg/day in the dog and 40 ml/kg/day in the cat [12].

Polyuric patients lose excessive amounts of water as urine. To counter this, polyuric patients often develop compensatory polydipsia or increased thirst. Polydipsic patients drink more than 90 ml/kg/day (dog) and 45 ml/kg/day (cat) [12].

Horses typically drink 5–10% of their body weight in water per day [27]. A 500 kg horse is expected to drink 25–50 liters of water daily [27]. A polydipsic horse would drink water in excess of this [27].

Common clinical conditions in companion animal practice that are associated with PU/PD include: [5]

- hypercalcemia
  - ○ chronic kidney disease (CKD)
  - ○ hypoadrenocorticism (Addison's disease)
  - ○ hypervitaminosis D
- endocrinopathies
  - ○ diabetes insipidus
    - central diabetes insipidus
    - nephrogenic diabetes insipidus
  - ○ diabetes mellitus
  - ○ hyperadrenocorticism (Cushing's disease or Cushing's syndrome)
  - ○ hyperthyroidism
- hepatopathy
- infectious disease
  - ○ pyometra
    - *Escherichia coli* endotoxins interfere with the nephron's ability to reabsorb sodium [28]
- neoplasia
  - ○ hypercalcemia of malignancy

- lymphoma
- anal sac apocrine gland adenocarcinoma
- multiple myeloma
- pharmaceutical agents
  - anticonvulsants
    - phenobarbital
    - phenytoin
    - primidone
  - diuretics
  - corticosteroids
- post-obstructive diuresis
- psychogenic polydipsia
- pyelonephritis.

Patients that exhibit PU/PD are likely to become dehydrated when urine production exceeds their capacity to drink enough water. At that point, if renal production is adequate, then low USG may transform into high USG.

Patients that have high USG are often dehydrated and/or azotemic.

Dehydrated patients are likely to display one or more of the following signs: [12, 29–31]

- cool extremities
- pallor
- prolonged capillary refill time (CRT)
- skin tenting
- tacky mucous membranes
- weak pulse.

Skin tenting is evaluated by grasping a generous fold of skin at the nape or between the shoulder blades. The skin fold is lifted up and then released [30]. In a euhydrated patient, skin elasticity causes the fold to return to its normal position almost immediately [30]. In other words, there is no persistent skin tent.

As the patient dehydrates, skin turgor is progressively lost. The fold of skin is sluggish. The time it takes to return to its original position is delayed. In cases of severe dehydration, the skin fold remains tented.

The extremely dehydrated patient may also display sunken globes and/or dehydrated corneas [30].

13.8 Clinical Case Example(s)

- A nine-year-old male castrated Labrador retriever dog is presented to you for evaluation of a four-month history of reported PU/PD. The dog has free rein of the house by day and is crated at night. The client offers water ad libitum. The client became concerned when the dog could no longer hold his urine overnight. Every morning for the past week, the client has awakened to find a large puddle of urine in the dog's crate. Last night, out of desperation, the client removed the water bowl from the crate, hoping that it would help. The dog still had a urinary accident overnight and the client is at their wit's end. They managed to obtain a "free catch" sample of urine from the dog on their morning walk and bring it with them to their appointment, 30 minutes later.

On physical examination, the dog is bright, alert, and responsive. Vital signs are within the reference ranges, and the patient appears to be euhydrated.

CBC and serum biochemistry profile are unremarkable.

The urine sample is greater than 10 ml in quantity and appears to be both clear (in terms of transparency) and colorlessness.

Urine pH is 6.5.

Urine dipstick is negative for protein, glucose, ketones, bilirubin, and blood (heme) (see Chapter 14).

USG is 1.005.

The patient's test results make the following causes of PU/PD unlikely:

- diabetes mellitus
- Fanconi syndrome
- hepatopathy
- hyperadrenocorticism
- hypercalcemia
- hypoadrenocorticism
- kidney disease.

Based upon the patient's history of PU/PD and the laboratory results, the following causes of PU/PD are most likely:
- diabetes insipidus
  - central
  - nephrogenic.

Psychogenic polydipsia is less likely because the patient would have been expected to concentrate his urine overnight given that his water source had been removed from the crate. The fact that his urine remained dilute in the absence of water prioritizes diabetes insipidus as the primary differential diagnosis.

Based upon your high index of suspicion, you discuss next steps with the client. You review the pros and cons of performing a modified water deprivation test to determine whether endogenous ADH is released in response to dehydration and whether the dog's kidneys can respond to the ADH. Due to the inherent risks of testing (e.g. dehydration and hypernatremia), the client consents to a desmopressin acetate trial instead.

You instruct the client to administer 1–2 drops of 0.01% desmopressin human intranasal spray to both conjunctival sacs of the patient every 12 hours. Seven days later, the patient returns for a recheck. The client reports a decrease in water consumption and no further house-soiling. You repeat the patient's urinalysis using a first morning voided sample. USG is now 1.022.

Based upon the patient's response to the trial, you confirm the diagnosis of central diabetes insipidus.

13.9   Add-On Tests That You May Need to Consider and Their Additive Value

USG represents just one isolated data point when it comes to assessing the patient's hydration status. In addition to measuring USG, the clinician should consider the following factors in making determinations about the patient's hydration:

- historical data, obtained from anamnesis
- physical examination findings
- packed cell volume (PCV) and/or complete blood count (CBC)
- chemistry panel or profile.

A decline in hydration status is clinically detectable on physical examination when the patient is 5% dehydrated [5, 32].

A patient is said to be 5% dehydrated when the skin tents slightly, meaning that the skin fold returns to its original position but less rapidly than anticipated [5, 32].

In addition, the patient's mucous membranes will be slightly tacky, that is, sticky to the touch [5, 32]. The veterinarian's finger does not "stick" to the gums, but the patient's gums are not as moist as they appear in health [5, 31, 32].

A patient is said to be 6–8% dehydrated when there is a moderate skin tent [5, 32]. The skin fold is sluggish to return to its proper anatomic location following an attempt to tent the skin [5, 32]. The patient's mucous membranes are now dry to the touch [5, 31, 32].

A patient is said to be 10–12% dehydrated when the skin remains tented [5, 32]. The veterinarian's fingers now stick to the patient's mucous membranes because they are bone dry [5, 32]. The eyes take on a sunken appearance [5, 32]. As a result, the nictitating membranes become prominent [5, 31, 32].

Note that dehydration is in actuality a continuum and these percentages are simply guidelines to help the clinician to prognosticate [5, 32].

In addition to assessing hydration status during the patient's physical examination, the following clinicopathologic data are supportive of dehydration when paired with an elevated USG [5, 32]:

- CBC
  ○ hemoconcentration with increased total solids
- chemistry panel
  ○ azotemia
    ▪ increased blood urea nitrogen (BUN)
    ▪ increased creatinine.

13.10   Key Takeaways

- USG is highest for the first urine sample of the morning [23, 24].
- USG is generally lower in the evening as compared with the morning [24].
- USG varies throughout the day in healthy dogs [24].
- USG should be interpreted in the context of dehydration: *is this patient's USG expected, given their hydration status?*
  ○ A dehydrated patient should have concentrated urine.
  ○ If a dehydrated patient does not have concentrated urine, then renal function is likely compromised.
- Interpretations about proteinuria should be made in the context of USG [1]
  ○ A patient with a USG of 1.060 and + 2 dipstick protein has mild proteinuria.
  ○ A patient with a USG of 1.007 and + 2 dipstick protein has marked proteinuria.

13.11   Clinical Pearls

- Neonates do not have the renal concentrating ability of adults; therefore, USG among neonates is low [1].
  ○ USG in neonatal kittens ranges from 1.006 to 1.007 [1].
  ○ By four weeks of age, kittens may achieve USG readings up to 1.038 [33].
  ○ By eight weeks of age, kittens may achieve USG readings up to 1.080 [33].
- USG decreases with age [24].
- USG is independent of patient sex [24].
- Glucosuria increases urine volume due to osmotic diuresis; however, the presence of glucose within the urine will increase USG [3].
- If a patient is dehydrated or azotemic yet has dilute urine, this is abnormal. Consider the following rule-outs [3]:
  ○ diabetes insipidus
  ○ hyperadrenocorticism
  ○ hypercalcemia
  ○ hypoadrenocorticism
  ○ kidney disease.

References

1 Reppas, G. and Foster, S.F. (2016). Practical urinalysis in the cat: 1: urine macroscopic examination 'tips and traps'. *Journal of Feline Medicine and Surgery* 18 (3): 190–202.

2 Polzin, D.J. and Osborne, C.A. (2012). Urinalysis in acutely and critically ill dogs and cats. In: *Advanced Monitoring and Procedures for Small Animal Emergency and Critical Care* (ed. J.M. Burkitt Creedon and H. Davis), 409–420. Chichester, West Sussex: Wiley-Blackwell.

3 Callens, A.J. and Bartges, J.W. (2015). Urinalysis. *The Veterinary Clinics of North America. Small Animal Practice* 45 (4): 621–637.

4 Reece, W.O. (2004). Kidney function in mammals. In: *Dukes' Physiology of Domestic Animals*, 12e (ed. H.H. Dukes and W.O. Reece), 73–106. Ithaca: Comstock Pub. Associates.

5 Englar, R.E. (2019). Polyuria and polydipsia. In: *Common Clinical Presentations in Dogs and Cats* (ed. R.E. Englar), 799–809. Hoboken, NJ: Wiley-Blackwell.

6 Nichols, R. (2001). Polyuria and polydipsia - diagnostic approach and problems associated with patient evaluation. *Veterinary Clinics of North America: Small* 31 (5): 833-+.

7 DiBartola, S.P. (1992). Disorders of sodium and water: hypernatremia and hyponatremia. In: *Fluid Therapy in Small Animal Practice* (ed. S.P. DiBartola). Philadelphia: WB Saunders.

8 Feldman, E.C. and Melson, R.W. (1996). Water metabolism and diabetes insipidus. In: *Canine and Feline Endocrinology and Reproduction* (ed. E.C. Feldman and R.W. Melson). Philadelphia: WB Saunders.

9 Hardy, R.M. (1982). Disorders of water metabolism. *The Veterinary Clinics of North America. Small Animal Practice* 12 (3): 353–373.

10 Verbalis, J.G. (2003). Disorders of water metabolism. In: *Contemporary Endocrinology: Handbook of Diagnostic Endocrinology* (ed. J.E. Hall and L.K. Nieman), 23–53. Totowa, NJ: Humana Press, Inc.

11 Marks, S.L. and Taboada, J. (1998). Hypernatremia and hypertonic syndromes. *The Veterinary Clinics of North America. Small Animal Practice* 28 (3): 533–543.

12 Tilley, L.P. and Smith, F.W.K. (2004). *The 5-Minute Veterinary Consult : Canine and Feline*, 3e, vol. lviii. Baltimore, MD: Lippincott Williams & Wilkins 1487 p.

13 Agarwal, S.K. and Gupta, A. (2008). Aquaporins: the renal water channels. *Indian Journal of Nephrology* 18 (3): 95–100.

14 Schoeman, J.P. (ed.) (2008). *Approach to Polyuria and Polydipsia in the Dog. Proceedings of the 33rd World Small Animal Veterinary Congress*. Dublin, Ireland: World Small Animal Veterinary Association (WSAVA).

15 Waddell, L.S. (2015). Colloid osmotic pressure and osmolality monitoring. In: *Small animal critical care medicine* (ed. D.C. Silverstein and K. Hopper), 978–981. St. Louis, Mo: Saunders/Elsevier.

16 Smart, L., Hopper, K., Aldrich, J. et al. (2009). The effect of hetastarch (670/0.75) on urine specific gravity and osmolality in the dog. *Journal of Veterinary Internal Medicine* 23 (2): 388–391.

17 Rudinsky, A.J., Wellman, M., Tracy, G. et al. (2019). Variability among four refractometers for the measurement of urine specific gravity and comparison with urine osmolality in dogs. *Veterinary Clinical Pathology* 48 (4): 702–709.

18 Grauer, G.F. and Pohlman, L.M. (2016). *Canine and Feline Urinalysis: From Collection to Interpretation*. Zaragoza, Spain: Grupo Asís Biomedia, S.L.

19 George, J.W. (2001). The usefulness and limitations of hand-held refractometers in veterinary laboratory medicine: an historical and technical review. *Veterinary Clinical Pathology* 30 (4): 201–210.

20 Tvedten, H.W. and Noren, A. (2014). Comparison of a Schmidt and Haensch refractometer and an Atago PAL-USG cat refractometer for determination of urine specific gravity in dogs and cats. *Veterinary Clinical Pathology* 43 (1): 63–66.

21 Tvedten, H.W., Ouchterlony, H., and Lilliehook, I.E. (2015). Comparison of specific gravity analysis of feline and canine urine, using five refractometers, to pycnometric analysis and total solids by drying. *New Zealand Veterinary Journal* 63 (5): 254–259.

22 Stockham, S.L. and Scott, M.A. (2002). Urinary system. In: *Fundamentals of Veterinary Clinical Pathology*, 1e (ed. S.L. Stockham and M.A. Scott), 416–449. Ames, Iowa: Iowa State Press.

23 Chew, D.J., DiBartola, S.P., and Schenck, P.A. (2011). Urinalysis. In: *Canine and Feline Nephrology and Urology*, 2e (ed. D.J. Chew, S.P. DiBartola, P.A. Schenck and D.J. Chew), 1–31. Elsevier/Saunders: St. Louis, Mo.

24 van Vonderen, I.K., Kooistra, H.S., and Rijnberk, A. (1997). Intra- and interindividual variation in urine osmolality and urine specific gravity in healthy pet dogs of various ages. *Journal of Veterinary Internal Medicine* 11 (1): 30–35.

25 Rishniw, M. and Bicalho, R. (2015). Factors affecting urine specific gravity in apparently healthy cats presenting to first opinion practice for routine evaluation. *Journal of Feline Medicine and Surgery* 17 (4): 329–337.

26 eClinpath (2020). Concentrating ability Ithaca, NY: Cornell University College of Veterinary Medicine; https://eclinpath.com/urinalysis/concentrating-ability.

27 Savage, C.J. (2008). Urinary clinical pathologic findings and glomerular filtration rate in the horse. *The Veterinary Clinics of North America. Equine Practice* 24 (2): 387–404, vii.

28 Bruyette, D.S. (2008). Diagnostic approach to polyuria and polydipsia. DVM 360 [Internet]. http://veterinarycalendar.dvm360.com/diagnostic-approach-polyuria-and-polydipsia-proceedings-0.

29 King, L.G. and Donaldson, M.T. (1994). Acute vomiting. *The Veterinary Clinics of North America. Small Animal Practice* 24 (6): 1189–1206.

30 Englar, R.E. (2017). *Performing the Small Animal Physical Examination*. Hoboken, NJ: Wiley pp. 29–30, 221–222.

31 DiBartola, S.P. and Bateman, S. (2006). Introduction to fluid therapy. In: *Fluid, Electrolyte, and Acid-Base Disorders in Small Animal Practice*, 3e (ed. S.P. DiBartola), 325–344. Saunders/Elsevier: St. Louis, Mo.

32 Englar, R.E. (2017). Assessing the big picture: the body, the coat, and the skin of the cat. In: *Performing the Small Animal Physical Examination* (ed. R.E. Englar), 24–51. Hoboken, NJ: Wiley/Blackwell.

33 Hoskins, J.D., Turnwald, G.H., Kearney, M.T. et al. (1991). Quantitative urinalysis in kittens from four to thirty weeks after birth. *American Journal of Veterinary Research* 52 (8): 1295–1299.

14

Chemical Evaluation of Urine

Urine Dipstick Analysis

Ryane E. Englar

14.1 Procedural Definition: What Is This Test About?

Chemical evaluation of urine involves the use of commercially available, colorimetric, reagent test strips to provide qualitative and/or semiquantitative measurements of the following chemical properties of urine [1–6]:

- pH
- protein
- glucose
- ketones
- occult blood (heme)
- bilirubin.

Test strips for the chemical evaluation of urine are commonly called dipsticks. By design, dipsticks have one or more pads that are impregnated with reagents [4]. These pads change color in the presence of the substance of interest [4]. How much of that substance is present in the urine sample will determine the degree of color change [4]. Color change is also time dependent. Manufacturers will provide specific instructions concerning how long to wait after soaking the pad with urine to interpret the test results [5].

Results are typically read manually by the members of the veterinary team who are tasked with performing urinalysis. However, automated urine chemistry test strip analyzers are available that will interpret and print results in lieu of personnel [4].

Many different brands of dipsticks are commercially available within human healthcare and veterinary practices. Dipsticks may be manufactured to test one or more chemical properties of urine.

Dipsticks that test for only one substance in the urine include:

Albustix®
- protein
Ketostix (see Figure 14.1.)
- ketones
Diastix® (see Figure 14.2.)
- glucose.

Dipsticks that test for two substances include:

- Keto-Diastix®
  - ketones and glucose.

Dipsticks that test for more than two substances include:

- Multistix® 10 SG (see Figure 14.3.)
  - glucose
  - bilirubin
  - ketone
  - urine specific gravity (USG)
  - blood (heme)
  - pH
  - protein
  - urobilinogen
  - nitrite (for detection of bacteria)
  - leukocyte esterase (for detection of white blood cells).

Human urine dipstick tests are also available over the counter to screen for the presence of drugs that are commonly abused. These commercially available test kits have been used off-label by veterinarians to successfully identify barbiturates, opiates, benzodiazepines, and amphetamines/methamphetamines within canine urine in emergency settings [7]. However, these are beyond the scope of

Low-Cost Veterinary Clinical Diagnostics, First Edition. Ryane E. Englar and Sharon M. Dial.
© 2023 John Wiley & Sons, Inc. Published 2023 by John Wiley & Sons, Inc.

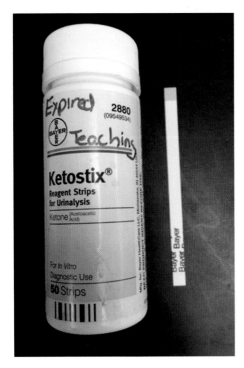

Figure 14.1 Example of reagent test strip that exclusively tests for urine ketones. *Source:* Courtesy of Ryane E. Englar, DVM, DABVP (Canine and Feline Practice).

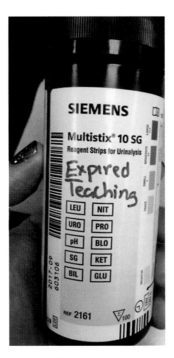

Figure 14.3 Example of a reagent test strip that assesses multiple chemical parameters within a urine sample. *Source:* Courtesy of Ryane E. Englar, DVM, DABVP (Canine and Feline Practice).

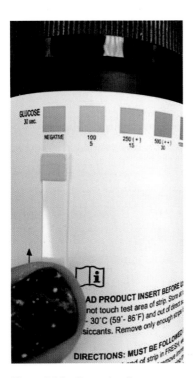

Figure 14.2 Example of reagent test strip that exclusively tests for urine glucose. *Source:* Courtesy of Ryane E. Englar, DVM, DABVP (Canine and Feline Practice).

this chapter, which will focus on routine rather than toxicological screening of urine.

For cost efficiency and the sake of completeness, most veterinary practices incorporate a multiple-test reagent strip into routine urinalysis.

Because strips such as Multistix® were developed as a diagnostic tool for human health care, it is important to note that not all tests that are provided on a multiple-test reagent strip are useful or reliable in veterinary species [4]. Specifically, the following test pads on the Multistix® are not advised for use in veterinary practice [1–4]:

- USG
- urobilinogen
- nitrite
- leukocyte esterase [8, 9].

USG is a measure of how concentrated or dilute the urine is. This is determined by the patient's renal tubular function and hydration status. The USG pad on commercially available dipsticks only measures up to 1.030. This is not an appropriate cutoff point for assessing the canine or feline patient's ability to concentrate urine [5, 10–12]. In addition, dilute urine is not always accurately identified by the USG pad [6]. Therefore, the gold standard method by which to measure USG is via refractometry. See Chapter 13 for additional details.

Urobilinogen is a metabolic byproduct of bilirubin. It is normal to excrete some urobilinogen in the urine. In people, an increased amount of urobilinogen can indicate elevated levels of serum bilirubin. Elevated bilirubin is supportive of hepatobiliary disease in people. However, in dogs and cats, there is not necessarily an association between increased levels of urobilinogen and hepatobiliary disease or hemolysis. Therefore, the urobilinogen pad is not diagnostically useful in veterinary species [6, 11–13].

The nitrite and leukocyte esterase pads are not diagnostically accurate for veterinary species [5, 10, 13].

The nitrite pad aims to detect certain Gram-negative bacteria that convert nitrate to nitrite [6]. These bacteria are commonly implicated in UTIs in people, hence the growing popularity of this test among over-the-counter products that screen people with lower urinary tract signs. However, detection is unpredictable among veterinary patients, even if the bacterial population is abundant [6].

The leukocyte esterase pad tends to produce false positive results for cats and false-negative results for dogs [3, 6]. Evaluating urine sediment is therefore a more appropriate method by which to accurately identify leukocytes in veterinary patients. See Chapter 15 for additional details.

14.2 Procedural Purpose: Why Should I Perform This Test?

Urine is an aqueous solution. Ninety-five percent of urine is water; however, knowledge of the chemical composition of its remaining 5% is essential because this recipe reflects the body's water and electrolyte balance and renal tubular function. In order of decreasing concentration, urine contains:

- urea
- chloride
- sodium
- potassium
- creatinine
- other
  - dissolved ions
  - inorganic compounds
  - organic compounds (e.g. glucose)
  - proteins
  - hormones
  - metabolites.

The presence/absence of these constituents and the relative abundance of each have implications for patient health. Being able to qualitatively and/or quantitatively identify chemical features of a urine sample contributes essential data to the diagnostic process. An understanding of chemical features of the urine can also facilitate case management by monitoring how a disease progresses and/or how the patient is responding to therapy.

14.3 Equipment

Examination of the chemical properties of a urine sample requires:

- exam gloves for handling biofluids
- a fresh sample of urine within a clean, clear collection container
- Multistix® or a comparable brand of multiple-test reagent strip
- timer to measure the color change according to the timetable outlined by the manufacturer. Note that many test pads require interpretation at different times, so you will have to use the timer more than once
- pipette (if pipetting the sample onto each test pad of the dipstick)
- paper towel to absorb spillage (if pipetting the sample onto each test pad of the dipstick) or comparable lab bench absorbent pad
- test chart provided by the manufacturer of the multiple-test reagent strip *or* an automated dipstick reader.

14.4 Procedural Steps

1) Collect urine sample.
2) Gather supplies (see Figure 14.4).
   a) Remove only one test strip from the bottle and replace the cap (see Figure 14.5).
   b) Avoid touching the test pads with your fingers.
3) Apply urine to the dipstick test pads in one of two ways [3]:
   a) Immersion method (see Figure 14.6):
      Start this process with urine in a collection container (e.g. a clear, conical centrifuge tube). This allows you to submerge the entire test strip in urine at once.
      After complete, but brief immersion, remove the dipstick.
      Tap the dipstick against the urine collection container or on an absorbent pad to remove excess urine (see Figure 14.7).
      Start the clock.
      Hold the strip against the test chart to manually read results.
      The manufacturer will provide recommendations concerning the timetable for reading results.

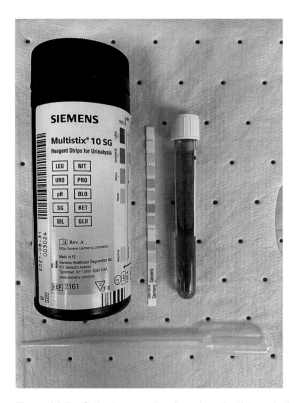

Figure 14.4 Gathering supplies for urine dipstick analysis. Courtesy of Jeremy Bessett, Inaugural Class of 2023, University of Arizona College of Veterinary Medicine. *Source:* Courtesy of Jeremy Bessett, Inaugural Class of 2023, University of Arizona College of Veterinary Medicine.

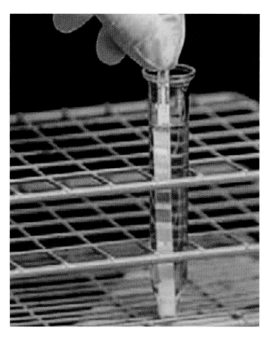

Figure 14.6 Immersing the dipstick within the patient's urine sample so as to saturate all reagent pads simultaneously. *Source:* Courtesy of Ryane E. Englar, DVM, DABVP (Canine and Feline Practice).

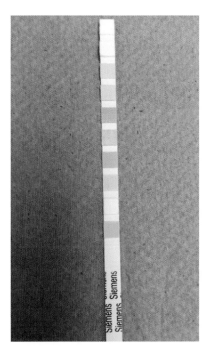

Figure 14.5 One individual Multistix® test strip. *Source:* Courtesy of Ryane E. Englar, DVM, DABVP (Canine and Feline Practice).

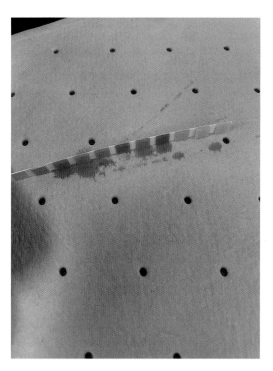

Figure 14.7 Removing excess sample from the reagent test pads immediately following immersion. *Source:* Courtesy of Jeremy Bessett, Inaugural Class of 2023, University of Arizona College of Veterinary Medicine.

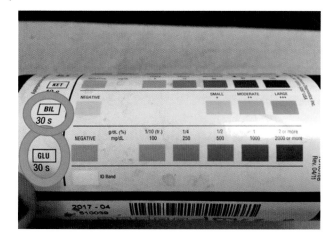

Figure 14.8 The label of the product contains the recommended times to read each reagent pad. This photograph displays the recommended time to report out the results for both glucose and bilirubin. *Source:* Courtesy of Ryane E. Englar, DVM, DABVP (Canine and Feline Practice).

Read each pad at the time shown on the label, beginning with the shortest time. For example, Multistix® reports the following schedule for manual interpretation of test pad color changes (see Figure 14.8):

- o glucose – 30 seconds
- o bilirubin – 30 seconds
- o ketones – 40 seconds
- o occult blood (heme) – 60 seconds
- o pH – 60 seconds
- o protein – 60 seconds.

Manually compare the color on your strip for each individual test pad to the corresponding row of color blocks on the test chart (see Figures 14.9 and 14.10).

See which color on the test chart is the closest match to the color on your strip (see Figures 14.11–14.14).

Document each result in the patient's medical record.

Sometimes a test pad produces an erroneous result: the color of the test pad does not match up against the test chart. In this case, it is reasonable to question the accuracy of the results and retest the urine sample using a new dipstick (see Figure 14.15).

b) Pipetting method [3, 4]:

Place a paper towel or a lab bench absorbent pad on the countertop where you will be performing chemical evaluation of the urine.

Lay a dipstick on top of the paper towel or absorbent pad.

Using a pipette, place one drop of urine on each pad of the dipstick (see Figures 14.16–14.18).

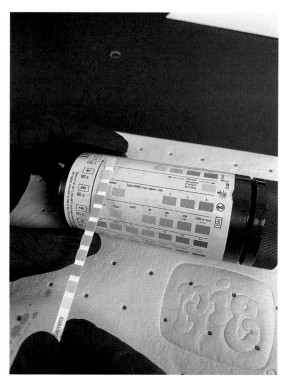

Figure 14.9 Manually reading the urine dipstick. *Source:* Courtesy of Jeremy Bessett, Inaugural Class of 2023, University of Arizona College of Veterinary Medicine.

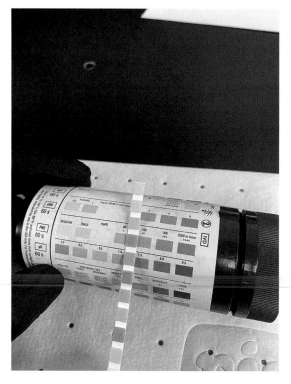

Figure 14.10 Manually reading the urine dipstick. *Source:* Courtesy of Jeremy Bessett, Inaugural Class of 2023, University of Arizona College of Veterinary Medicine.

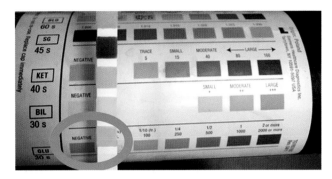

Figure 14.11 This photograph demonstrates how you would read the test pad for glucose. This patient's sample is negative for glucosuria. *Source:* Courtesy of Ryane E. Englar, DVM, DABVP (Canine and Feline Practice).

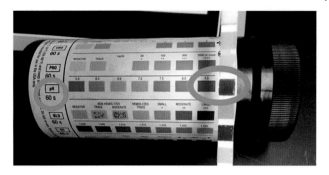

Figure 14.14 This photograph demonstrates how you would read the test pad for urine pH. This patient has alkalinuria. *Source:* Courtesy of Ryane E. Englar, DVM, DABVP (Canine and Feline Practice).

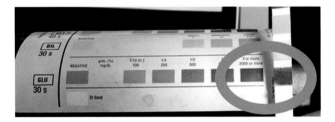

Figure 14.12 This photograph demonstrates how you would read the test pad for glucose. This patient's sample is positive for glucosuria. *Source:* Courtesy of Ryane E. Englar, DVM, DABVP (Canine and Feline Practice).

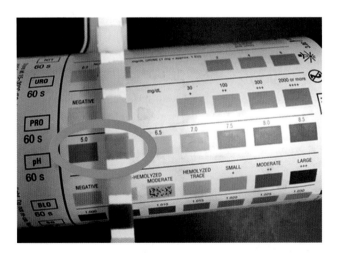

Figure 14.13 This photograph demonstrates how you would read the test pad for urine pH. This patient has aciduria. *Source:* Courtesy of Ryane E. Englar, DVM, DABVP (Canine and Feline Practice).

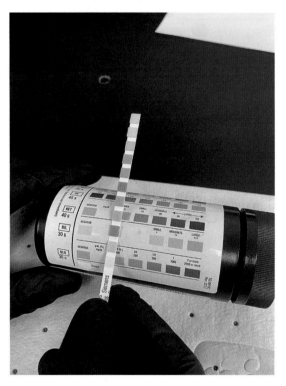

Figure 14.15 Manually reading the urine dipstick. Note that the bilirubin test pad has produced a vibrant orange color. This is not a viable option if we compare the test pad color against the test chart. In this case, we need to consider retesting the sample to get a valid result concerning the presence or absence of bilirubinuria. *Source:* Courtesy of Jeremy Bessett, Inaugural Class of 2023, University of Arizona College of Veterinary Medicine.

Allow each droplet to fully coat the test pad.

Tap the dipstick against the urine collection container or on the paper towel or absorbent pad to remove excess urine.

Start the clock.

Hold the strip against the test chart to manually read results.

The manufacturer will provide recommendations concerning the timetable for reading results.

Read each pad at the time shown on the label, beginning with the shortest time.

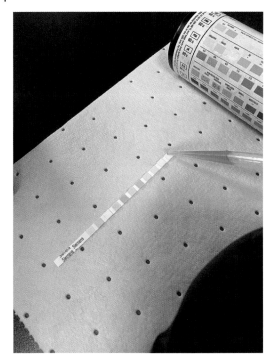

Figure 14.16 Pipetting urine droplets onto each test pad. *Source:* Courtesy of Jeremy Bessett, Inaugural Class of 2023, University of Arizona College of Veterinary Medicine.

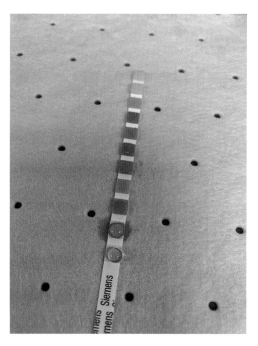

Figure 14.18 Close-up of test strip after urine has been applied to all reagent pads. *Source:* Courtesy of Jeremy Bessett, Inaugural Class of 2023, University of Arizona College of Veterinary Medicine.

Manually compare the color on your strip for each individual test pad to the corresponding row of color blocks on the test chart.

See which color on the test chart is the closest match to the color on your strip.

Document each result in the patient's medical record.

Sometimes a test pad produces an erroneous result: the color of the test pad does not match up against the test chart. In this case, it is reasonable to question the accuracy of the results and consider retesting the urine sample using a new dipstick.

14.5 Time Estimate to Perform Test

Less than five minutes.

14.6 Procedural Tips and Troubleshooting

14.6.1 Regarding the Urine Sample

- The sample should ideally be fresh and sealed, meaning that the lid of the urine collection container is closed (while the urine sample is awaiting analysis) to prevent evaporation of ketones [3].

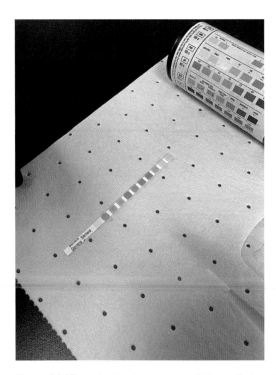

Figure 14.17 Urine has been successfully applied to all reagent test pads. *Source:* Courtesy of Jeremy Bessett, Inaugural Class of 2023, University of Arizona College of Veterinary Medicine.

- If the sample had to be refrigerated due to delays in processing, allow the sample to warm to room temperature before performing chemical evaluation of the urine [3].
- If the sample is turbid, centrifuge the urine prior to chemical analysis [1]. Apply the resulting supernatant to the test pads so that turbidity does not influence the color change on test pads [1, 12].
- If the sample is heavily pigmented, centrifuge the urine prior to chemical analysis [1, 2]. Apply the resulting supernatant to the test pads so that pigmenturia does not influence the color change on test pads [1].

14.6.2 Regarding the Test Strips

- Test strip containers should be sealed to prevent prolonged exposure of the dipsticks to room air [12]. The glucose and occult blood (heme) pads are particularly sensitive to oxidation [3].
- Test strip containers should be sealed to prevent prolonged exposure of the dipsticks to light [3]. The glucose and occult blood (heme) pads are particularly sensitive to oxidation [3].
- Test strip containers should not be exposed to moisture [1]. Maintain supplies in a cool, dry place [12].
- Visually examine the test strip before use. If the strip has test pads that are discolored or darkened prior to use, then avoid using that strip.
- Check expiration dates of test strips. Avoid using expired test strips because accuracy of results is questionable. In particular, the glucose test pad is likely to report false-negative reactions if the dipstick is out-of-date [3] (see Figure 14.19).

- Oil and debris from your fingers may influence the results that are displayed by the test pads. Therefore, do not touch the test pads with your bare fingers.

14.6.3 Regarding the Procedure

- Do not oversaturate test pads with urine. Remove excess urine. Tap the strip against the urine collection container if you are immersing the dipstick in urine. Otherwise, reagent run-off may influence test results from adjacent pads [3].
- The pipetting method avoids reagent run-off as opposed to the immersion method.
- You can reuse the pipette used in the pipetting method to load the stage during refractometry to determine the sample's USG [3].

14.6.4 Regarding Color Change Interpretations

- Do not attempt to interpret color changes on test pads without adequate lighting.
- Be cognizant of any visual acuity barriers or color blindness that may impair detection of color changes [14]. For instance, if you have been diagnosed with deuteranopia, a type of red-green color blindness, it may be difficult for you to accurately interpret the glucose, ketones, occult blood, pH, and protein test pads. In this case, you will want to partner with a colleague for their aid in interpreting or confirming test results, or you may wish to invest in an automated analyzer (see Figures 14.20 and 14.21).
- Make sure that you are reading the dipstick from the correct end. The easiest way to tell which end of the Multistix® test strip contains the glucose test pad is that the glucose test pad appears light blue before use. (Note that a negative result for this test pad will also be light blue.)

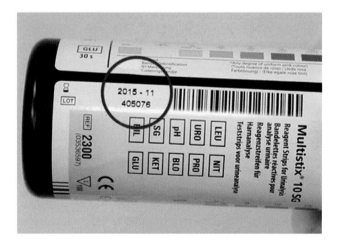

Figure 14.19 Checking the expiration date on a container of urine dipsticks. This container expired in November of 2015. Therefore, the entire container needs to be tossed. Results from these test strips are not guaranteed to be accurate. *Source:* Courtesy of Ryane E. Englar, DVM, DABVP (Canine and Feline Practice).

>	pH	8.0	
>	Urine Protein	30	mg/dL
>	Glucose	neg	
>	Ketones	neg	
>	Blood / Hemoglobin	neg	
>	Bilirubin	neg	

Figure 14.20 Dipstick reading printout from an automated analyzer that evaluated a urine sample from a two-year-old male castrated Poodle dog. *Source:* Courtesy of Ryane E. Englar, DVM, DABVP (Canine and Feline Practice).

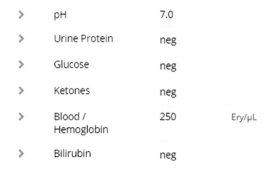

➤	pH	7.0	
➤	Urine Protein	neg	
➤	Glucose	neg	
➤	Ketones	neg	
➤	Blood / Hemoglobin	250	Ery/μL
➤	Bilirubin	neg	

Figure 14.21 Dipstick reading printout from an automated analyzer that evaluated a urine sample from a four-year-old male castrated Ragdoll cat. The positive finding of microscopic hematuria in this case was believed to be iatrogenic, secondary to cystocentesis. *Source:* Courtesy of Ryane E. Englar, DVM, DABVP (Canine and Feline Practice).

- Begin your manual interpretation of the dipstick from the end that contains the glucose test pad. This end contains the test pads with the shortest time elapses. By starting here, you can simply read up the strip and in this way, keep pace with the timetable outlined by the manufacturers. For instance, for the Multistix® test strip, you will read glucose and bilirubin first, followed by ketones, then occult blood (heme), pH, and protein.

14.7 Interpreting Test Results

Each test pad will be interpreted individually by comparing its color change to the corresponding row of color blocks on the test chart that appears on the bottle's label.

For all test pads except pH, no color change implies that the result is negative [4].

14.7.1 For Glucose

The renal threshold for glucose is >180 mg/dl in most species and 260–310 mg/dl in cats [1, 5]. In health, because the patient's blood glucose level does not exceed the renal threshold, all filtered glucose is reabsorbed in the proximal renal tubules [1].

If the patient's blood glucose level does exceed the renal threshold, then glucosuria will result [1].

When glucose in a urine sample touches the test pad, it reacts with glucose oxidase–peroxidase [1, 6]. This causes a change from blue to green to brown depending upon the quantity of glucose within the sample. Samples that contain 250 mg/dl of glucose will change the test pad from green to blue; samples that contain 500–1000 mg/dl of glucose will change the test pad to a green-brown; samples

that contain greater than or equal to 2000 mg/dl of glucose will change the test pad to a medium brown.

Glucosuria can result from [1, 2, 13]:

- intravenous fluid therapy that is spiked with dextrose
- stress hyperglycemia, particularly in feline patients
- diabetes mellitus
- pituitary pars intermedia dysfunction in horses [15]
- excessive endogenous glucocorticoids, as from hyperadrenocorticism
- excessive exogenous glucocorticoids
- proximal renal tubular defect
  - ○ Fanconi syndrome
    - more commonly seen in Basenjis
  - ○ primary renal glucosuria
- tubular injury secondary to acute kidney injury (AKI).

14.7.1.1 Tips Regarding the Glucose Test Pad

- Some test pads for glucose require you to apply urine to the side of the test pad rather than the top [6]. This means that to obtain an accurate result for the glucose test pad, you may have to adjust how you apply urine to the test pad with your dropper or pipette.
- Pigmenturia will impact accuracy of test results [6].
- A false-negative result may occur if the urine that is used to test for glucose is cold [6].
- A false-negative result may also occur if the urine contains high concentrations of ascorbic acid (vitamin C), ketones, and/or pronounced bilirubin [1, 6].
- Contamination of the urine sample with hydrogen peroxide, chlorine, or bleach may cause a false positive result [1, 6].
- A false positive may also result in canine patients that are receiving cephalexin and/or enrofloxacin [16].

14.7.2 Bilirubin

Bilirubin is a byproduct of the degradation of hemoglobin [1]. Specifically, the heme portion of hemoglobin is converted to bilirubin [1]. Within the liver, bilirubin is conjugated [1]. Some of it is excreted in bile [1]. Some of it is excreted in the urine after filtration at the level of the glomerulus [1].

In addition to this metabolic pathway, the canine kidney can also produce bilirubin from hemoglobin [5]. Therefore, we are more likely to see bilirubinuria in small amounts in the healthy canine patient whereas the presence of bilirubin in the urine of a feline patient typically is suggestive of underlying pathology [5].

When bilirubin in a urine sample touches the test pad, it reacts with a diazonium salt [6]. This produces a color change from beige to variations of a muddy light brown.

It can be normal to see some bilirubin in canine urine, particularly if the urine is concentrated [13].

However, bilirubinuria may be indicative of [1, 2, 13]:

- hemolysis
- hepatopathy
- extrahepatic biliary obstruction
- fever
- starvation.

14.7.2.1 Tips Regarding the Bilirubin Test Pad

- When urine is left at room temperature or exposed to light for an extended period, any bilirubin that is contained within will convert into biliverdin [12]. The bilirubin test pad cannot detect biliverdin [6]. The presence of biliverdin will produce a false negative.
- A false-negative result may also result from urine that contains ascorbic acid [6].
- A false positive may result if patients are being treated with synthetic blood products, such as Oxyglobin®, rifampin, and some sulfa drugs [12].

14.7.3 Ketones

Ketones are a byproduct of fatty acid metabolism [1]. There are three types of ketones of clinical significance [1]:

- acetone
- acetoacetic acid
- beta-hydroxybutyrate (β-hydroxybutyrate).

The ketone test pad *cannot* detect β-hydroxybutyrate.

The ketone test pad detects primarily acetoacetate and some acetone. A positive result is signified by a color change from a rosy beige to rose, deep rose, and ultimately, burgundy maroon.

Ketonuria signifies that the patient is in a state of negative energy balance that is causing production of excess ketones as from [1, 2, 13]:

- diabetic ketoacidosis (DKA)
- primary ketosis in ruminants
- consumption of low-carbohydrate, high-fat diets
- prolonged fasting or starvation in immature patients
- glycogen storage disease.

14.7.3.1 Tips Regarding the Ketone Test Pad

- Heat, light, and moisture will impair accuracy of test results for the ketone test pad [6]. Storage of test strips in accordance with manufacturer recommendations is paramount to the accuracy of the diagnosis.

- The ketone test pad cannot detect β-hydroxybutyric acid [6]. This means that a handful of ketotic patients will test negative for ketones using this test pad [5].
- Pigmenturia will impact accuracy of test results [6].

14.7.4 Occult Blood (Heme)

The source of blood in hematuria can originate from anywhere within the urogenital tract [17]:

- nonrenal disease
  - ureter
    - E.g. ureterolith
  - urinary bladder
    - E.g. cystitis, urolithiasis, bladder tumor
  - prostate
    - E.g. prostatitis
  - urethra
- renal disease
  - cystic disease
  - glomerulonephropathy
  - nephroliths
  - pyelonephritis
  - renal tumors.

In addition, hematuria can be iatrogenic, as from cystocentesis or urethral catheterization.

When blood in a urine sample touches the test pad, its heme group (porphyrin ring plus iron) reacts with peroxidase [6]. Hemoglobin, methemoglobin, and myoglobin will produce positive results [1, 6]. A positive result is signified by a color change from mustardy-yellow to yellow with green speckling to lime-green to green to dark green.

The most common explanation for a positive result in clinical practice is the presence of erythrocytes (RBCs) in urine [13]. This could be due to the method of collection (e.g. cystocentesis) or underlying pathology [13].

Hemoglobinuria may result from [2]:

- heatstroke
- immune-mediated hemolytic anemia (IMHA)
- disseminated intravascular coagulation (DIC)
- severe hypophosphatemia
- splenic torsion
- transfusion reaction
- zinc toxicosis
- rare deficiencies in RBC enzymes (e.g. phosphofructokinase, pyruvate kinase).

Myoglobinuria results from severe rhabdomyolysis, as from [2]:

- heatstroke
- high-intensity exertion (e.g. racing greyhound or horse)
- vehicular crushing injury (e.g. hit-by-car dog)

- protracted state of status epilepticus
- severe hypokalemia (primarily cats).

14.7.4.1 Tips Regarding the Occult Blood (Heme) Test Pad

- If the urine sample is a "free catch" and becomes contaminated with flea feces, then it is possible to see a false positive result on the occult blood (heme) test [2].
- A false positive test result is possible if the urine sample is contaminated by semen or seminal fluid [18].

14.7.5 pH

The reportable range of pH by Multistix® dipsticks is 5.0–8.5.

- Samples that are acidic produce a color change of orange (pH 5.0) to yellow (pH 6.5).
- Samples that have a neutral pH (7.0) produce a color change of light yellow-green.
- Samples that are alkaline produce a color change of green (pH 8.0) to Caribbean blue (pH 8.5).

The pH of urine is affected by the following factors [2, 13]:

- diet
  - A meat-based diet is associated with acidic urine. Therefore, urine is typically acidic among carnivores.
  - An exception occurs immediately after eating.
  - Increased secretion of hydrochloric acid (HCl) into the stomach triggers a postprandial alkaline tide. The body produces alkaline urine in response to a meal to buffer gastric acid secretion [19].
  - This causes transient alkalinity of the urine.
  - A plant-based diet is associated with alkaline urine. Therefore, urine is typically alkaline among grazing animals.
  - Urine pH reportedly ranges from 7.0 to 8.7 in dairy and beef cows [20].
  - Urine pH of most horses in health ranges from 7.5 to 8.5 [15].
  - When horses consume large amounts of grain or sweet feed in their diet, urine pH decreases to a range of somewhere between 6 and 7.5 [15].
  - Young herbivores that are receiving milk as a large part of their diet tend to have acidic urine.
- freshness of urine sample
  - Older samples have a slightly higher pH due to loss of carbon dioxide in the air.
- presence/absence of urease-positive bacteria
  - *Streptococcus*, *Ureaplasma*, and *Proteus* spp. can form ammonia from urea.
  - Ammonia raises urine pH, making urine that contains urease-positive bacteria more alkaline.

- medications [1, 2]
  - Ammonium chloride and DL-methionine are prescribed to acidify urine. Therefore, patients that are receiving these medications should produce acidic urine.
  - Furosemide therapy has been linked to aciduria [19].
  - Potassium citrate is prescribed as an alkalinizing agent. Therefore, patients that are receiving this medication should produce alkaline urine.
- acid–base balance [2]
  - Metabolic acidosis and respiratory acidosis are associated with acidic urine.
  - Metabolic alkalosis and respiratory alkalosis are associated with alkaline urine.
- catabolism [2]
  - Catabolic states, such as starvation, are associated with acidic urine.

The pH of urine is important because it may promote the formation of certain types of uroliths [6]. For instance, struvites prefer alkaline urine. Therefore, canine and feline patients that chronically produce alkaline urine may be at increased risk of struvite urolithiasis. On the other hand, cystine crystals preferentially form in acidic urine [1]. Patients with acidic urine may be at greater risk for formation of cystine uroliths.

The pH of urine is equally important from the monitoring aspect of case management. Let's say that we have a patient with a history of struvite urolithiasis and that we have taken measures to acidify the patient's urine. Measuring the pH of that patient's urine sample repeatedly over time can help us see if we are on the right track. In other words, are our adjustments to the patient's diet and/or medication(s) effective?

14.7.5.1 Tips Regarding the pH Test Pad

- Urine pH may be overestimated by the pH test pad in dogs [5].
- Run-off of the reagent from the adjacent protein test pad may result in an inaccurately low pH [6].
- Pigmenturia will impact accuracy of test results [6].

14.7.6 Protein

Most of the protein that is filtered through the glomerulus is effectively reabsorbed by the proximal renal tubular epithelial cells [19]. Therefore, dipstick analysis of urine from healthy patients typically contains little to no detectable protein [19].

When a urine sample that contains protein touches the test pad, it reacts with tetrabromophenol blue [1, 6]. Negatively charged proteins will bind to the pad [6]. This produces a color change from a light yellow-green to a muddy green to a forest green.

The reagent pad more readily detects albumin than globulin [19].

Some types of protein go undetected altogether [19]. These include so-called Bence–Jones proteins, which are free immunoglobulin light chains [19].

Proteinuria is typically categorized as being present in trace amounts, +1 (30 mg/dl), ++ (100 mg/dl), +++ (300 mg/dl), or ++++ (2000 mg/dl or greater).

Small amounts of albumin may appear in the urine of healthy dogs and cats [13]. Highly concentrated urine magnifies this [2]. An estimate of 100 mg/dl (++) for protein in the urine in a sample that exceeds 1.060 for USG is *not* considered pathological [2].

When proteinuria does occur, it may be prerenal, renal, or post-renal s [1].

Prerenal proteinuria results from large concentrations of small proteins in plasma that overwhelm the glomerulus. Because these proteins are small, they are readily filtered by the glomerulus. If present in plasma in high concentrations, they will also appear in the glomerular filtrate in high concentrations. Because they are abundant, not all will be resorbed by renal tubules. The excess will be excreted in urine.

Prerenal proteinuria may be due to [1, 21]:

- dehydration
- excitement
- fever
- strenuous exercise
- stress.

Other causes of prerenal proteinuria are [13, 19]:

- colostral ingestion, due to abundant circulating antibodies
- inflammation, due to the release of acute phase proteins
- intravascular hemolysis, due to hemoglobinuria
- severe rhabdomyolysis, due to myoglobinuria.

Multiple myeloma also causes prerenal proteinuria; however, because Bence–Jones proteins are not detected by the protein test pad, these patients will have a false-negative test.

Renal proteinuria may be caused by [1, 13, 19]:

- ○ glomerular disease
  - ○ renal amyloidosis
  - ○ glomerulonephritis
- ○ proximal tubular disease
  - ○ Fanconi syndrome
  - ○ renal ischemia
  - ○ nephrotoxins

- ○ aminoglycosides (e.g. gentamicin, amikacin)
- ○ both glomerular and proximal tubular disease.

Proteinuria may also stem from postrenal causes, including, but not limited to [1, 13, 19]:

- urinary tract infection (UTI), inflammation, and/or hemorrhage
- reproductive tract inflammation and/or hemorrhage
- blood contamination secondary to urine collection method (e.g. cystocentesis).

14.7.6.1 Tips Regarding the Protein Test Pad

- Pigmenturia will impact accuracy of test results [6].
- The protein test pad is more likely to detect albumin than globulin [6].
- Prolonged exposure of urine to the protein test pad (e.g. beyond that which is recommended by the manufacturer of the test strip) can cause a false positive for proteinuria.
- A pH of 8.0 or greater may produce a false positive result indicating some degree of proteinuria [13].
- A false positive test result is possible if the urine sample is contaminated by semen or seminal fluid [18].
- This test pad does not detect Bence–Jones proteins [6]. Patients with Bence–Jones proteins, namely those with multiple myeloma, will have a false-negative test result.

14.8 Clinical Case Example(s)

A 10-year-old spayed female mixed breed dog presented for evaluation of a two-day history of dysuria and pollakiuria. Other than palpating a small, tense urinary bladder on abdominal palpation, physical examination was unremarkable. A urine sample was obtained by cystocentesis. The urine was peach in color, turbid, and had a foul odor. After centrifugation, the supernatant was used for urine dipstick analysis. The test pad for pH disclosed a test result of 8.0. The owner confirmed that the patient last ate over four hours ago; therefore, the elevation in urine pH cannot be explained by postprandial alkaline tide. The patient's history in combination with alkalinuria and abnormal urine color, turbidity, and odor raised suspicion of UTI. Subsequent examination of the urine sediment disclosed pyuria, hematuria, crystalluria (struvites), and cocci. Urine was submitted for culture and susceptibility testing. The urine culture was positive for *Staphylococcus* spp. Recall that urease-producing bacteria produce ammonia, which increases the urine pH. Urine alkalinity promotes struvite crystal formation. The patient was prescribed a seven-day course of antibiotics based on the culture and susceptibility results.

Urinalysis was repeated the day after cessation of antibiotic therapy. At the recheck appointment, the owner shared that the patient's urinary signs had resolved by the third morning of antibiotic therapy. The urinalysis that was performed at this recheck visit disclosed clear, yellow urine. Sediment was inactive, and the urine pH was 6.5.

14.9 Add-On Tests That You May Need to Consider and Their Additive Value

Evaluation of the chemical features of urine is a vital diagnostic tool; however, it is just one of many components of the urinalysis. In addition to considering urine pH, protein, glucose, ketones, occult blood (heme), and bilirubin, we must also explore the physical properties of urine (e.g. volume, color, turbidity, odor), including USG. Collective results from a comprehensive urinalysis can then be compared with the patient history and physical exam findings to determine what, if any abnormalities, align and what those abnormalities require in terms of further investigation. Sometimes that investigation is merely a commitment to recheck urinalysis at predetermined intervals to establish if one or more chemical features (e.g. proteinuria) is increasing in significance. On other occasions, that investigation may require blood tests (e.g. complete blood count and/or chemistry profile) or diagnostic imaging (e.g. abdominal radiographs or ultrasonography).

14.9.1 Improving the Accuracy of Data Concerning the Sample's Glucose

It is not possible to differentiate the cause of glucosuria using dipstick analysis. Feline patients are prone to stress hyperglycemia; therefore, it is difficult to determine if glucosuria is secondary to stress or secondary to true pathology [1, 2, 13]. In cases where diabetes mellitus is suspected, it may be advisable to perform a serum fructosamine test. This test reflects the patient's blood glucose over an extended period [5]. A clinically healthy patient that is stressed in the clinic during urine collection and has resultant glucosuria should have a normal fructosamine test as compared with a patient with diabetes mellitus, whose fructosamine test results will be elevated [5].

14.9.2 Improving the Accuracy of Data Concerning the Presence or Absence of Ketones

The ketone test pad cannot detect β-hydroxybutyric acid [6]. Those patients that are ketotic secondary to β-hydroxybutyric acid will test negative for ketones using the Multistix® or

equivalent dipstick [5]. If you suspect that the patient is ketotic but the result on the Multistix® is negative, then add a few drops of hydrogen peroxide (H_2O_2) to the urine sample [5]. This addition will convert β-hydroxybutyric acid to acetoacetate, which is detectable [5]. Then repeat the dipstick analysis. This specific subset of patients will test positive now that their sample contains ketones that are detectable by the reagent pad.

14.9.3 Distinguishing Hematuria, Hemoglobinuria, and Myoglobinuria if the Occult Blood (Heme) Tests Positive

The occult blood test will test positive in the presence of hemoglobin, methemoglobin, myoglobin, and, to a lesser extent, erythrocytes [1, 6]. Once you have a positive test, you need to determine which substance triggered the test to test positive. Start by examining the urine sediment for evidence of erythrocytes [5]. If these are present on urine sediment analysis (see Chapter 15), then the patient has microscopic hematuria [5]. The same is true if ghost cells are present on urine sediment analysis [5]. In the absence of erythrocytes on sediment analysis, the patient either has hemoglobinuria or myoglobinuria [5].

To distinguish hemoglobinuria from myoglobinuria, take a blood sample from the patient and spin it down to examine the patient's plasma [1]. When hemoglobinuria is due to intravascular hemolysis, the patient's plasma will appear pink to red [1]. Myoglobin, on the other hand, is cleared rapidly from plasma, therefore the plasma of patients with myoglobinuria is clear [1].

14.9.4 Improving the Accuracy of Data Concerning the Sample's pH

Accuracy of the pH test pad reading is said to fall within $+/- 0.5$ pH units [1]. This means that the actual urine pH may fall between 6.0 and 7.0 if the test pad produces a reading of 6.5 [1]. That being said, there is immense variability in results from reading the pH test pad more so than any other [22]. If accuracy is critical to the diagnostic process, then pH should be determined by a pH meter. This will improve accuracy of the test result, particularly for canine urine [5, 23].

14.9.5 Improving the Accuracy of Data Concerning Proteinuria

If proteinuria is present based upon dipstick analysis, the next step is to examine the urine sediment for evidence of post-renal inflammation, hemorrhage, and/or infection [1].

If present, as in the case of UTI, the patient should be treated for the underlying issue. Appropriate medical intervention should eliminate proteinuria on follow-up exam, assuming that the underlying issue is resolved with treatment.

If, on the other hand, the sediment is inactive, then post-renal causes of proteinuria are unlikely. In this case, it is important to consider how much protein is being lost in the urine and from where [1]. This requires advanced testing, most typically in the form of the protein–creatinine ratio [1, 24]. This test is not usually performed in-house; a urine sample is sent to an outside diagnostic lab for analysis. The diagnostic lab will divide the urine protein concentration (UP) by the urine creatinine concentration (UC) [1]. This ratio (UP : UC) estimates the quantity of protein that is being lost in the urine [1, 24]. The result helps to determine whether the patient's proteinuria is significant [1] and whether the proteinuria is glomerular or tubular in origin [24]. High UP : UC (greater than 2.0–2.5) points toward a glomerular source of proteinuria [5, 24].

The urine protein–creatinine ratio is usually <0.5 in healthy dogs [24]. Non-azotemic dogs that have a UP : UC between 0.5 and 1.0 are borderline and should be monitored for progressive proteinuria [24]. A UP : UC greater than 1.0 is abnormal in a non-azotemic dog and will require further investigation [24].

Feline patients track similarly; however, it is important to note that UP : UC of some healthy male cats may reach 0.6 [24].

14.10 Key Takeaways

- Perform dipstick analysis on fresh samples, within 30 minutes of sample collection. When sample processing is delayed, preserve the sample by refrigerating it.
- Prior to performing dipstick analysis on a refrigerated sample, allow the urine to warm to room temperature. This will reduce the number of inaccurate results.
- Prior to performing dipstick analysis on any sample, mix the urine well. This will ensure that you are testing a representative sample. Failure to mix urine is a commonly observed technique error [14].
- Dipsticks are sensitive to room air, light, heat, and moisture. Only take what you need from the dipstick container and recap the container tightly to preserve the integrity of the testing strips for future use.
- Avoid touching the dipstick test pads with your bare fingertips. Doing so can lead to inaccurate results.
- Always check the expiration date of your dipsticks! Expired dipsticks are not guaranteed to produce accurate results.

- Turbidity and pigmenturia will impact accuracy of test results [6]. Centrifuge heavily pigmented and/or turbid urine prior to dipstick analysis; use the supernatant for analysis.
- More urine is not always better! Remove excess urine from the dipsticks after soaking the test pads to avoid reagent run-off. Run-off from one test pad can contaminate another, influencing color change with unintended consequences.
- Read the test strip according to the timetable that is outlined in the manufacturer's instructions. Reading a test pad prematurely can alter test results. Failure to time readings is a commonly observed technique error [14].
- Always consider method of urine collection when there is macroscopic hematuria and/or when the occult blood (heme) test pad yields a positive result. Iatrogenic hematuria may result from cystocentesis and/or urethral catheterization [12]. If this is the case, then bleeding is minimal. The urine sediment should reflect no more than 10–20 erythrocytes (RBCs) per high powered field (HPF) [12].
- If hematuria is present in both a free-catch sample and a sample obtained by cystocentesis, then you need to consider one or more of the following sites to be your source [25]:
  - kidneys
  - ureters
  - urinary bladder
  - proximal urethra
  - prostate gland.
- If hematuria is present in a free-catch sample, but not in a sample from the same patient that was obtained by cystocentesis, then the source of bleeding is distal to the urinary bladder [12]. This means that you should consider the distal urogenital tract to be the source of the frank blood [25]:
  - vagina
  - distal urethra
  - penis.
- Dipstick test results provide vital information to the diagnostic work-up of any patient; however, they are not intended to be standalone. Always perform urine dipstick analysis as part of a comprehensive urinalysis. This requires evaluation of urine's physical properties (e.g. volume, color, turbidity, odor), including USG and examination of the urine sediment. Sediment is particularly essential when it comes to detection of pyuria [8]. The leukocyte esterase pad on dipsticks for routine urinalysis is nonspecific and cannot replace the sediment [8].

- Manual dipstick analysis may suffer from poor technique, poor reading of the results, or both [26].
- Automated readers improve precision of dipstick analysis [14]. However, lack of sample mixing remains a commonly observed technique error for automated readers [14].

14.11 Clinical Pearls

14.11.1 Regarding Glucosuria

- Read the instructions that come with the dipsticks in your clinic. If you do, you will find that Multistix®, Diastix®, and Petstix® absorb urine from the side of the pad rather than from the top. You will get a false negative for glucose if you only apply droplets of urine to the top of the reagent pad.
- Many countertop and cage cleaners contain hydrogen peroxide, bleach, and/or chlorine [12]. These can cause the glucose test pad to test positive [12]. Therefore, be cautious of positive test results for glucose when countertop and bottom-of-the-cage urine samples are used for analysis [12]. These results are likely to be spurious.

14.11.2 Regarding Bilirubinuria

- It is normal to see some bilirubin in canine urine, particularly if the urine is concentrated [13].
- Male dogs excrete more bilirubin than females [12].
- Neutered male dogs excrete less bilirubin than intact male dogs [12].
- Puppies excrete little bilirubin, if any, in their urine [12].
- Feline kidneys cannot conjugate bilirubin, which means that any degree of bilirubinuria in cats requires investigation [12].
  The feline renal threshold for the excretion of bilirubin is significantly higher in cats than dogs [5, 27]. To be exact, it is nine times higher [5, 27]. This means that you are able to detect bilirubinuria in cats before you see evidence of icterus on the physical exam [5] (see Figure 14.22).

14.11.3 Regarding the Impact of Urine pH on the Sediment

- Cells and casts tend to break down in alkaline urine (pH >8.0). Therefore, the urine sediment may appear relatively quiet in the presence of alkalinuria when in fact erythrocytes and leukocytes may be present [13]. Do not rule out inflammation and/or infection if the urine pH is 8.0 and the sediment looks unremarkable.

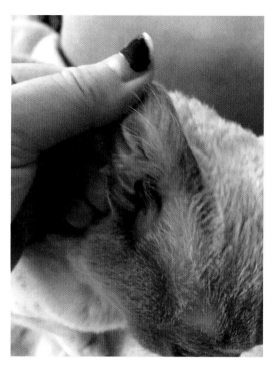

Figure 14.22 Peri-aural icterus in a feline patient with underlying hepatopathy. *Source:* Courtesy of Ryane E. Englar, DVM, DABVP (Canine and Feline Practice).

- Crystalluria does not guarantee the presence of urolithiasis. Crystals merely precipitate in supersaturated urine. Their precipitation is highly dependent upon urine pH:
  - alkaline urine promotes the precipitation of struvite crystals [13]
  - acidic urine promotes the precipitation of cystine crystals [1].

14.11.4 Proteinuria

- The UP : UC ratio should be assessed in dogs with a dipstick test result of +1 for proteinuria if USG is less than or equal to 1.012 [28].
- Dogs that have a dipstick test result of +1 for proteinuria and a USG that exceeds 1.012 are unlikely to be proteinuric [28].

14.11.5 Other

- Dipsticks are inaccurate when it comes to measuring USG. Invest in a refractometer [11].
- If you need to know the exact pH of a urine sample, invest in a pH meter [11]. The test pad for pH gets you in the right ballpark but pH determination by dipstick is error-prone.

References

1 Callens, A.J. and Bartges, J.W. (2015). Urinalysis. *The Veterinary Clinics of North America. Small Animal Practice* 45 (4): 621–637.

2 Chew, D.J., DiBartola, S.P., and Schenck, P.A. (2011). Urinalysis. In: *Canine and Feline Nephrology and Urology*, 2e (ed. D.J. Chew, S.P. DiBartola, P.A. Schenck and D.J. Chew), 1–31. St. Louis, MO: Elsevier/Saunders.

3 Reppas, G. and Foster, S.F. (2016). Practical urinalysis in the cat: 1: urine macroscopic examination 'tips and traps'. *Journal of Feline Medicine and Surgery* 18 (3): 190–202.

4 Rizzi, T.E. (2014). Urinalysis in companion animals – part 2: evaluation of Urine Chemistry & Sediment. *Today's Veterinary Practice* 86–91.

5 Polzin, D.J. and Osborne, C.A. (2012). Urinalysis in acutely and critically ill dogs and cats. In: *Advanced Monitoring and Procedures for Small Animal Emergency and Critical Care* (ed. J.M. Burkitt Creedon and H. Davis), 409–420. Chichester, West Sussex: Wiley Blackwell.

6 Grauer, G.F. and Pohlman, L.M. (2016). *Canine and Feline Urinalysis: From Collection to Interpretation*. Zaragoza, Spain: Grupo Asís Biomedia, S.L.

7 Teitler, J.B. (2009). Evaluation of a human on-site urine multidrug test for emergency use with dogs. *Journal of the American Animal Hospital Association* 45 (2): 59–66.

8 Holan, K.M., Kruger, J.M., Gibbons, S.N., and Swenson, C.L. (1997). Clinical evaluation of a leukocyte esterase test-strip for detection of feline pyuria. *Veterinary Clinical Pathology* 26 (3): 126–131.

9 Vail, D.M., Allen, T.A., and Weiser, G. (1986). Applicability of leukocyte esterase test strip in detection of canine pyuria. *Journal of the American Veterinary Medical Association* 189 (11): 1451–1453.

10 Osborne, C.A. and Stevens, J.B. (1999). *Urinalysis: A Clinical Guide to Compassionate Patient Care*. Shawnee Mission, Kansas: Bayer Corporation.

11 Osborne, C.A. (ed.) (2009). *Urine strips: Maximizing the diagnostic value*. FetchDVM dvm360.

12 Pressler, B. (ed.) (2010). Advanced interpretation of the urine dipstick FetchDVM, dvm360.

13 eClinpath (2020). Chemical constituents Ithaca. NY: Cornell University College of Veterinary Medicine. https://eclinpath.com/urinalysis/chemical-constituents.

14 Ferreira, M.D.F., Garcia Arce, M., Handel, I.G. et al. (2018). Urine dipstick precision with standard visual and automated methods within a small animal teaching hospital. *The Veterinary Record* 183 (13): 415.

15 Savage, C.J. (2008). Urinary clinical pathologic findings and glomerular filtration rate in the horse. *The Veterinary Clinics of North America. Equine Practice* 24 (2): 387–404, vii.

16 Rees, C.A. and Boothe, D.M. (2004). Evaluation of the effect of cephalexin and enrofloxacin on clinical laboratory measurements of urine glucose in dogs. *Journal of the American Veterinary Medical Association* 224 (9): 1455–1458.

17 Englar, R.E. (2019). Grossly abnormal urine. In: *Common Clinical Presentations in Dogs and Cats* (ed. R.E. Englar), 821–830. Hoboken, NJ: Wiley Blackwell.

18 Prober, L.G., Johnson, C.A., Olivier, N.B., and Thomas, J.S. (2010). Effect of semen in urine specimens on urine protein concentration determined by means of dipstick analysis. *American Journal of Veterinary Research* 71 (3): 288–292.

19 Piech, T.L. and Wycislo, K.L. (2019). Importance of urinalysis. *The Veterinary Clinics of North America. Small Animal Practice* 49 (2): 233–245.

20 Herman, N., Bourges-Abella, N., Braun, J.P. et al. (2019). Urinalysis and determination of the urine protein-to-creatinine ratio reference interval in healthy cows. *Journal of Veterinary Internal Medicine* 33 (2): 999–1008.

21 Welles, E.G., Whatley, E.M., Hall, A.S., and Wright, J.C. (2006). Comparison of Multistix PRO dipsticks with other biochemical assays for determining urine protein (UP), urine creatinine (UC) and UP:UC ratio in dogs and cats. *Veterinary Clinical Pathology* 35 (1): 31–36.

22 Boag, A.M., Breheny, C., Handel, I., and Gow, A.G. (2019). Evaluation of the effect of urine dip vs urine drip on multi-test strip results. *Veterinary Clinical Pathology* 48 (2): 276–281.

23 Athanasiou, L.V., Katsoulos, P.D., Katsogiannou, E.G. et al. (2018). Comparison between the urine dipstick and the pH-meter to assess urine pH in sheep and dogs. *Veterinary Clinical Pathology* 47 (2): 284–288.

24 eClinpath (2020). Urinalysis Ithaca, NY: Cornell University College of Veterinary Medicine. https://www.vet.cornell.edu/animal-health-diagnostic-center/testing/protocols/urinalysis.

25 Forrester, S.D. (2004). Diagnostic approach to hematuria in dogs and cats. *The Veterinary Clinics of North America. Small Animal Practice* 34 (4): 849–866.

26 Bauer, N., Rettig, S., and Moritz, A. (2008). Evaluation the Clinitek status automated dipstick analysis device for semiquantitative testing of canine urine. *Research in Veterinary Science* 85 (3): 467–472.

27 Wamsley, H. and Allerman, R. (2007). *Complete Urinalysis*, 2e. Gloucester, UK: British Small Animal Association.

28 Zatelli, A., Paltrinieri, S., Nizi, F. et al. (2010). Evaluation of a urine dipstick test for confirmation or exclusion of proteinuria in dogs. *American Journal of Veterinary Research* 71 (2): 235–240.

15

Urine Sediment Examination

Sharon M. Dial

15.1 Procedural Definition: What Is This Test About?

The urine sediment examination identifies and provides a semiquantitative estimate of the number of erythrocytes, leukocytes, urinary casts, crystals, and bacteria present in a standard volume of urine. Urine sediment examination is necessary to fully interpret the urine reagent strip findings and can assist in identifying underlying causes for abnormalities found in a concurrent CBC and chemistry profile. In most cases, urine contains a relatively low concentration of the formed elements (cells, crystals, and casts). As a result, urine is centrifuged to assist in finding and identifying any formed elements that relate to underlying disease processes. A consistent protocol for urine sediment preparation is necessary to make this in-house laboratory test semiquantitative rather than simply qualitative.

15.2 Procedural Purpose: Why Should I Perform This Test?

Urinalysis is a component of the "minimum" database often requested when presented with an ill patient. The complete urinalysis includes gross evaluation of the urine color and turbidity, urine specific gravity, reagent strip chemical reactions, and urine sediment examination. The findings in each of these components are essential in interpreting the others. It may be tempting in some cases to just perform the gross examination and reagent strip chemistry test and forego the sediment examination if no abnormalities are seen. However, this can result in missing a significant number of abnormalities on the sediment examination. Approximately 12% of canine urine samples and 6% of feline urine samples with no abnormalities in gross appearance or chemical analysis will have significant abnormalities in the urine sediment, including abnormal numbers of erythrocytes (hematuria), leukocytes (pyuria), and bacteria (bacteriuria) (Barlough et al., 1981). This is especially true in patients with endocrine disease, such as hyperadrenocorticism, where there is increased susceptibility to bacterial cystitis and inhibition of leukocyte movement into tissues.

Urine sediment examination is essential in the interpretation of the gross appearance of the urine and any increased protein concentration noted on the chemical analysis. Red urine can be the result of hematuria, hemoglobinuria, or (less commonly) myoglobinuria. Hematuria is usually associated with a change in clarity from clear to cloudy. Identification of erythrocytes on the urine sediment is necessary to confirm hematuria. Both pyuria and significant crystalluria can result in a grossly cloudy urine sample. Identification of crystalluria or pyuria differentiate between these two causes of change in clarity. Any sample with a significant amount of protein identified on the chemical analysis requires evaluation of the sediment to determine if inflammation of the urinary tract versus glomerular or tubular loss are the cause of the increased proteinuria.

It is unfortunate that many veterinarians choose to send out urinalysis rather perform this valuable test in-house. By making urinalysis a routine and commonly used diagnostic test, the general practitioner and their well-trained veterinary technician can develop the necessary skills and the confidence needed to evaluate urine sediment. In addition, there are newer in-clinic instruments dedicated to urine analysis, such as the IDEXX SediView™, that can assist in performing this valuable procedure. The in-house instruments still require a good level of skill by the user in identifying formed elements as an internal control for the instrument.

The primary reason for performing urine sediment examination in-house is the changes that occur when urine is stored prior to analysis. It is optimum to perform a urinalysis within one hour of collection. If a sample cannot be analyzed in this time frame, it can be refrigerated. If left at room temperature for longer than one hour, significant changes can occur in both the chemical and sediment analysis. The primary changes in urine sediment findings seen with prolonged time between collection and analysis include:

- lysis of erythrocytes in dilute urine
- degeneration of cellular elements
- dissolution and precipitation of crystals
- changes between types of crystals (dihydrate calcium oxalate versus monohydrate calcium oxalate)
- degeneration of crystals
- bacterial growth.

These changes can occur during refrigeration but at a slower rate. If the sample is refrigerated, it should be analyzed within 4–6 hours to prevent significant changes in the sediment. The urine sample should be warmed to room temperature and mixed very well before analysis. Warming to room temperature is essential for the chemical analysis. Some crystal that may have precipitated out during storage may redissolve at room temperature.

The use of a stain with a sediment examination is a controversial issue. Because of the artifacts and alteration in concentration of formed elements that are introduced with the use of a stain such as SediStain™, it is best to refrain from using a stain. If there is concern for whether the operator is seeing bacteria, if the cells present are leukocytes versus erythrocytes, or if there are atypical transitional cells present, a cytological preparation using the "line preparation" method is preferable.

Table 15.1 lists reference intervals for urine sediment formed elements (Rizzi et al., 2017).

Table 15.1 Reference intervals for urine sediment formed elements.

	Expected quantity (5 ml of urine)
Erythrocytes	<5/hpf
Leukocytes	<5/hpf
Epithelial cells	<2/lpf
Bacteria	None
Casts	Occasional hyaline/rare granular casts
Crystals	Variable[a]

[a] Dihydrate calcium oxalate and triple phosphate (struvite) crystals can be found in urine from healthy dogs and cats.

15.3 Equipment

Equipment used in this test include:

- centrifuge
- conical or round bottom centrifuge tubes
- pipettes
- glass microscope slides
- 25 × 25 mm coverslips
- quick Romanowski stain set up
- a fresh urine sample collected in a sterile container at room temperature.

15.4 Procedural Steps: How Do I Perform This Test?

- Gather the equipment and supplies for the test (see Figure 15.1).
- Gently mix the urine sample before aliquoting a standard volume into a conical or round bottom centrifuge tube. The recommended volume for a urinalysis is 5–10 ml. It is important to use the same sample size in each procedure in order to achieve consistent results (see Figure 15.2).
  - If the standard volume of urine is not available, record the volume used. Semiquantitative interpretation of the formed elements in the sediment examination will be negatively affected and interpretation of the findings should be done with that consideration.
- Place the centrifuge tube in the centrifuge with an appropriate balance tube containing the same volume of fluid (see Figure 15.3).
- Centrifuge for five minutes at 250 or 480 relative centrifugal force (RCF), or 2000 rotations per minute (RPMs) if the centrifuge does not provide for adjustment using RCF (see Figure 15.4a and b).
- Once the centrifuge has completely stopped. Decant the supernatant by pouring it off or by removing it using a pipette. Using a pipette allows more control for retaining a standard volume for resuspension of the sediment (see Figures 15.5 and 15.6).
  - Approximately 0.5 mL of fluid should be retained for resuspension of the sediment. Consistency in how much fluid is used for resuspending the sediment is necessary to allow semiquantitative evaluation of the sediment. The sample can be resuspended by gently "flicking" the tube or by using a pipette (see Figure 15.7a and b).
- Once the sediment is resuspended, place a drop of the sediment on a glass microscope slide and cover it with a 25 × 25 mm coverslip. This size of the coverslip should be used for consistency (see Figure 15.8a and b).

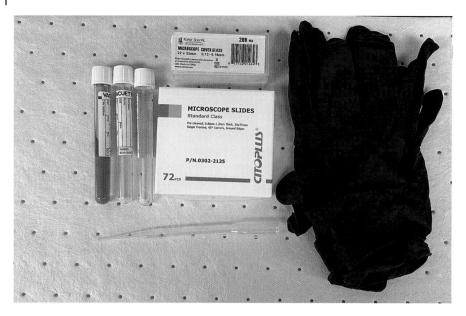

Figure 15.1 Equipment needed for a urine sediment analysis includes a centrifuge, conical or round bottom centrifuge tubes, pipettes, glass microscope slides, 25 × 25 mm coverslips, a fresh urine sample at room temperature. Not included in this picture are the centrifuge and conical centrifuge tubes. *Source:* Courtesy of Jeremy Bessett.

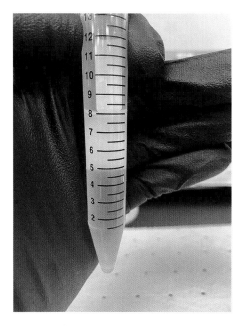

Figure 15.2 Calibrated conical centrifuge tubes are helpful in consistently measuring out the volume of urine indicated in the clinic's standard operating procedure for urine sediment examination. In this case, 8 ml is the volume used. *Source:* Courtesy of Jeremy Bessett.

- After placing the microscope slide on the stage, to best view the elements in an unstained wet mount, lower the condenser on your microscope, or, if your microscope does not have an adjustable condenser, close the iris diaphragm slightly. This will increase the contrast and make the unstained elements visible (see Figure 15.9).

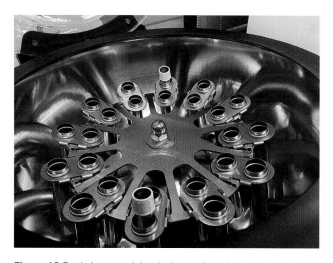

Figure 15.3 It is essential to balance the tubes by using the same type of tube and same volume when centrifuging the samples. *Source:* Courtesy of Jeremy Bessett.

The initial evaluation of the sediment is done using the 10x objective to quantify the number of large formed elements, such as epithelial cells, crystals, and casts.

- ○ The average number of each of these elements/10x field is recorded as number/low power field (lpf).
- Next the sediment is evaluated using the 40x objective to identify the presence and number of RBCs, leukocytes, small epithelial cells, and microorganisms (bacterial and fungal agents).
- ○ The average number for each of these elements is recorded as number/high power field (hpf).

(a)

(b)

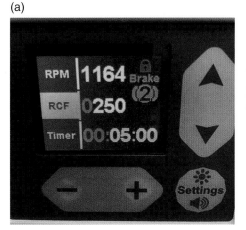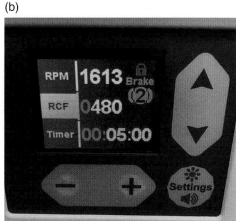

Figure 15.4 (a) The centrifuge is set for five minutes at 250 RCF, which, with this centrifuge, correlates to 1164 RPM. *Source:* Courtesy of Jeremy Bessett; (b) in this case, the centrifuge is set at 480 RCF, which correlates to 1613 RPM. Notice that the RCF and RPMs do not have a linear correlation. *Source:* Courtesy of Jeremy Bessett.

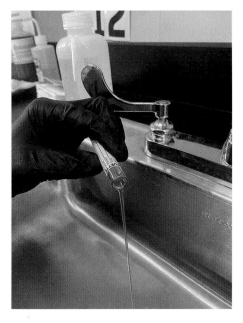

Figure 15.5 The supernatant can be poured off the sediment. It may be difficult to retain a standard amount of fluid for sediment suspension when using this method. *Source:* Courtesy of Jeremy Bessett.

- A line preparation for staining can be prepared if microorganisms and atypical cells are seen in the sediment examination. The line preparation will concentrate formed elements in a single line providing a smaller more concentrated area to review.
  - Place a drop of sediment or, if the urine has high cellularity, nonsedimented urine on a microscope slide.
  - Using a spreader slide, draw the spreader slide back to the drop of urine and allow the sample to spread out along the edge of the spreader slide (see Figure 15.10).

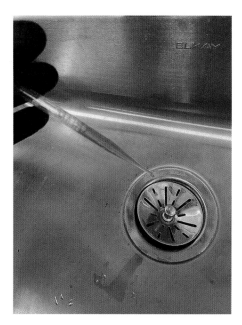

Figure 15.6 Conversely, a pipette can be used to remove the sediment from the tube. *Source:* Courtesy of Jeremy Bessett.

  - Push the spreader slide toward the end of the microscope slide (see Figure 15.11).
  - About 1/2 to 2/3 of the way to the end, abruptly lift the spreader slide (see Figure 15.12).
  - The formed elements of the urine will be carried to a line formed as the spreader slide is lifted (see Figure 15.13).

15.5 Time Estimate to Perform Test

Ten to twenty minutes.

(a)

(b)

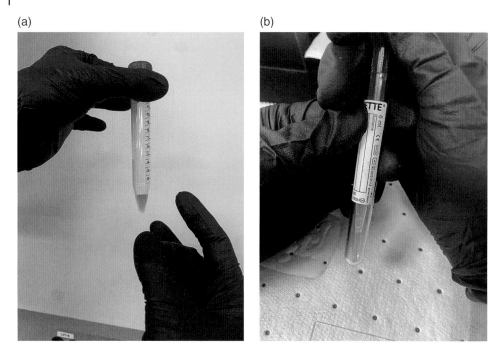

Figure 15.7 (a) Once the supernatant has been removed, the sediment can be resuspended by gently "flicking" the bottom of the tube. *Source:* Courtesy of Jeremy Bessett; (b) a pipette can also be used to resuspend the sediment. *Source:* Courtesy of Jeremy Bessett.

(a)

(b)

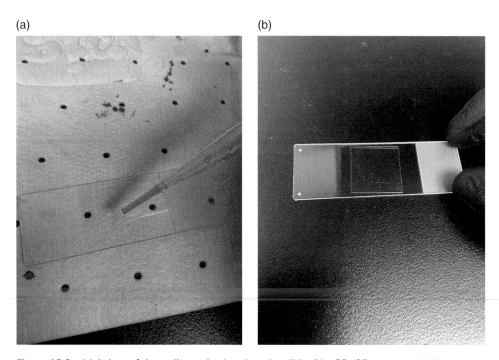

Figure 15.8 (a) A drop of the sediment is placed on the slide; (b) a 25 × 25 mm coverslip is placed on the slide. *Source:* Courtesy of Jeremy Bessett.

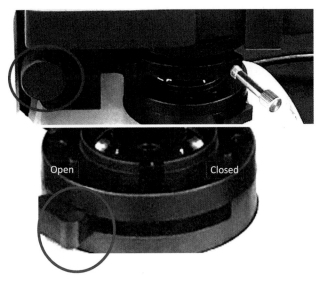

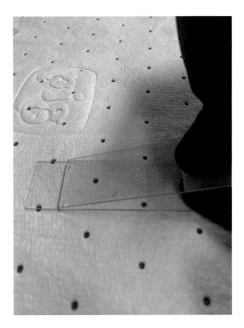

Figure 15.9 Microscopes with an adjustable condenser have a knob below the stage (red circle) that will allow it to be lowered when viewing wet mounts of urine or other fluids. The iris diaphragm is located below the condenser and can be closed using the sliding knob (blue circle) to increase contrast if the condenser cannot be lowered. *Source:* Courtesy of Jeremy Bessett.

Figure 15.11 Push the spreader slide toward the end of the slide. *Source:* Courtesy of Jeremy Bessett.

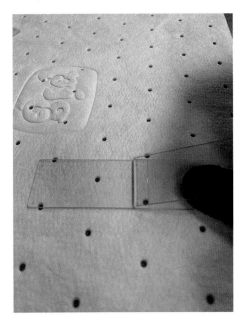

Figure 15.10 Using the same technique for making a blood film, draw the spreader slide back into the drop of urine and allow it to spread along the edge of the spreader slide. *Source:* Courtesy of Jeremy Bessett.

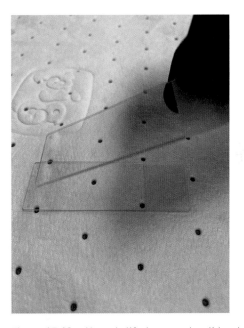

Figure 15.12 Abruptly lift the spreader slide when it reaches about two-thirds of the way to the end of the microscope. *Source:* Courtesy of Jeremy Bessett.

15.6 Procedural Tips and Troubleshooting

A urine sediment analysis is considered semiquantitative because the formed elements seen in the sediment are reported as #/hpf or lpf. In order to provide a good semiquantitative analysis, the procedure for performing the sediment preparation and examining the slide must be consistent. The most important aspects to consider are:

- performing the urinalysis within a specific time frame
- bringing the sample to room temperature prior to analysis

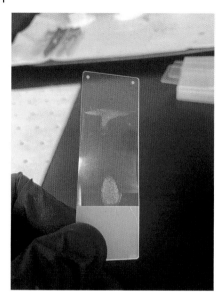

Figure 15.13 The formed elements will be concentrated to the area where the slide was lifted. *Source:* Courtesy of Jeremy Bessett.

- using a standard volume of urine for preparation of the urine sediment
- using a consistent RPM or RCF and length of centrifugation
- resuspending the sediment into a consistent volume of residual supernatant
- using the same pipette when dispensing the drop of urine; different pipettes will have a different volume of urine/drop
- consistently using a 25 × 25 mm coverslip
- evaluating a consistent number of low power (10×) and high power (40x) fields to determine the average number/field.

Having a good urine sediment atlas or urinalysis text beside the microscope is essential to assist in identifying formed elements that may be less common (see Suggested Bench-Side References).

It is worth the additional cost to have a microscope with an adjustable condenser. An adjustable condenser will provide the best contrast for examining wet mounts.

Perform urine sediment examination as quickly as possible after obtaining the sample. The sample can be refrigerated if needed but must be allowed to return to room temperature before the urinalysis is performed (this is especially true for performing the chemical analysis). Urine crystals can degenerate or, in the case of calcium oxalate crystals, change forms. Bacterial contaminants can increase significantly in number. Epithelial cells and crystal can deteriorate as well.

15.7 Interpreting Test Results

As with all clinical pathology diagnostic testing, interpretation of urine sediment findings should be done in the context of the patient's history and clinical exam findings. A complete blood count and serum chemistry profile are often necessary follow-up tests for a full evaluation of a urine sediment examination. Minimally, a packed cell volume, plasma total protein, and plasma color should accompany any urinalysis.

15.7.1 Cellular Element: Erythrocytes, Leukocytes, Epithelial Cells

15.7.1.1 Erythrocytes

Erythrocytes are the smallest cell found in the urine sediment. They are round and often have a slight red color. Their biconcave shape may be evident in canine samples and they may be more refractive than the other cellular elements.

Small numbers of erythrocytes (<5/hpf) can be seen in urine samples from healthy dogs and cats. Samples obtained by cystocentesis may result in a slightly increased number of erythrocytes. It is important to record the method of urine collection since it will affect the interpretation of sediment examination.

Increased numbers of erythrocytes indicate hemorrhage into the urinary tract and can be seen with inflammatory, neoplastic, and defects in coagulation. Microscopic hematuria can be seen with any of these conditions involving the kidney, ureter, and bladder. Macroscopic (grossly) visible hematuria is suggestive of hemorrhagic cystitis, neoplasia, or coagulation abnormalities including hereditary and acquired coagulopathies.

Although uncommon, renal hemorrhage due to glomerular or tubular damage can result in the formation of red cell casts in the urine (see section on casts).

Increased numbers of erythrocytes indicate hemorrhage within the urinary tract from the kidney to the bladder if the sample is collected via cystocentesis. If the sample is free catch, the hemorrhage could be from the kidney to the distal urethra and portions of the genital tract.

If the urine sample has a low urine specific gravity, erythrocytes will lyse over time and artifactual hemoglobinuria will be present. In most cases, some intact erythrocytes will be present to support hemorrhage. In addition, true hemoglobinuria should be associated with hemoglobinemia evident on evaluation of a spun microhematocrit tube (see Figure 15.14).

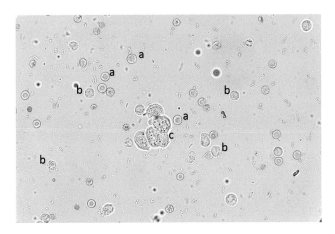

Figure 15.14 This image of an active sediment reveals several erythrocytes (a); leukocytes (b); and a small cluster of transitional epithelial cells (c). *Source:* Courtesy of Jeremy Bessett.

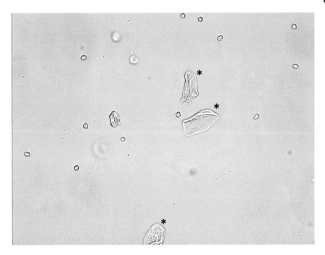

Figure 15.15 Several large squamous epithelial cells (*) and a few scattered erythrocytes are present in this sediment preparation from a free-catch midstream sample. *Source:* Courtesy of Jeremy Bessett.

15.7.1.2 Leukocytes

The most common leukocytes seen in urine sediment are neutrophils. They are larger than erythrocytes but smaller than most transitional cells. They have a granular "glittering" appearance to the cytoplasm and close examination at 40x usually reveal their segmented nuclear shape. Occasionally, other cell types, lymphocytes, monocytes/macrophages, and eosinophils, may be seen in the urine. When significant numbers of leukocytes are seen, a cytological sample using the line preparation is recommended. This will help identify other leukocytes that may be present and help confirm the presence of microorganisms. Since it can be difficult to differentiate the leukocytes from small transitional cells on a wet preparation, the line preparation will also help distinguish these two cell types.

Like the erythrocytes, small numbers of leukocytes can be seen in the urine of healthy dogs and cats. Increased numbers of leukocytes indicate an inflammatory process within the urinary tract from the kidney to the bladder if the sample is collected via cystocentesis. If the sample is free catch, the inflammatory process could be from the kidney to the distal urethra and portions of the genital tract (see Figure 15.15).

15.7.1.3 Transitional Epithelial Cells

Transitional cells are the cells that line the urinary outflow tract from the renal pelvis to the urethra. These cells are slightly to moderately larger than leukocytes and usually have a round nuclei and small to moderate amount of cytoplasm that is less granular then a neutrophil.

Small numbers (<2/hpf) of transitional cells can be seen in the urine from healthy dogs and cats. Inflammation with secondary mucosal hyperplasia is the most common cause of increased numbers of transitional epithelial cells in urine sediment collected by cystocentesis or free catch. In catheterized samples, increased numbers of transitional cells (as well as erythrocytes and leukocytes) can be seen if the catheterization was traumatic. In fact, purposefully traumatic catheterization is a method that can be used to collect samples for cytology in cases of suspected neoplasia. Neoplasia can also cause increased numbers of transitional cells. Significant atypical cell morphology can be seen with mucosal hyperplasia and neoplasia. Submission of urine cytology for a pathology review is recommended if neoplasia is suspected.

15.7.1.4 Squamous Epithelial Cells

A small number of squamous epithelial cells can be seen in the catheter and free-catch sample collection. These cells originate from the distal urethra and are considered insignificant (see Figure 15.16).

15.7.2 Casts: Hyaline Casts, Granular Casts, Cellular Casts, Waxy Casts

Urinary casts are formed within the renal tubular lumen and their size and shape reflect the size of the tubule in which they form. They are elongate with parallel sides and rounded to irregular ends. They can be straight or curved. The presence of significant numbers of casts in the urine indicates renal tubular damage or significant proteinuria. Casts are shed intermittently into the urine. The lack of casts does not rule out significant renal injury. Significant showering of casts can be seen in dogs after strenuous exercise, following rehydration of a dehydrated patient, and

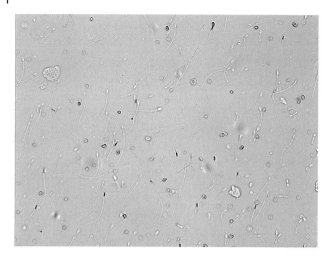

Figure 15.16 While not common, spermatozoa can be incidental findings in the urine of both male and female dogs. This image shows numerous normal spermatozoa throughout the background with refractile heads and long tails. *Source:* Courtesy of Jeremy Bessett.

posturinary tract obstruction. While the type of cast can suggest a specific mechanism, such as red cell casts (hemorrhage into the nephron), leukocyte casts (inflammation within the nephron), and hyaline casts (proteinuria), other types of casts do not indicate a specific mechanism or location of formation.

Most casts are colorless (except red cell casts); however, casts in urine samples with significant pigmenturia can take on the color of the pigment; yellow with bilirubinuria and pink or red with hemoglobin or myoglobinuria.

15.7.2.1 Hyaline Casts

Hyaline casts are transparent and can be difficult to see unless lipid droplets are incorporated into the protein matrix. Having the contrast adjusted appropriately is imperative to finding hyaline casts. These casts are formed from the mucoprotein found in urine (Tamm–Horsfall protein). They are occasionally found in the urine of healthy dogs and cats. When present in increased numbers, they are indicative of increased urine protein and suggest glomerular protein loss and, less often, tubular protein loss.

15.7.2.2 Granular Casts

Granular casts are casts with fine to coarse granulation. They form in the renal tubule from sloughed renal tubular epithelial cells. The granulation becomes finer the longer the granular cast travels in the nephron. They are uncommon in urine from healthy dogs and cats. When present in increased numbers, granular casts indicate renal tubule injury (see Figure 15.17).

Figure 15.17 A single coarsely granular cast is present in this urine sediment. *Source:* Sharon M. Dial (Author).

15.7.2.3 Cellular Casts

Cellular casts are casts in which individual cells can be appreciated. Cellular casts are always considered abnormal findings and should not be present in the urine of healthy dogs and cats. Red cells, leukocytes, and epithelial cells within the renal tubular lumen combine with the Tamm–Horsfall protein and form casts that preserve the cellular components. Red cell casts indicate hemorrhage into the nephron at the glomerular or tubular level. Leukocyte casts indicate inflammation at the glomerular or tubular level. Epithelial casts indicate active tubular injury and necrosis.

15.7.2.4 Waxy Casts

Waxy casts are large transparent casts and often have fractures forming small cracks in their edges. They are uncommon and usually seen in association with chronic renal disease. They are thought to be formed primarily in the collecting ducts of the nephron as a consolidation of other casts.

15.7.3 Crystals: Ammonium Biurates, Bilirubin, Calcium Oxalate, Cystine, Struvite, Tyrosine, Uric Acid

Crystalluria is a common finding in the urine of healthy dogs and cats. The most common crystal types are struvite and the dihydrate form of calcium oxalate. Cystine, tyrosine, and ammonium biurate crystals are not considered normal findings in most healthy dogs and cats. These crystals are associated with hereditary enzyme abnormalities. The most common condition associated with these crystals is increased ammonium biurate crystalluria in Dalmatian dogs.

The presence and number of crystals does not correlate with the presence of uroliths. While the type of crystal can suggest the type of stone present if urolithiasis is suspected, it is important to remember that more than one type of crystal can be present. In addition, the pH of the urine can affect the type of crystal present; struvite crystal can be found in urine with a pH > 7.0 and calcium oxalate crystals can be found in urine with a pH < 7.0.

15.7.3.1 Ammonium Biurate

Ammonium biurate crystals are dense brown irregular to round crystals with irregularly spaced spicules. They are considered abnormal findings in dog and cat urine. They are associated with increased blood ammonia in patients with hepatic disease including portosystemic shunts. They are seen in some breeds of dogs with abnormal purine metabolism such as the Dalmatian. In these breeds, uric acid crystals may also be seen.

15.7.3.2 Bilirubin

Bilirubin crystals are most commonly seen as needle-like crystals with a golden color. They are common in the urine of healthy dogs (especially male dogs). They are not considered normal in the urine of cats. Cats have a much higher renal threshold for bilirubin. The presence of bilirubinuria is indicative of hyperbilirubinemia in the cat. Bilirubinuria and bilirubin crystals are associated with all causes of hyperbilirubinemia and should prompt evaluation for liver function and hemolytic anemia.

15.7.3.3 Calcium Oxalate

Calcium oxalate crystal can be present in two forms in the urine of dogs and cats, the dihydrate and monohydrate forms. Dihydrate calcium oxalate crystals are square with a cross from corner to corner. This form is often called the "maltese cross" form (see Figure 15.18). The dihydrate

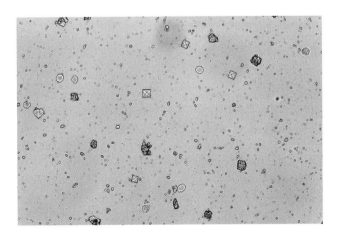

Figure 15.18 Several small square "maltese cross" dihydrate calcium oxalate crystals are present in this urine sediment from a healthy dog. A few red cells, leukocytes, and amorphous debris are present in the background. *Source:* Courtesy of Jeremy Bessett.

form of calcium oxalate can be seen in the urine of healthy dogs and cats. This crystal can also be seen in sick animals with calciuria, indicative of possible hypercalcemia. The presence of dihydrate calcium oxalate in healthy patients does not infer the presence or likelihood of developing calcium oxalate uroliths.

Monohydrate calcium oxalate crystals are elongate crystals with pointed ends, often resembling the pickets in a picket fence. They can occasionally have small "daughter" crystals that grow from the main crystal. The monohydrate form of calcium oxalate, when present in urine sediment from freshly collected urine is not considered a normal finding in healthy dogs and cats. In stored urine or urine left too long at room temperature, small numbers of monohydrate calcium oxalate crystals can precipitate out. When found in urine sediment from fresh urine, they are associated with hypercalcemia and ethylene glycol toxicity. Oxalic acid is one of the toxic metabolites from ethylene glycol that forms monohydrate calcium oxalate crystals within the renal tubules.

15.7.3.4 Cystine

Cystine crystals are flat transparent six-sided crystals. They are not considered a normal finding in urine from healthy dogs and cats. When present, they are indicative of proximal renal tubular dysfunction. Cystine is an amino acid that is usually reabsorbed from the urine filtrate in the proximal tubule. Diseases like Fanconi syndrome result in amino aciduria and promote the formation of cystine crystals.

15.7.3.5 Struvite

Struvite crystals are variably sized rectangular crystals with a "coffin-lid" appearance. Struvite crystals are commonly found in the urine of healthy dogs and cats. They can be associated with cystitis in both species. In dogs, they are often associated with bacterial cystitis, while in cats, there is no association with the presence of bacteria in the urine (see Figure 15.19).

15.7.3.6 Tyrosine

Tyrosine crystals are colorless to slightly yellow needle-like crystals. Like cystine, tyrosine is an amino acid that should be cleared from the urine filtrate in the proximal tubule. When present in the urine, tyrosine crystals indicate a renal tubular defect such as Fanconi syndrome.

15.7.3.7 Uric acid

Uric acid crystals are rhomboid flat transparent colorless crystals. They are often associated with the same disease processes and seen with ammonium biurate crystals. They are not considered normal in the urine of healthy dogs and cats. As with ammonium biurate crystals, they

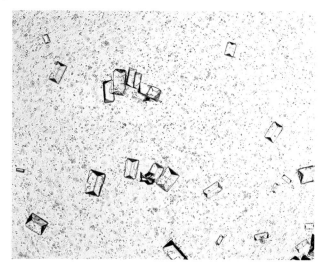

Figure 15.19 Numerous struvite crystals are present along with a large amount of amorphous crystalline debris in urine sediment from a healthy dog. *Source:* Courtesy of Jeremy Bessett.

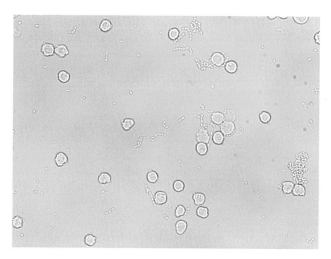

Figure 15.20 Numerous coccoid bacteria in variably sized chains are present along with leukocytes in this urine sediment preparation. *Source:* Sharon M. Dial (Author).

are seen in dogs with defective purine metabolism or liver dysfunction.

15.7.4 Microorganisms

Urine should be sterile. When collected by cystocentesis or catheterization using appropriate sterile technique, no microorganisms should be seen. When collected by free catch, midstream, only rare bacteria are usually found. When found in a free-catch sample, a sterile sample should be obtained for further evaluation. When microorganisms are found in a sterile sample, a urine culture should be submitted.

An inflammatory response should accompany a urinary tract infection; there are instances where concurrent disease, such as hyperadrenocorticism, or concurrent administration of immune suppressant drugs can inhibit an appropriate cellular response. If a sample has been obtained using the appropriate sterile technique, the presence of microorganisms should be considered an abnormal finding that should be addressed even when no evidence of an inflammatory response is seen.

It can be difficult to differentiate background amorphous debris from coccoid bacteria. Finding coccoid bacteria in variably sized chains will help identify true bacteriuria due to coccoid species (see Figure 15.20). Brownian motion of granular debris can mimic motility. Rod-shaped bacteria are more easily identified because of their shape and their prominent forward motility (see Figure 15.21). If there is any concern about whether bacteria are present, a line preparation can be made and evaluated to confirm the presence of the bacteria, especially if intracellular bacteria are found in the cytologic preparation.

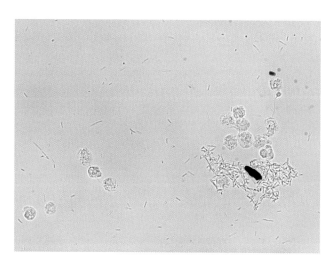

Figure 15.21 A large aggregate of rod-shaped bacteria and scattered individual rods and rods in short chains are present along with several leukocytes in this urine sediment preparation. *Source:* Sharon M. Dial (Author).

It is not uncommon to find significant contamination of urine samples collected by free catch or collected off of surfaces. These saprophytic contaminants can grow readily in urine if allowed to sit at room temperature or stored for long periods in the refrigerator (see Figure 15.22).

While uncommon in urine sediment, occasional parasite eggs can be seen in dogs and cats with bladder worms. Ova of nematodes of the genus Pearsonema (*Pearsonema plica*, dog; *Pearsonema feliscati*, cat) are an incidental finding in most cases. They may be accompanied by mild pyuria and hematuria or in urine with no cellular abnormalities. When the adult worms are present in large numbers, they can result in transitional cell hyperplasia, inflammation, and

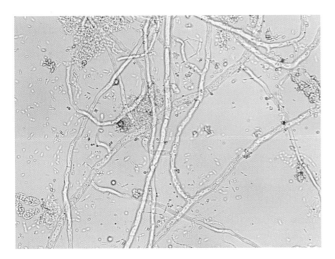

Figure 15.22 Large numbers of branching fungal hyphae, bacteria, amorphous debris, and small numbers of epithelial cells are seen in the urine sediment from urine that was collected from an environmental surface and allowed to sit at room temperature overnight before being submitted for a urinalysis. *Source:* Sharon M. Dial (Author).

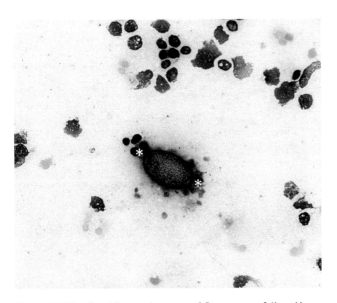

Figure 15.23 One bioperculate ova of *Pearsonema feliscati* in a urine cytology from a cat. Note the opercula (*). *Source:* Sharon M. Dial (Author).

obstruction of one or both ureters. The ova of *Pearsonema* spp. are oval and bioperculate with internal granularity and a thick refractile shell. The ova are approximately 60 μm long and 25 μm wide (see Figure 15.23).

15.8   Clinical Case Example(s)

15.9   Add-On Tests That You May Need to Consider and Their Additive Value

The presence of increased WBCs with or without identification of bacteria or other microorganisms should prompt submission of a urine culture. Most cases of cystitis are secondary to bacterial infection in the dog. While it is true that most cases of cystitis in the cat are sterile, culture to rule out infectious disease is still important. In addition, finding bacteria without an increase in leukocytes can be seen with immunocompromised patients. If the sample was appropriately obtained and the patient is being treated with immunosuppressants or has underlying disease associated with immunosuppression, urine culture is warranted.

The presence of abnormal crystals (ammonium biurate, cystine, tyrosine, uric acid, bilirubin [in cats], monohydrate calcium oxalate) should prompt additional evaluation for underlying disease or inherited defects in purine metabolism. A serum chemistry profile for evaluation of liver and renal function is warranted.

The presence of a significant number of casts should prompt full evaluation of renal function and be interpreted in the context of the serum chemistry and results of the chemical analysis of the urine.

15.10   Key Takeaways

- The urine sediment evaluation can be semiquantitative if standard protocol is used in its preparation.
- Urine sediment findings are affected by the collection method, especially in relationship to the findings of increased cellularity and the presence of microorganisms.
- Urine sediment examination should be done on fresh urine since storage of urine (even at refrigeration temperature) can alter the composition of formed elements. Cell and casts may degenerate. Crystals may form or dissolve when stored. Bacteria can increase in number.
- The presence of crystals in the urine does not equate to the presence of or increase the possibility of urolith formation.

Reference

Barlough, J.E., Osborne, C.A., and Stevens, J.B. (1981). Canine and feline urinalysis: value of macroscopic and microscopic examinations. *Journal of the American Veterinary Medical Association* 178 (1): 61–63.

Suggested Bench-Side References

Rizzi, T.E. et al. (2017). *Atlas of Canine and Feline Urinalysis.* New York: John Wiley & Sons, Incorporated.

Sink, C.A. and Weinstein, N.M. (2011). *Practical Veterinary Urinalysis.* Wiley.

Osborne, C.A., Stevens, J.B., and Ulrich, L.K. (1999). *Urinalysis: A Clinical Guide to Compassionate Patient Care.* Bayer AG.

Part 4

Quick Assessment Tests (QATS) Involving Feces

16

Assessing the Physical Properties of Fecal Matter
Ryane E. Englar

16.1 Procedural Definition: What Is This Test About?

Fecal analysis is a diagnostic test that involves both macroscopic and microscopic examination of the patient's sample. Fecal samples are routinely obtained via "free catch," meaning that a fresh sample is collected after the patient defecates. In dogs, this is most often achieved by picking up after the patient on leashed walks. Stool samples may be gathered with gloved hands or through a baggie that has been turned inside out to facilitate collection. Because we are essentially picking up the stool from the ground, samples frequently contain plant material, sand, dirt, or pebbles (see Figures 16.1 and 16.2).

In cats, feces are obtained by scooping the litterbox, in which case, the resultant sample is often encased with litter (see Figure 16.3).

Diarrheic samples from either species are more difficult to gather and may require serial collection to obtain sufficient material for testing (see Figure 16.4).

Occasionally, veterinarians elect to obtain fresh samples of feces during the physical examination with the assistance of a fecal loop (see Figure 16.5) [1]. This pencil-sized polyethylene wand has a slotted end that is lubricated prior to insertion into the rectum. The looped end traps fecal material if it is present within the rectum. Following extraction of the tool from the rectum, the trapped fecal matter can be analyzed. Alternatively, veterinarians may sample feces by inserting a gloved finger into the rectum during rectal palpation. Fecal matter that adheres to the gloved finger can be evaluated following rectal examination for both macroscopic and microscopic features.

Fecal analysis begins with a macroscopic assessment of the sample. The sample is characterized in terms of its physical properties. This chapter will concentrate on the following physical properties of feces:

- consistency
- color
- presence/absence of blood
- presence/absence of mucus
- gross parasitism
- odor.

Subsequent chapters (see Chapters 17 and 18) will introduce microscopic assessment of feces, that is, what is traditionally thought of as fecal analysis.

16.2 Procedural Purpose: Why Should I Perform This Test?

The evaluation of feces is a critical diagnostic tool that is used in the detection and management of a variety of medical conditions ranging from localized gastrointestinal disease (e.g. small and large bowel endoparasitism) to metabolic dysfunction (e.g. exocrine pancreatic insufficiency [EPI]).

Physical characteristics of feces also provide clues about the health of seemingly unrelated body systems. For example, rock hard fecal balls may reflect prolonged retention of feces within the lower digestive tract due to orthopedic challenges that make posturing to defecate difficult (e.g. osteoarthritis).

Fecal analysis is an essential part of screening patients, especially puppies and kittens, for endoparasites, many of which are zoonotic [2, 3].

In 2018, a research team led by Caroline Sobotyk analyzed 4692 fecal flotation test results from 10 veterinary diagnostic laboratories in nine states in the United States [4]. Samples came from client-owned dogs as well as research and shelter dogs [4]. One-fifth of samples were positive for one or more parasites [4]. Giardiasis was confirmed in 8.33% of samples followed by parasites within the

Low-Cost Veterinary Clinical Diagnostics, First Edition. Ryane E. Englar and Sharon M. Dial.
© 2023 John Wiley & Sons, Inc. Published 2023 by John Wiley & Sons, Inc.

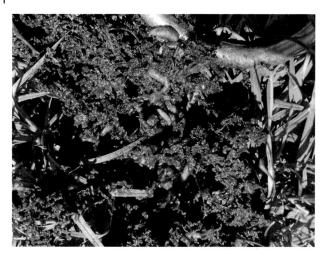

Figure 16.1 Example of loose canine feces prior to being sampled. Note that this sample contains maggots and is seated against a backdrop of grass. Once gathered from the ground, this sample is likely to contain plant material as an incidental finding. *Source:* Courtesy of Ryane E. Englar, DVM, DABVP (Canine and Feline Practice).

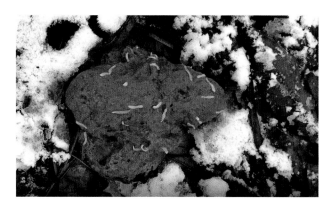

Figure 16.2 Example of semi-formed canine feces prior to being sampled. Note that this sample contains tapeworms and is seated against a backdrop of snow and decaying leaves. Once gathered from the ground, this sample is likely to contain plant material as an incidental finding. *Source:* Courtesy of Michelle Lugones, DVM.

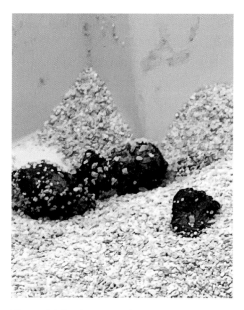

Figure 16.3 Example of formed feline feces prior to being sampled. Note that this sample is contained within a litterbox. Once sampled, this sample will contain litter as an incidental finding. *Source:* Courtesy of Ryane E. Englar, DVM, DABVP (Canine and Feline Practice).

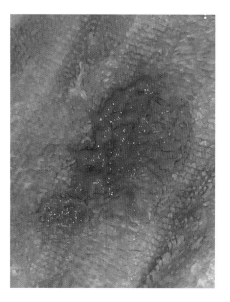

Figure 16.4 Example of diarrheic feces from a puppy. This gelatinous fecal matter will be challenging to sample and may require multiple attempts to obtain sufficient volume for analysis. *Source:* Courtesy of Ryane E. Englar, DVM, DABVP (Canine and Feline Practice).

family Ancylostomatidae, *Cystoisospora* spp., *Toxocara canis*, and *Trichuris vulpis*, in order of prevalence [4].

A 2020 study by Stafford et al. specifically studied fecal samples from canine patients that frequent dog parks within the United States [5]. Stafford found that, again, one-fifth of the sample population was infected with one or more intestinal parasites [5]. Moreover, of the dog parks that were studied by the research team, 85% were contaminated with intestinal parasites [5].

Identification of endoparasites, particularly within asymptomatic patients, is of utmost importance when managing public health and maintaining the human–animal bond.

The zoonotic potential associated with ascarids is a significant concern [6–12]. At least 750 cases of uveitis, vision loss, and blindness in people in the United States are attributed to toxocariasis annually [7, 9, 11]. Children are particularly at risk because they are more likely to play in and ingest dirt [7].

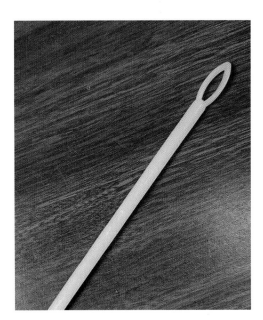

Figure 16.5 Example of a polyethylene fecal wand. *Source: Courtesy of Ryane E. Englar, DVM, DABVP (Canine and Feline Practice).*

Tapeworms are also zoonotic. People become infected when they ingest whole fleas that contain *Dipylidium caninum* [12–15]. Affected human patients may develop perianal pruritus as they produce tapeworm segments [7].

People may also become infected with tapeworms of *Taenia* spp. through accidental ingestion of tapeworm eggs after handling contaminated canine feces [7]. Infections are rare but can lead to cyst formation within the central nervous system (CNS), eye, muscle, or subcutaneous tissue [7].

Infection of people with *Echinococcus granulosus* is also of great concern because this tapeworm causes the development of cystic lesions within viscera [7].

Diagnosis of endoparasitism within companion animals is key to reducing the risk that their owners will contract disease. Furthermore, diagnosis paves the way for parasite treatment and preventative measures to reduce risk of recurrence [2].

According to the 2020 guidelines from the Companion Animal Parasite Council (CAPC), fecal analysis should take place at least four times during the first year of life [16]. However, it is critical to understand that parasite prevention and control does not end once puppies and kittens become adults. CAPC advises that canine and feline patients undergo fecal examinations at least twice per year throughout adulthood [16]. Patient health and lifestyle as well as parasite prevalence within the geographical residence of the patient may further influence frequency of fecal examination [16].

Beyond routine screening, fecal analysis also plays an essential part of the diagnostic workup for those patients that present with aberrant defecation histories and/or clinical presentations including, but not limited to [12]:

- constipation – prolonged retention of feces within the colon, resulting in infrequent or difficult evacuation of the feces
- coprophagia – ingestion of fecal matter [17]
- diarrhea – loose, liquid bowel movements
- dyschezia – difficult or painful defecation
- hematochezia – the presence of fresh (red) blood in the stool from lower gastrointestinal bleeds
- Melena – dark-colored (often black) tarry feces containing digested blood from upper gastrointestinal bleeds
- obstipation – inability to evacuate accumulated, dry, hard feces due to diminished or absent function of the large bowel, causing impaction that may extend the entire length of the colon
- pica – the intentional consumption of nonfood items [18]
- tenesmus – straining to defecate.

In addition to playing an essential role in diagnosis, fecal analysis allows us to monitor the patient's response to case management and/or make assessments concerning disease progression. In the ideal world, patients with known endoparasites re-present for follow-up examination and feces are resubmitted until samples retest as "negative," meaning that no ova or parasites are seen. This allows the veterinary team to shift focus from treatment onto parasite prevention.

Routine fecal analysis involves multiple steps:

1) assessment of stool's physical features
2) microscopic examination of feces
   - direct smear/fecal cytology/wet mount (see Chapter 17)
   - fecal flotation (see Chapter 18)
     - passive (gravitational)
     - centrifugal.

There are also a variety of add-on fecal tests that may be considered on a case-by-case basis, depending upon the clinician's list of differential diagnoses and index of suspicion. For instance,

- Fecal cultures evaluate the microbial composition and make determinations about treatment in patients that are experiencing dysbiosis.
- The Baermann technique evaluates patient samples for free-living parasitic nematode larvae, including, but not limited to, lungworms (in cats, horses, and ruminants primarily) and the canine intestinal threadworm, *Strongyloides stercoralis* [19].

These add-on tests are beyond the scope of this text and specifically this chapter, which will concentrate on macroscopic analysis as a guide to characterizing stool based on its physical features.

Gross observations about fecal matter include consistency, color, presence/absence of blood, presence/absence of mucus, gross parasitism, and odor.

16.2.1 Sample Consistency

Fecal consistency is a useful feature because it is one of many indicators of whole-body hydration and gut transit time. Although each patient has their own version of what constitutes "normal" fecal consistency, in general, canine and feline feces should feel a bit like Play-Doh – compact with a shape, yet squishable, moist, and easy to pick up. As fecal matter becomes increasingly loose, as from increased water content, it loses shape and leaves a residue behind when it is sampled. At the other extreme is stool that is too firm. As fecal matter dries out, it loses its ability to become compressed. It may become impossible to indent and may trade its log shape for individual pebbles or so-called fecal balls.

We can discuss fecal consistency with members of the veterinary team, including clients, when we assign a fecal score to the patient's sample [20]. Because there is no universal fecal scoring system in veterinary practice, many nutritional companies have developed their own [20]. Scores provide accompanying descriptions and an assortment of visual aids that are user-friendly and get veterinary clients and clinicians on the same page. An example of the Nestlé–Purina fecal scoring system has been provided for your review here (see Figure 16.6).

How to read the fecal score for any given patient sample and what each fecal score might mean in terms of potential etiologies will appear under the subheader, interpretation of test results.

16.2.2 Sample Color

Fecal color is a useful feature because it is one of the many indicators of gastrointestinal health. For example, feces that are yellow-to-orange in color may reflect underlying hepatic or biliary dysfunction, whereas feces that are gray and greasy may point toward EPI.

Refer to the subsection below, "Interpreting Test Results," to consider what various colors of feces may indicate.

16.2.3 Presence/Absence of Blood

Evaluating feces for gross evidence of blood is a useful feature because the presence or absence of blood and whether that blood appears to be fresh or digested localizes disease within the gastrointestinal tract [12].

Refer to the subsection below, "Interpreting Test Results," to consider how to localize gastrointestinal tract lesions based upon the presence/absence of blood and whether that blood appears to have been digested.

16.2.4 Presence/Absence of Mucous Coating

Evaluating feces for a heavy mucous coating is a useful feature because excessive mucous may be indicative of colonic inflammation, that is, colitis.

Refer to the subsection below, "Interpreting Test Results," to consider the significance of mucus.

16.2.5 Presence/Absence of Gross Parasitism and Other "Content"

Finding evidence of endoparasites or larvae that can be seen with the naked eye is diagnostic.

Canine and feline fecal samples may contain proglottids (segments) from *Dipylidium caninum* and *Taenia pisiformis*, two common tapeworm species [19].

Adult helminths, such as *Parascaris equorum*, can be found whole in equine feces.

Finding evidence of nonfood items is indicative of pica, that is, the patient is ingesting material that they should not be.

16.2.6 Sample Odor

Clients may present a patient for evaluation of a particularly fetid fecal odor. Alternatively, veterinary team members might smell something unusual in a patient's sample during fecal analysis that prompts further investigation. It is important not to discount fecal odor because a variety of scents that we are only just now beginning to explore as a profession may indicate a change in the patient's gastrointestinal health.

Refer to the subsection below, "Interpreting Test Results," to consider the relevance of odor to fecal analysis.

16.3 Equipment

Gross examination of a fecal sample requires minimal "supplies." You need only:

- exam gloves for handling biosamples
- a fresh sample of feces
- your eyes to see
- your fingertips to feel
- your nose to smell.

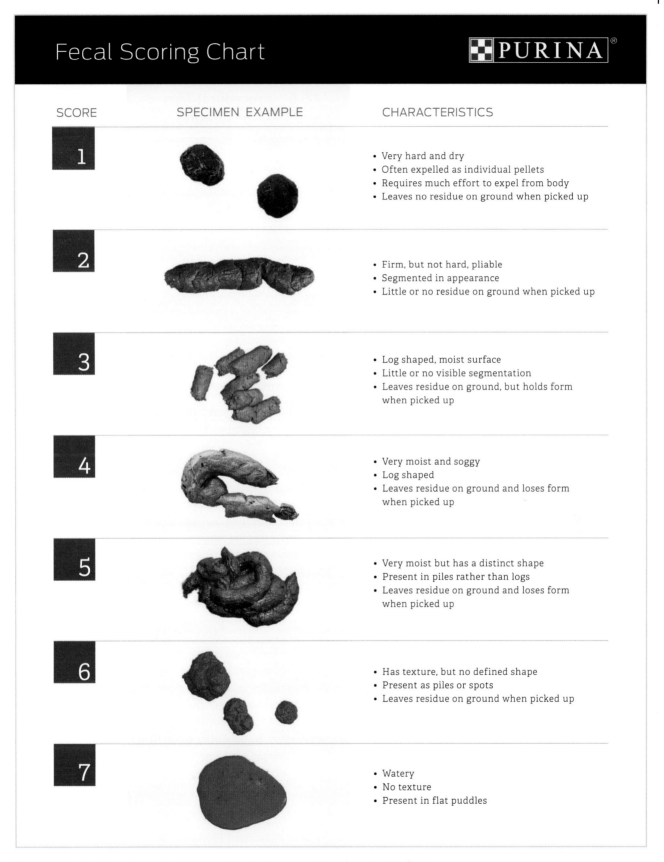

Figure 16.6 Fecal scoring system for dogs. *Source:* Courtesy of Nestlé–Purina PetCare.

16.4 Procedural Steps

1) Obtain a fecal sample from the patient either by "free catch," rectal examination, or via fecal loop.
2) Place the fecal sample in an airtight, leak-proof container with the following details:
   - animal identification (e.g. name and case number)
   - owner identification: (e.g. client last name)
   - date and time of sample collection.
3) Analyze the fecal sample as quickly as possible but not later than 24 hours after collection to maximize accuracy of the results [19].

   If fecal analysis must be delayed beyond two hours after collection, then refrigerate the sample to slow sample degradation [19, 21].

   Refrigerated samples should not be analyzed beyond 24 hours after collection.
4) Identify and record the patient's fecal consistency using the scoring system of your choice.

   Refer to the subsection below, "Interpreting Test Results," to consider what fecal consistency may indicate.
5) Identify and record the color of the fecal sample using an appropriate descriptor, including but not limited to:
   a) white
   b) pale to light gray to clay-colored yellow
   c) yellow, yellow-orange, orange
   d) green, green-blue, blue
   e) brown
   f) brown and spotted with white/white speckled/polka dotted
   g) black
   h) red streaks
   i) raspberry jam color.

   Refer to the subsection below, "Interpreting Test Results," to consider what each color may indicate.
6) Evaluate the fecal sample for the presence/absence of blood.

   Refer to the subsection below, "Interpreting Test Results," to differentiate melena from hematochezia and to consider what either may indicate.
7) Evaluate the fecal sample for the presence/absence of mucus.

   Refer to the subsection below, "Interpreting Test Results," to consider the significance of fecal mucus.
8) Evaluate the fecal sample for the presence/absence of macroscopic endoparasites and any other unusual contents.

   Refer to the subsection below, "Interpreting Test Results," to differentiate common endoparasites that you may see when you assess the fecal sample macroscopically.
9) Smell the fecal sample and record any unusual features.

16.5 Time Estimate to Perform Test

Less than five minutes.

16.6 Procedural Tips and Troubleshooting

16.6.1 Patient-Specific Considerations: Important Clues from History-Taking

Fecal analysis is performed to obtain data about gastrointestinal health; however, results should be considered within the context of the patient's history and physical exam findings. Historical and physical exam data are especially vital in sick or otherwise unhealthy patients. We may need to encourage the client to share their observations with us using open-ended questions that ask the client to expand upon the patient's bowel habits [22]. Examples of open-ended questions include [20, 22]:

- "Tell me what you're noticing at home with respect to your pet's stool."
- "Describe what you're seeing."

You may need to clarify key details within the client's story using closed-ended questions [22]:

- "When did the problem begin?"
- "How long has the problem been going on for?"
- "What is the problem's frequency?"
- "Has this happened before?"
- "How often does the patient produce a bowel movement?"
- "When was the patient's last bowel movement?"
- "Does your pet strain when passing stool?"
- Is any stool at all passed?
  - What does the stool look like?
  - What is the stool's shape and has it changed?
    - Dogs with prostate disease often develop ribbon-like stools.
- Is the stool coated with mucus?
- Is the stool coated with fresh red blood?
- What is the color of the stool today?
- What is the color of the stool typically?
- What is the patient's fecal score today?
- What is the patient's "usual" fecal score?
- Has the pet's fecal score changed? If so, how?

If the patient is presenting for evaluation of diarrhea, then the history can help to localize disease.

Large bowel diarrhea is characterized by [12, 23]:

- gelatinous semi-formed stool
- high volume of fecal mucus
- increased frequency of defecation

- increased urgency of defecation
- tenesmus
- ± hematochezia.

Small bowel diarrhea tends to be voluminous and is associated with weight loss [12, 20, 24, 25]. It typically does *not* involve fecal mucus, increased frequency of defecation, tenesmus, or dyschezia [12, 24–26].

Diet contributes to fecal output, so it is important that we broaden history-taking to consider what the patient is eating [22, 27]:

- How is the pet's appetite?
  - Is the pet still eating?
  - Is the pet's appetite increased, decreased, or the same?
- What does the pet eat in terms of food?
- What does the pet eat in terms of snacks?
- Has the pet's diet changed? If so, how?
- Is the pet unsupervised outdoors?
- Does the pet have a history of eating plants, dirt, other animals, or other animals' stool?
- Does the pet have a history of eating nonfood items?
- Could the pet have gotten into anything?

Because gastrointestinal health involves both ends of the dog or cat, it is important that history-taking include whether the pet is keeping food down [22]. Consider asking [22]:

- Is the pet vomiting?
  - If yes, then ask the client to describe the vomiting:
  - Is the pet really vomiting or is the pet regurgitating?
    - When does vomiting occur relative to eating?
    - When did the vomiting start?
    - What is the frequency? How many times has the pet vomited?
    - Is vomiting productive? Does anything come up?
    - What is the pet vomiting?
    - What color is the vomitus?
    - Does the vomitus contain blood?

Because the act of defecation involves posture, you need to also inquire about the pet's overall orthopedic health [22]. Past orthopedic disease, such as limb dislocations or pelvic fractures, and ongoing orthopedic disease, including osteoarthritis, may make posturing to defecate challenging [22]. This may lead to incomplete evacuation of feces and constipation [22].

16.6.2 Patient-Specific Considerations: Important Clues from Physical Examination

A physical examination may provide insight into the likelihood of any orthopedic considerations that may potentiate bowel issues.

Another key feature of the physical examination that should be considered in the context of an elimination history is the patient's body condition score (BCS). We estimate a veterinary patient's composition in terms of body fat by assigning them a BCS. There are several different scales for BCS. The author prefers the Purina 9-point system of body condition scoring (see Figure 16.7). This scale determines BCS by assessing visible and palpable landmarks [28].

According to the Purina 9-point system [28]:

- A dog that has a BCS of 1 is emaciated. These dogs have visually prominent ribs, lumbar vertebrae, and pelvic bones that are evident without palpation. There is no palpable body fat and muscle mass is overwhelmingly poor. The waistline is exaggerated. The patient takes on a skeletal appearance.
- A dog that has a BCS of 2 is moderately underweight, with easily visible ribs, lumbar vertebrae, and pelvic bones; however, when compared with dogs with a BCS of 1, dogs with a BCS of 2 have adequate muscle mass. The abdominal tuck remains pronounced, and there is still no palpable fat.
- A dog that has a BCS of 3 is mildly underweight. The ribs may or may not be visible, but they are easy to palpate without overlying fat. The pelvic bones, such as the wings of the ilia, are prominent, and the tips of the spinous processes of the lumbar vertebrae are visible. Overall, there is minimal body fat. The waistline is obvious.
- A dog that has a BCS of 4 may be considered by some to be a "lean normal" or what the author refers to as an "athletic build." This patient has easily palpable, but not visible ribs, with minimal fat coverage, and a prominent abdominal tuck.
- A dog that has a BCS of 5 is ideal. These patients are well-proportioned. They have a visible waist and palpable ribs without an excess of fat coverage.
- A dog that has a BCS of 6 is slightly overweight. There is a slight excess of fat covering otherwise palpable ribs. One can discern the waist, but it is not prominent.
- A dog that has a BCS of 7 is mildly overweight. It is possible but challenging to feel the ribcage due to heavy fat coverage, and fat deposits may be starting to accumulate over the lumbar region and tail base. The waist is absent as is the abdominal tuck.
- A dog that has a BCS of 8 is moderately overweight. It is not possible to feel the ribcage due to heavy fat coverage, and there is no waistline. Fat deposits are easily seen and palpable in the lumbar region bilaterally as well as at the tail base. There may also be visible rounding of the ventral abdomen due to fat deposition.

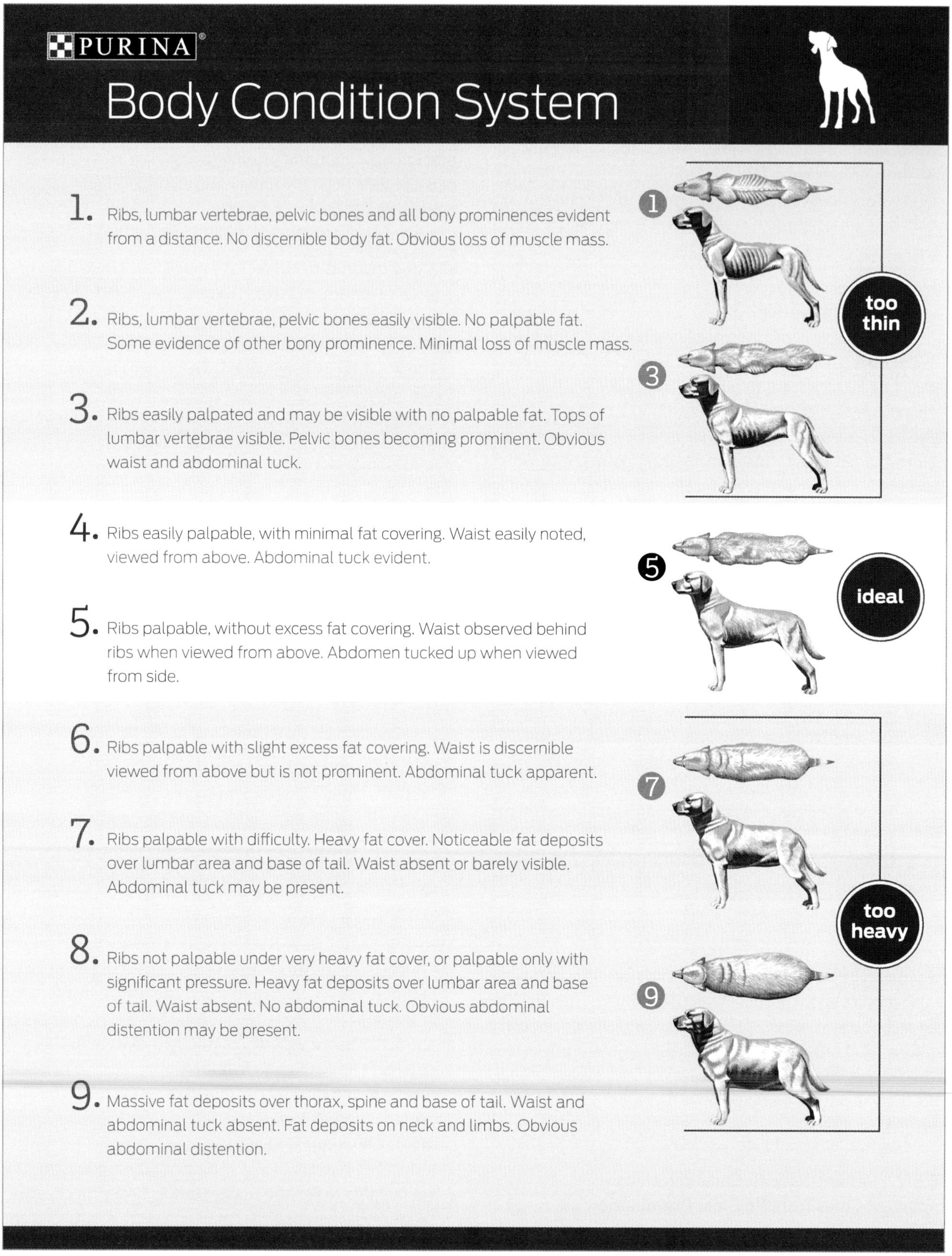

PURINA®

Body Condition System

1. Ribs, lumbar vertebrae, pelvic bones and all bony prominences evident from a distance. No discernible body fat. Obvious loss of muscle mass.

2. Ribs, lumbar vertebrae, pelvic bones easily visible. No palpable fat. Some evidence of other bony prominence. Minimal loss of muscle mass.

3. Ribs easily palpated and may be visible with no palpable fat. Tops of lumbar vertebrae visible. Pelvic bones becoming prominent. Obvious waist and abdominal tuck.

4. Ribs easily palpable, with minimal fat covering. Waist easily noted, viewed from above. Abdominal tuck evident.

5. Ribs palpable, without excess fat covering. Waist observed behind ribs when viewed from above. Abdomen tucked up when viewed from side.

6. Ribs palpable with slight excess fat covering. Waist is discernible viewed from above but is not prominent. Abdominal tuck apparent.

7. Ribs palpable with difficulty. Heavy fat cover. Noticeable fat deposits over lumbar area and base of tail. Waist absent or barely visible. Abdominal tuck may be present.

8. Ribs not palpable under very heavy fat cover, or palpable only with significant pressure. Heavy fat deposits over lumbar area and base of tail. Waist absent. No abdominal tuck. Obvious abdominal distention may be present.

9. Massive fat deposits over thorax, spine and base of tail. Waist and abdominal tuck absent. Fat deposits on neck and limbs. Obvious abdominal distention.

too thin

ideal

too heavy

Figure 16.7 Assessing canine BCS using the Purina 9-point system. *Source:* Courtesy of Nestlé–Purina PetCare.

- A dog that has a BCS of 9 is extremely obese. Fat deposits are extensive: in addition to prominent lumbar "love handles," fat is present over the neck, thorax, spine, tail, and limbs.

Cats have a similar BCS scoring system through Nestlé–Purina (see Figure 16.8).

BCS is underutilized by the veterinary team [29], yet it is an important screening tool [30] that assists the team in documenting trends. The cat that was once described as being "big-boned" with a BCS of 7 and is now a BCS of 3 on physical exam, without any identifiable changes in diet or feeding routine at home, requires an extensive diagnostic workup.

Similarly, BCS is an important consideration when the patient presents with an aberrant elimination history. A diarrheic dog or cat that is losing body condition is important data to consider as we perform fecal analysis. In other words, fecal analysis is one of many diagnostic tools that provides clues as to digestive and overall health. However, it needs to be considered in addition to other information so that the clinician has a complete clinical portrait of the patient.

16.6.3 Sample Collection

Encourage that the client observe the patient defecating so that they can disclose the following details [12, 19]:

- patient's elimination site
  - normal/as expected
  - abnormal, as in house-soiling (see Figure 16.9)
- patient's elimination behavior
  - normal/as expected
  - abnormal, as in new or unusual circling or nonproductive squats
- patient's posture during defecation
  - normal (see Figure 16.10)
  - abnormal
- patient's demeanor
  - normal and relaxed
  - abnormal and sense of urgency
- vocalization during defecation
- ease of defecation
  - normal
  - multiple attempts to produce stool
  - dyschezia
  - tenesmus (see Figure 16.11)
- anatomy of the perineum
  - normal
  - abnormal (e.g. redness, swelling, fistulation and/or abscessation, discharge)

- patient's interest in perineum
  - normal
  - abnormal (e.g. licking, grooming, chewing, and/or biting excessively).

If the patient appears to be exhibiting tenesmus, are they straining to defecate or are they actually straining to urinate?

Feline posture for urination is often distinct from feline posture for defecation; however, not all clients are familiar with elimination postures in cats since cats tend to eliminate in privacy without spectators (see Figures 16.12 and 16.13).

It is helpful when the client witnessed the act of defecation especially in multi-pet households so that you know the sample is truly associated with the patient in question [1, 19]. Sometimes owners will present a fecal sample that they gathered from the yard or litterbox. It may be grossly abnormal in appearance and/or microscopically, yet if more than one patient has access to the yard or litterbox, then it becomes a diagnostic challenge to know who the sample belongs to. If the fecal sample were to turn up positive in any regard [e.g. (+) for parasitism, (+) for blood, (+) for excessive mucus], then who do we treat and how? Diagnostic next steps are significantly more challenging when we must investigate everyone in the household.

16.6.4 Sample Collection Containers

Provide owners with a sterile collection cup and lid in advance of their next visit. This encourages compliance by training owners to bring in a fecal sample.

However, sometimes clients find themselves unexpectedly needing to sample fecal matter at home. In this case, they may reach for any container that is handy, including those that once housed food, detergent, or other residues. Instruct owners who find themselves in this position to use clean storage containers. The author has had fecal samples submitted to her in jam and jelly jars, many of which were not cleaned prior to filling. This impeded accurate observations about that sample's physical properties because it was impossible to determine if the fecal matter was truly gelatinous or if that texture was the result of feces being added to a jar that contained jelly.

It is also important to note to members of the veterinary team that gloves should not be used as primary storage "containers" for fecal samples. When clinicians perform rectal examinations, they often extract feces in the process. It may be tempting for the clinician to invert the glove upon the gloved finger's exit from the rectum, tie a knot in the glove, and consider that to be an appropriate sample holder. Although this is convenient for the clinician, feces stored

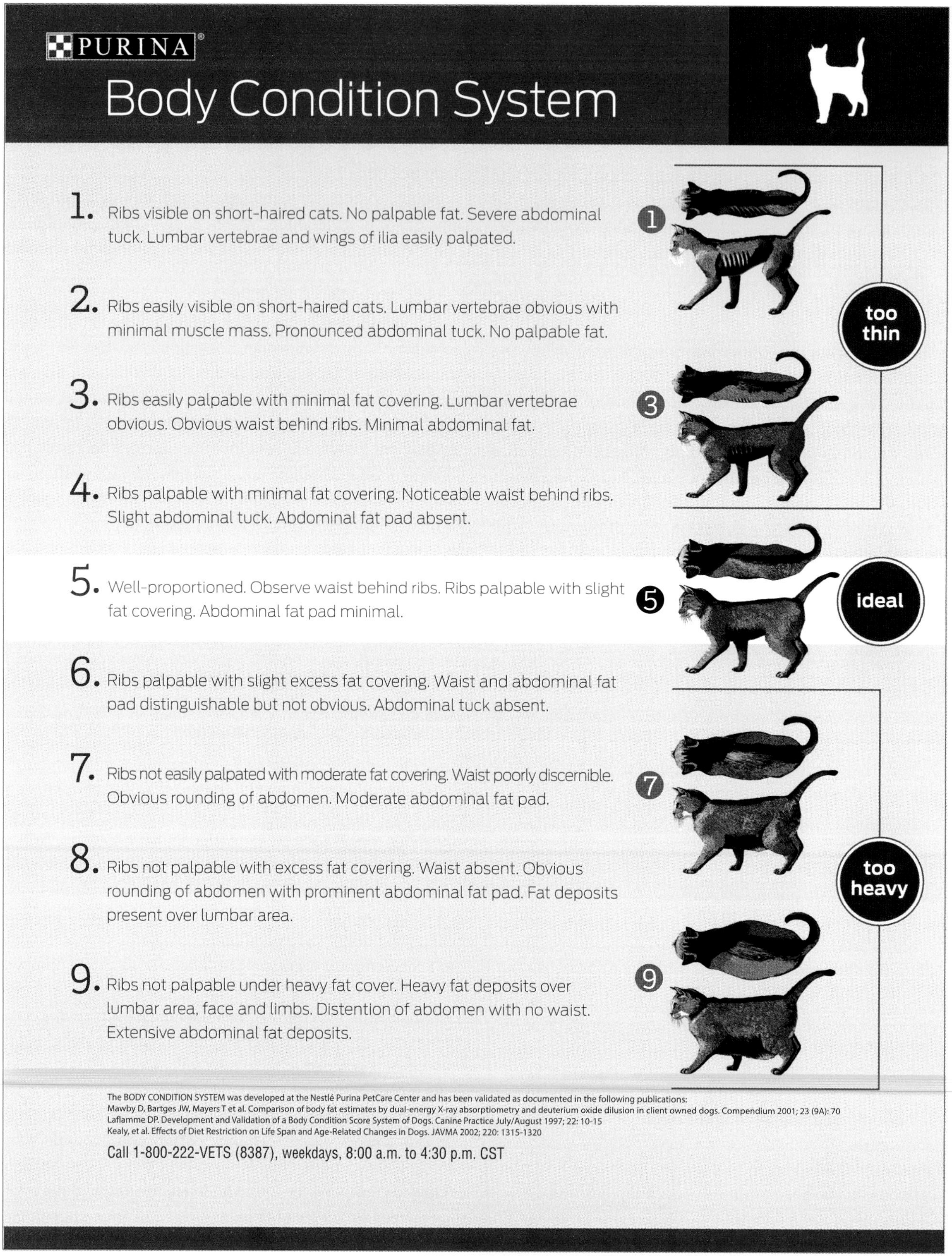

Body Condition System

PURINA®

1. Ribs visible on short-haired cats. No palpable fat. Severe abdominal tuck. Lumbar vertebrae and wings of ilia easily palpated.

2. Ribs easily visible on short-haired cats. Lumbar vertebrae obvious with minimal muscle mass. Pronounced abdominal tuck. No palpable fat.

3. Ribs easily palpable with minimal fat covering. Lumbar vertebrae obvious. Obvious waist behind ribs. Minimal abdominal fat.

4. Ribs palpable with minimal fat covering. Noticeable waist behind ribs. Slight abdominal tuck. Abdominal fat pad absent.

5. Well-proportioned. Observe waist behind ribs. Ribs palpable with slight fat covering. Abdominal fat pad minimal.

6. Ribs palpable with slight excess fat covering. Waist and abdominal fat pad distinguishable but not obvious. Abdominal tuck absent.

7. Ribs not easily palpated with moderate fat covering. Waist poorly discernible. Obvious rounding of abdomen. Moderate abdominal fat pad.

8. Ribs not palpable with excess fat covering. Waist absent. Obvious rounding of abdomen with prominent abdominal fat pad. Fat deposits present over lumbar area.

9. Ribs not palpable under heavy fat cover. Heavy fat deposits over lumbar area, face and limbs. Distention of abdomen with no waist. Extensive abdominal fat deposits.

too thin (1)

ideal (5)

too heavy (9)

The BODY CONDITION SYSTEM was developed at the Nestlé Purina PetCare Center and has been validated as documented in the following publications:
Mawby D, Bartges JW, Mayers T et al. Comparison of body fat estimates by dual-energy X-ray absorptiometry and deuterium oxide dilusion in client owned dogs. Compendium 2001; 23 (9A): 70
Laflamme DP. Development and Validation of a Body Condition Score System of Dogs. Canine Practice July/August 1997; 22: 10-15
Kealy, et al. Effects of Diet Restriction on Life Span and Age-Related Changes in Dogs. JAVMA 2002; 220: 1315-1320

Call 1-800-222-VETS (8387), weekdays, 8:00 a.m. to 4:30 p.m. CST

Figure 16.8 Assessing feline BCS using the Purina 9-point system. *Source:* Courtesy of Nestlé–Purina PetCare.

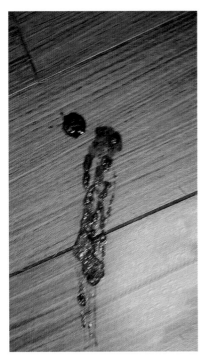

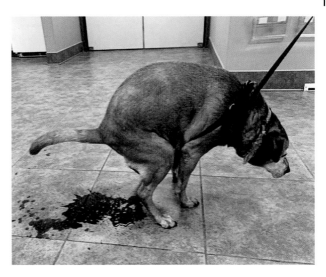

Figure 16.11 Tenesmus in a dog with hematochezia. *Source:* Courtesy of Danelle Capobianco.

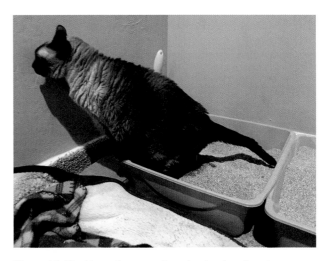

Figure 16.12 Normal posture for urination in a female cat. *Source:* Courtesy of Ryane E. Englar, DVM, DABVP (Canine and Feline Practice).

Figure 16.9 Example of house-soiling in a dog with diarrhea. The patient demonstrated urgency to defecate but did not make it outside in time to release its bowels. This patient was subsequently diagnosed with colitis. *Source:* Courtesy of Frank Isom, DVM.

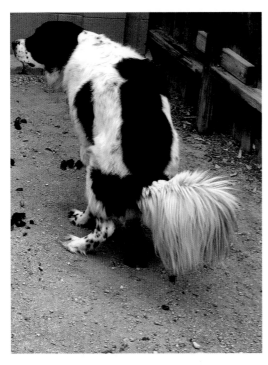

Figure 16.10 Normal canine posture for defecation. *Source:* Courtesy of Lisa Hallam, BS, CVT.

within an inverted glove make a mess for the individual who must analyze the sample.

16.6.5 Sample Size

Clients should be instructed on how much of a sample is needed to perform fecal analysis. On one hand, clients may be reluctant to bring in a sample for fear that they do not have "enough." At the other extreme are those clients who may run out of space within their collection container to stow an entire log of feces.

Giving clients a visual with regard to size streamlines the sample submission process. Most in-house fecal diagnostic tests can be run with 2–5 g of feces. For reference, one

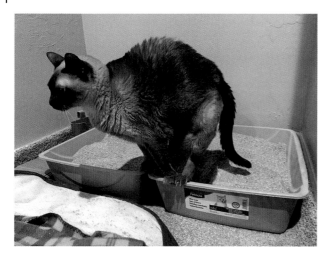

Figure 16.13 Normal feline posture for defecation. *Source:* Courtesy of Ryane E. Englar, DVM, DABVP (Canine and Feline Practice).

Hershey's Kiss weighs roughly 4.6 g. This amount is less than the size of an adult's thumb and is roughly the size of a quarter's surface.

Note that most fecal loops only extract, on average, 0.5 g of feces; therefore, unless this sample is being augmented by another source, it will not be sufficient for fecal flotation.

16.6.6 Age of Sample

- Prolonged storage of feces will age the sample. As fecal samples age, they desiccate. This will artificially change the sample's fecal score. You may inadvertently assign a low fecal score (if using the Nestlé–Purina scale) to a sample, implying that it is too dry when in fact it may have had an appropriate moisture content at time of collection.
- Similarly, sample color may change over time. Aged feces do not retain the classic brown color that is associated with healthy digestion. Instead, aged feces discolor to gray, gray-white, or even white. This process is hastened if samples are gathered from an enclosed yard in which fecal matter is exposed to intense sunlight. Sunlight will break down the normal pigments in stool. Humid environments may also trigger mold growth that discolors feces.
- Aged feces may harbor maggots, that is, fly larvae [19] (see Figure 16.1). These are not parasitic. They do not reside within the digestive tract of canine or feline patients. They develop from hatching eggs that were laid on the feces by free-living adult flies [19]. Some species of flies do not deposit eggs on feces; they deposit larvae directly [19]. These include flesh flies of the genus, *Sarcophaga* [19].
- Prolonged storage of feces is also likely to potentiate false negative results during fecal analysis. That is, no ova or parasites may be seen. Identification of parasites

microscopically (see Chapter 17) is often based upon their distinctive movement [19]. Parasites that would have been present and motile in fresh fecal samples may become immotile and/or they may die as feces age [19].

- Finally, prolonged storage of feces may also complicate microscopic diagnosis (see Chapter 17) in that parasites rapidly develop through their various life stages [19]. In other words, parasite eggs do not remain eggs forever. They will hatch into larvae [19]. When they do, eggs will no longer be present in the sample.

16.7 Interpreting Test Results

16.7.1 Fecal Consistency

Fecal scores were introduced earlier in this chapter as a means by which to describe consistency of stool. Such scoring systems pair a description with a visual aid to engage clients in dialogue with veterinary team members about fecal hardness, dryness, shape, and "scoopability" – that is, fecal ability to retain form, and whether any residue is left behind (see Figure 16.6).

Scores facilitate conversations about which fecal scores are "normal" for any given patient as well as how, if at all, the patient's fecal score has changed. In other words:

- What is the patient's fecal score today in comparison to what it has been previously?
- If there is a change in fecal score, is it intentional?
  For instance, maybe you evaluated a patient that presented with diarrhea and recommended a prescription diet. At a recheck appointment with that patient, you want to know if the stool is trending in the right direction. You can ask the client what the patient's fecal score is today. Even better yet, if the client brought in a stool sample, you can evaluate it and assign it a fecal score. If the diet is effective and the stool is indeed firming up, then you would expect to see stool produced that had a lower fecal score in comparison with its previous diarrheic state.
- If a change in fecal score is not intentional, then what could it mean?

According to the Nestlé–Purina fecal scoring system, normal feces should score a 2 or 3. Feces that are scored at a 1 are too firm. Any sample that scores higher than a 3 is too loose.

Let us begin by considering how we might interpret fecal scores of 1.

A fecal score of 1 indicates that feces are dried out and hardened [12]. This typically occurs when stool is retained in the colon [12, 31]. Prolonged retention enhances water resorption across the bowel wall [12, 31]. Fecal matter desiccates as water is reabsorbed over an extended period [12, 31] (see Figure 16.14).

Feces may be retained within the colon for a variety of reasons, including [12, 31–41]:

- decreased exercise
- dehydration
- drugs
  - anticholinergics
  - kaolin pectin or Kaopectate®
  - opioids
- excess dietary fiber
- environmental factors
  - dirty litter box, causing the patient to hold its bowels
  - hospitalization, causing the patient to hold off on elimination until returning home
  - increased ambient temperatures, causing increased water resorption
- foreign body ingestion, especially bones and/or fur
- mechanical obstruction
  - Manx cat deformities
  - neoplasia
  - pelvic fracture or other cause of narrowed pelvic canal
  - perineal hernia
  - prostatomegaly
  - rectal prolapse
  - rectal polyp
  - sublumbar lymphadenopathy
- metabolic disease
  - hypercalcemia
  - hyperparathyroidism
  - hypokalemia secondary to chronic kidney disease (CKD)
  - hypothyroidism
- neuromuscular disease
  - intervertebral disk disease (IVDD)
  - megacolon
  - paraplegia
  - spinal cord disease
  - tail pull injury and associated sacral nerve damage
- pain during defecation
  - painful posturing
    - dislocated limb(s)
    - fractured limb(s) or pelvis
    - osteoarthritis
  - painful evacuation of stool
    - anal sacculitis
    - anal stricture
    - perianal fistula
- supplements
  - iron
- toxicosis
  - lead.

Patients that experience one or more of the clinical scenarios outlined above may produce stool with a fecal score of 1 [12]. These patients are often constipated. Constipation is characterized by infrequent and/or incomplete passage of stool [12, 31, 33–35, 40–44]. If constipation is protracted and/or recurrent, patients may become obstipated [12, 31, 33, 43–45]. Obstipation implies that colonic function has become permanently compromised, as is the case for many cats with megacolon [12, 33, 44, 45] (see Figure 16.15).

Now let us consider those patients with fecal scores greater than 3. As fecal score climbs from 4 to 6, stool is increasingly loose due to excessive moisture content [12] (see Figures 16.16 and 16.17).

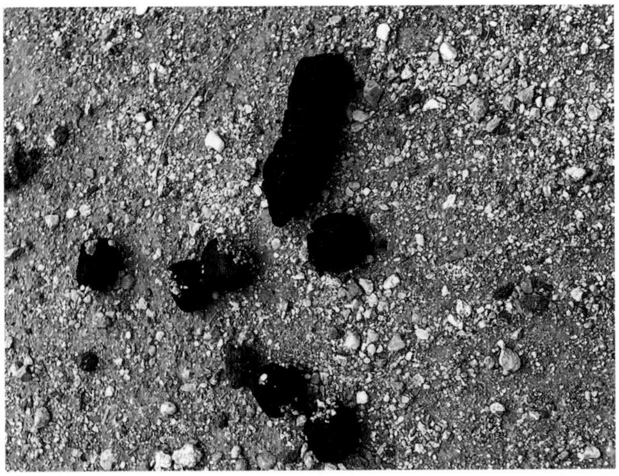

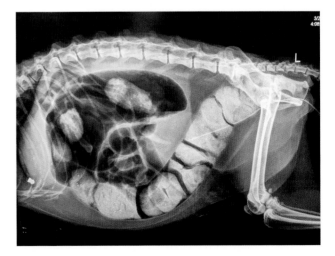

Figure 16.14 Canine sample with a fecal score of 1. *Source:* Courtesy of Lisa Hallam, BS, CVT.

Figure 16.15 Left lateral radiograph of a cat with megacolon. Note the significant distension within the descending colon. *Source:* Courtesy of Dr. Marina Kviker.

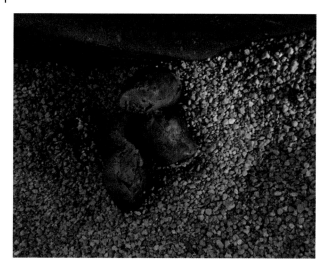

Figure 16.16   Feline sample with a fecal score of 4. The stool is moist and soggy. It leaves residue on the ground and loses form when it is picked up. *Source:* Courtesy of Ryane E. Englar, DVM, DABVP (Canine and Feline Practice).

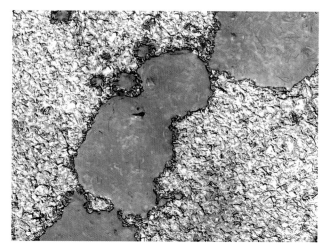

Figure 16.18   Canine sample with a fecal score of 7. The stool is watery and lays in puddles. *Source:* Courtesy of Simone Conwell.

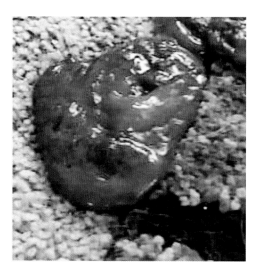

Figure 16.17   Feline sample with a fecal score of 6. The stool has texture but lacks defined shape. It presents as piles and leaves a residue on the ground when picked up. *Source:* Courtesy of Ryane E. Englar, DVM, DABVP (Canine and Feline Practice).

Feces that score a 7 have become liquified [12] (see Figure 16.18).

Stool liquifies when transit time through the gut is reduced [12, 31]. When digesta moves through the gut more quickly than the time that is required for digestion to be complete, the body cannot sufficiently reabsorb nutrients within the small bowel and water across the colonic wall [12]. As more water is retained within feces, the stool becomes soupier, and the patient is said to be diarrheic [12].

Diarrhea often results from hypermotility of the gut. In addition, diarrhea may develop as a response to [12, 31, 46, 47]:

- administration of medications that are osmotically active, but poorly digested (e.g. lactulose, magnesium sulfate, and sugar alcohols including mannitol, sorbitol, and xylitol)
- bacterial toxins
- impaired electrolyte absorption
- increased gut wall permeability from gut inflammation: the gut becomes leaky and excess fluid is lost via the digestive tract
- ingestion of food that is osmotically active, but poorly digested (e.g. high-fiber diets)
- overstimulation of the parasympathetic nervous system
- reduced absorptive surface, as might occur secondary to parvovirus (transient) and secondary to gut resection (permanent).

Recall from earlier in this chapter that diarrhea can also be classified in terms of whether it originates from the small or large bowel.

Small bowel diarrhea tends to be produced in large quantities and is often associated with weight loss [12, 20, 24, 25]. Common causes of small bowel diarrhea in companion animal patients include, but are not limited to [12, 20, 24–26, 48–54]:

- dietary indiscretion
- enteritis
  - bacterial
  - parasitic
    - hookworms

■ protozoa
■ roundworms
■ tapeworms
○ viral
■ canine parvovirus type 1 (CPV-1, minute virus)
■ canine parvovirus type 2 (CPV-2)
■ coronavirus
■ feline immunodeficiency virus (FIV)
■ feline leukemia virus (FeLV)
■ feline panleukopenia virus, otherwise referred to as feline parvovirus
● EPI
● food allergy or intolerance
● hypoadrenocorticism
● hyperthyroidism
● pancreatitis
● portosystemic shunt
● protein-losing enteropathy (PLE)
○ inflammatory bowel disease (IBD)
○ intestinal neoplasia (e.g. lymphoma)
● small intestinal bacterial overgrowth (SIBO) as from malabsorptive small bowel disease.

Large bowel diarrhea tends to involve small quantities of semi-formed or gelatinous stool due to excessive mucus. The patient does not typically lose weight when diarrhea of this nature is chronic; however, the patient commonly exhibits increased frequency and urgency of defecation, with tenesmus and/or hematochezia.

Large bowel diarrhea may result from [12, 20, 31, 52, 55–57]:

● dietary indiscretion
● infectious colitis
○ *Campylobacter* spp.
○ *Clostridium* spp.
○ *Cryptosporidium* spp.
○ *Entamoeba histolytica*
○ *Escherichia coli*
○ *Giardia* spp.
○ *Histoplasma capsulatum*
○ *Salmonella* spp.
○ *Prototheca*
● endoparasitism
○ hookworms
○ *Tritrichomonas*
○ whipworms
● food allergy or intolerance
● histiocytic ulcerative colitis
● IBD
● neoplasia.

16.7.2 Fecal Color

Feces contain undigested material, bacteria, sloughed epithelial cells that line the lumen of the gut, and metabolic waste, including urobilinoids [12, 58, 59]. Urobilinoids are bile pigments that are formed when intestinal bacteria metabolize heme that is released from hemoglobin [59]. Heme is converted into biliverdin, which is converted into bilirubin [59]. Bilirubin is secreted into bile [59]. When bile enters the intestinal lumen, bilirubin is converted by intestinal bacteria into four main urobilioids: urobilinogen, urobilin, stercobilinogen, and stercobilin [59]. Whereas urobilinogen is primarily transported to the kidney for excretion in the urine, stercobilinogen and its oxidized form, stercobilin, are excreted in feces [59]. These two pigments are responsible for coloring normal feces a chocolate brown (see Figure 16.19).

Abnormal fecal color results from endogenous or exogenous pigments [12].

Fecal color may be disguised in the litterbox by cats who cover up their waste. However, fecal color is readily apparent among cats that exhibit aberrant elimination behaviors. Clients are quick to seek veterinary advice when cats eliminate outside of litterboxes, particularly if the fecal residue stains.

Fecal color is also easily identified by observant owners who leash-walk dogs and pick up after their dogs by collecting waste.

Because fecal discoloration is such a visible characteristic and because abnormal pigmentation can be associated with so many diseased states, it is critical that clinicians familiarize themselves with the many shades of feces [12] (see Table 16.1).

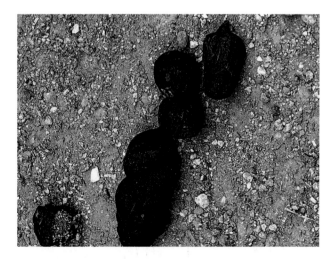

Figure 16.19 Canine fecal sample demonstrating normal color (brown). *Source:* Courtesy of Lisa Hallam, BS, CVT.

Table 16.1 The many shades of feces in cats and dogs and what each may be indicative of when identified during the macroscopic component of fecal analysis.

Color of feces	Possible explanation(s) for color	Accompanying photograph
White	Aged feces	See Figure 16.20
	Liquid barium passing through the digestive tract following oral administration for a radiographic contrast study.	
	High calcium diets (especially high calcium raw diets)	
	Hepatopathy	
	Bile duct obstruction	
Pale to light gray to clay-colored	When stool is pale to light gray, it is said to be acholic. Acholic feces most typically result from:	See Figure 16.21
	• bile duct obstruction	
	• exocrine pancreatic insufficiency (EPI) [12].	
	EPI is characterized by insufficient production of digestive enzymes by pancreatic acinar cells [12, 60]. Ingesta is not properly broken down into absorbable nutrients [12, 60]. The resultant stool may also appear greasy, because it contains excessive amounts of undigested fat [12, 20]. This end-product of digestion is referred to as steatorrhea [12].	
Yellow, yellow-orange, orange	Biliary disease	See Figures 16.22–16.24
	Hepatopathy	
	Reduced transit time through gastrointestinal tract	
Green, green-blue, blue	Eating excessive amounts of foliage that contains chlorophyll	See Figures 16.25–16.28
	Eating excessive amounts of green-colored treats (e.g. Greenies)	
	Biliary dysfunction	
	Rodenticide ingestion	
Brown	Normal	See Figure 16.19
Brown, but spotted with white/white speckled/polka dotted	• Tapeworm infestation, with proglottid segments visible	See Figures 16.29–16.31
Black	• Melena, as from an upper gastrointestinal bleed	See Figures 16.32–16.34
Red streaks	Hematochezia, as from a lower gastrointestinal bleed	See Figures 16.35–16.37
	Perianal or perineal bleeding, as from perianal fistulation	
Raspberry or strawberry jam	• Hemorrhagic gastroenteritis (HGE) [61, 62]	See Figures 16.38–16.40

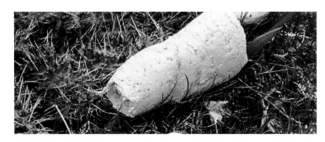

Figure 16.20 The color of this fecal sample (white) is attributed to the fact that these feces are aged. *Source:* Courtesy of Ryane E. Englar, DVM, DABVP (Canine and Feline Practice).

16.7.3 Presence/Absence of Blood

Evaluating feces for macroscopic evidence of blood is a useful feature because the presence or absence of blood and whether that blood appears to be fresh or digested helps to localize disease within the gastrointestinal tract [12].

Blood from esophageal lesions, the stomach, and/or the upper small bowel will undergo digestion [12]. This process causes the feces to appear dark and tarry [12]. The patient is said to exhibit melena [12] (see Figures 16.32–16.34).

On the other hand, streaks of fresh red blood in the feces are suggestive of colonic, rectal, or anal involvement [12] (see Figures 16.35–16.37).

Hemorrhagic gastroenteritis (HGE) is an extreme clinical condition in which affected dogs experience acute onset of severe bloody diarrhea and vomiting. Diarrhea is often explosive and voluminous. The consistency of the diarrhea is often likened to that of raspberry or strawberry jam due to the large numbers of clotted erythrocytes within the sample. These patients demonstrate superficial mucosal hemorrhagic necrosis of the intestines on histopathology of tissue samples. Patients very quickly develop

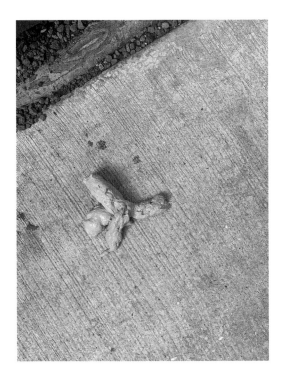

Figure 16.21 Acholic feces in a canine patient. *Source:* Courtesy of Dr. Lynda Perez.

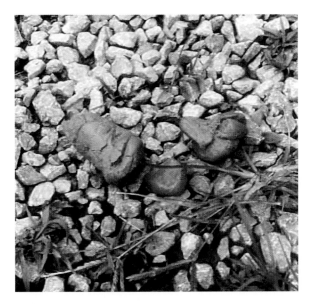

Figure 16.22 The color of this fecal sample is abnormal. The feces are yellow. *Source:* Courtesy of Ryane E. Englar, DVM, DABVP (Canine and Feline Practice).

hypovolemia and succumb to shock without rapid medical intervention.

16.7.4 Presence/Absence of Mucus

Mucus is naturally produced by goblet cells to lubricate the colon and facilitate passage of stool through the gut. Mucus

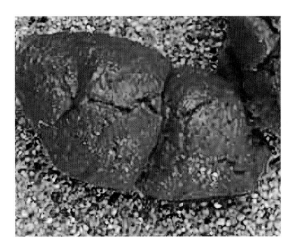

Figure 16.23 Orange feces in a canine patient. *Source:* Courtesy of Ryane E. Englar, DVM, DABVP (Canine and Feline Practice).

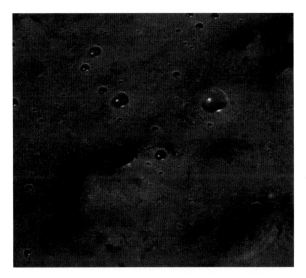

Figure 16.24 Deep orange diarrhea in a canine patient. *Source:* Courtesy of Ryane E. Englar, DVM, DABVP (Canine and Feline Practice).

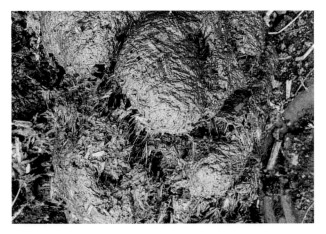

Figure 16.25 Stool from a horse to emphasize that the chlorophyll from a foliage-based diet produces stool that is pigmented green. *Source:* Courtesy of Ryane E. Englar, DVM, DABVP (Canine and Feline Practice).

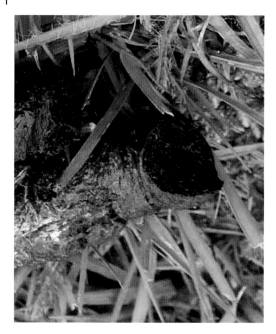

Figure 16.26 Green stool from a canine patient that ate excessive amounts of plant matter. *Source:* Courtesy of Ryane E. Englar, DVM, DABVP (Canine and Feline Practice).

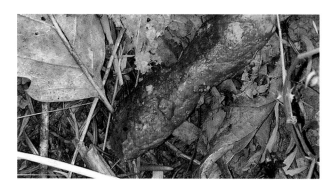

Figure 16.27 Green stool from a canine patient that ingested rodenticide. *Source:* Courtesy of Ryane E. Englar, DVM, DABVP (Canine and Feline Practice).

is clear and jelly-like; however, under normal circumstances, it mixes with the stool so as not to be readily apparent.

Patients that are experiencing colonic inflammation (colitis) may produce excessive amounts of mucus that coats their stool (see Figures 16.41 and 16.42).

Excessive mucus may envelop the stool, taking on the appearance of a sausage casing (see Figure 16.43).

Excessive mucus may be secondary to endoparasitism (e.g. whipworm infestation) or metabolic dysfunction (e.g. EPI ± SIBO).

16.7.5 Gross Parasitism

The majority of endoparasites will not be detected until the microscopic portion of fecal analysis because that

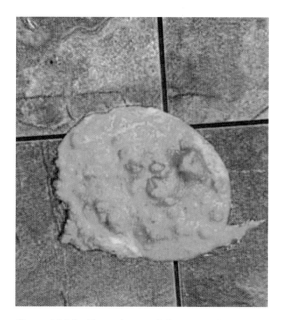

Figure 16.28 Turquoise vomit from a canine patient that had ingested rodenticide. This photograph serves as a reminder that if a patient presents with a history of ingesting rodenticide within two hours of the appointment, induce emesis to reduce the amount of poison that is absorbed by the body. By the time rodenticide is metabolized and appears in the stool, as in Figure 16.27, the patient has already been exposed to and is likely to be experiencing ill effects. *Source:* Courtesy of Ryane E. Englar, DVM, DABVP (Canine and Feline Practice).

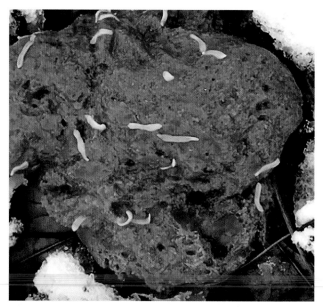

Figure 16.29 Stool of pudding-like consistency dotted with proglottid segments from a tapeworm. *Source:* Courtesy of Michelle Lugones, DVM.

technique allows us to visualize ova [19]. However, some parasites or portions of parasites are visible with the naked eye [19]. The most common of these that we can appreciate

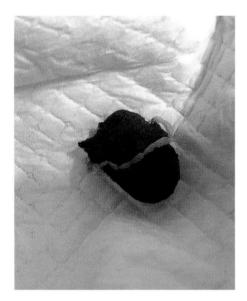

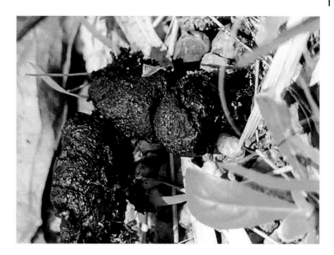

Figure 16.32 Example of melena produced by a canine patient. This stool is solid. This stool was produced by a patient to whom activated charcoal had been administered per os as medical management to treat toxicosis. *Source:* Courtesy of Ryane E. Englar, DVM, DABVP (Canine and Feline Practice).

Figure 16.30 Solid, formed stool that contains a ribbon of proglottid segments. *Source:* Courtesy of Michelle Lugones, DVM.

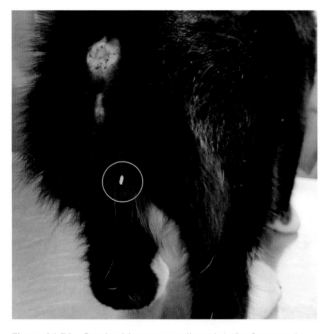

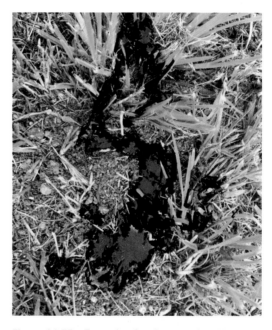

Figure 16.31 Proglottid segment adhered to the fur near the perineum of a feline patient. This photograph serves as a reminder that a comprehensive physical examination can augment findings from fecal analysis. *Source:* Courtesy of Michelle Lugones, DVM.

Figure 16.33 Example of melena produced by a canine patient. *Source:* Courtesy of Beki Regan Cohen, DVM.

on gross inspection of feces are tapeworms and adult roundworms [19].

Tapeworms are parasitic flatworms or cestodes [8, 12]. The most common tapeworms that we see in dogs and cats are *Dipylidium caninum and Taenia* spp. [12, 52] Recall that fleas are vectors of *Dipylidium caninum* [12, 13, 63–75],

whereas *Taenia* spp. cause disease when hosts ingest infected rodents or hares [8, 12].

Adult tapeworms attach themselves to small intestinal walls of their host [12]. As they mature, eggs are produced and stored within terminal segments known as proglottids [12]. Each proglottid contains egg capsules or packets of roughly 5–30 ova [8, 12] (see Figure 16.44).

Once a proglottid is full of eggs, it detaches to be shed in the host's feces [12]. Proglottids are visible to the naked

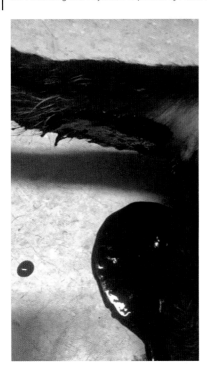

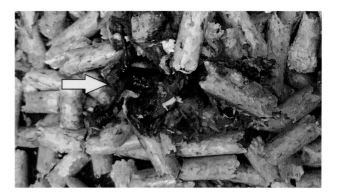

Figure 16.36 Example of hematochezia from a feline patient. *Source:* Courtesy of Ryane E. Englar, DVM, DABVP (Canine and Feline Practice).

Figure 16.34 Example of melena that has just been passed by a laterally recumbent patient. Only the patient's tail is visible in this photograph. *Source:* Courtesy of Chloe Bush.

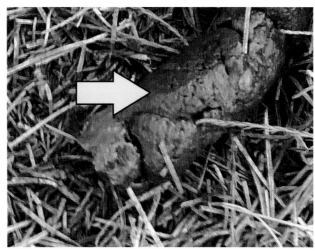

Figure 16.37 Example of hematochezia from a canine patient. Note that the stool is solid and formed, but there is a hint of red discoloration along its surface. *Source:* Courtesy of Ryane E. Englar, DVM, DABVP (Canine and Feline Practice).

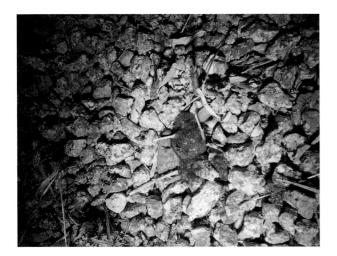

Figure 16.35 Example of canine diarrhea. Note the presence of a few fresh drops of blood dotting the surface of the sample. *Source:* Courtesy of Lisa Hallam, BS, CVT.

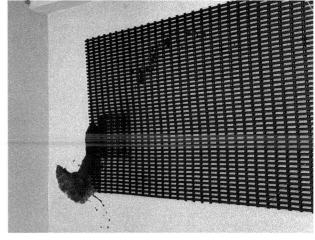

Figure 16.38 A sample from a canine patient with hemorrhagic gastroenteritis (HGE). *Source:* Courtesy of Ryane E. Englar, DVM, DABVP (Canine and Feline Practice).

eye [12]. They have been likened to grains of white rice or cucumber seeds [8, 12, 76] (see Figures 16.45–16.47).

Roundworms are a different type of endoparasite. Sometimes they are referred to as ascarids, a type of zoonotic helminth [6–8, 12]. Roundworms are present in the soil [12]. Eggs can be ingested if/when dogs and cats ingest dirt [12]. Pups may also become infected through the placenta [12]. In addition, both pups and kittens can

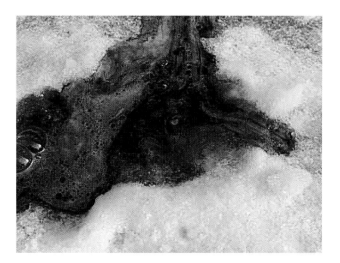

Figure 16.39 A sample from a canine patient with hemorrhagic gastroenteritis (HGE). *Source:* Courtesy of Ryane E. Englar, DVM, DABVP (Canine and Feline Practice).

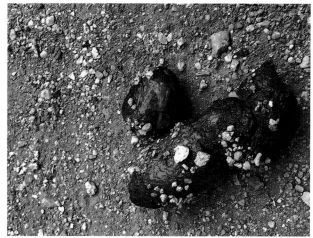

Figure 16.41 Canine feces with a slime-like coating of mucus. *Source:* Courtesy of Lisa Hallam, BS, CVT.

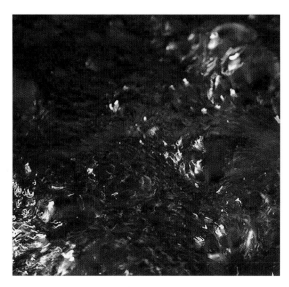

Figure 16.40 A sample from a canine patient with hemorrhagic gastroenteritis (HGE). *Source:* Courtesy of Ryane E. Englar, DVM, DABVP (Canine and Feline Practice).

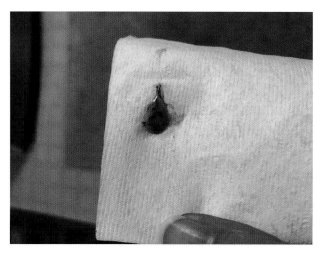

Figure 16.42 A sample of fecal mucus from a feline patient. This mucus is tinged red. This patient had concurrent hematochezia. *Source:* Courtesy of Tim Gregory.

develop ascariasis by ingesting infected milk [6–8]. Because of vertical transmission, puppies and kittens are assumed to have roundworms at and shortly after birth, and prophylactic deworming is considered routine [6–8, 12, 77].

Clinically important roundworms in dogs and cats include [6–8, 12]:

o *Toxocara canis*
o *Toxocara cati*
o *Toxocara leonina*.

Affected patients present with a characteristically round or prominent belly [12]. They may experience poor weight

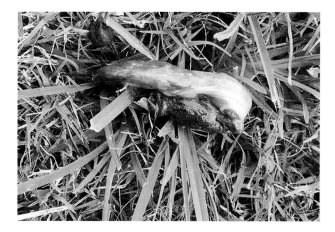

Figure 16.43 Appreciable mucus coating a canine fecal sample. *Source:* Courtesy of Ryane E. Englar, DVM, DABVP (Canine and Feline Practice).

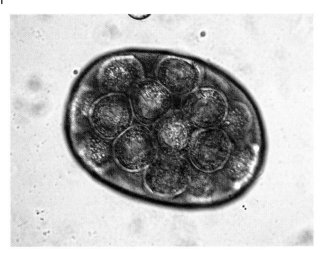

Figure 16.44 *Dipylidium caninum* egg packet, 20×. *Source:* Courtesy of Dr. Araceli Lucio-Forster, Cornell University College of Veterinary Medicine.

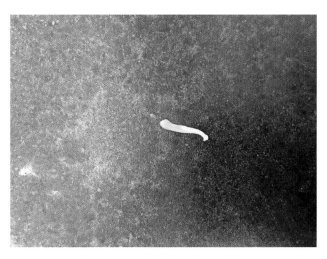

Figure 16.46 *Dipylidium caninum* proglottid. *Source:* Courtesy of Sarah Bashaw, DVM.

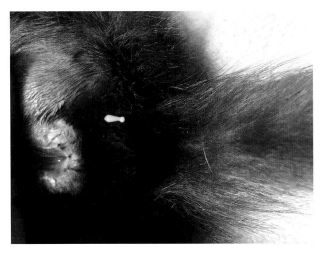

Figure 16.45 *Dipylidium caninum* proglottid, grossly visible to the naked eye as it scoots across the perineal fur of this canine patient. *Source:* Courtesy of Frank Isom, DVM.

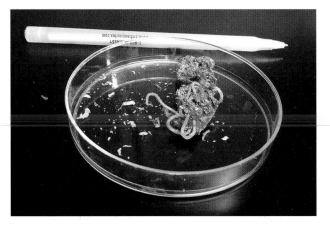

Figure 16.47 *Dipylidium caninum* proglottids. *Source:* Courtesy of Daria Turchenkova.

gain and stunted growth [12]. Sometimes, on account of this, affected patients are described as unthrifty. They may develop dull coats, vomiting, and/or diarrhea.

Although diagnosis is typically via the detection of ova through fecal flotation, gross observation of adult roundworms in the feces or vomitus is possible (see Figures 16.48 and 16.49).

16.7.6 Odor

Fecal odor is derived from the degradation of endogenous and undigested proteins by gastrointestinal flora [78]. This process yields ammonia, aliphatic amines, branched chain fatty acids, indoles, phenols, and volatile sulfur-containing

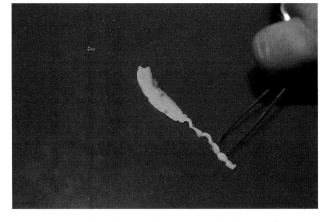

Figure 16.48 Adult *Toxocara cati* in a stool sample. *Source:* Courtesy of Dr. Araceli Lucio-Forster, Cornell University College of Veterinary Medicine.

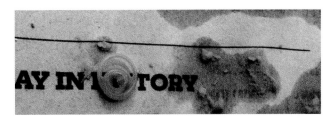

Figure 16.49 Adult roundworm in vomitus. *Source:* Courtesy of Ryane E. Englar, DVM, DABVP (Canine and Feline Practice).

compounds [78]. Feline feces contain 3-mercapto-3-methyl-1-butanol (MMB) [79]. This is similar to the sulfur-containing amino acid, felinine, in feline urine that is thought to play a role in territory-marking [79]. Feces from male cats contain greater levels of MMB than female cats [79]. Canine feces lack this sulfurous compound [79]. This could explain why feline feces often smells more pungent than canine feces [79]. This is considered normal.

What we are looking for when we appreciate the odor profile of a patient's fecal sample is a distinct change. For instance, samples from patients infected with canine parvovirus often smell metallic. This is attributed to the iron-containing heme groups in the blood that is sloughed into the lumen of the digestive tract of dogs with parvovirus.

If we smell something that is atypical and/or prompts pattern recognition, then we need to factor that into the diagnostic process.

16.8 Clinical Case Example(s)

- A 10-year-old castrated male toy poodle dog is presented for evaluation of acute onset of "dark" stool. The client initially reports that the patient has been "slowing down" but describes the patient as otherwise "healthy." Prior to taking a detailed patient history, you perform fecal analysis. On gross inspection, the patient's stool is tarry. You recall that melena is indicative of upper gastrointestinal bleeds, but that you have not prescribed the common offenders, nonsteroidal anti-inflammatory (NSAID) drugs. You ask the client if they have been administering any over-the-counter medications. The client discloses that they began administering 200 mg of ibuprofen twice daily for presumptive osteoarthritis. You attribute the patient's melena to NSAID administration. Although ibuprofen produces the desired clinical effect of reduced pain associated with osteoarthritis by decreasing prostaglandin synthesis, it also interferes with the protective capacity of the gastrointestinal mucosa.

- A two-year-old female spayed Akita dog is presented for evaluation of a three-month history of unintentional weight loss and diarrhea. During history-taking, the client reports that the patient's diarrhea is voluminous and pale in color, and rancid in odor. The client is particularly distressed because they are being asked by neighbors why they are not feeding the dog enough, but they report that the dog has a "hearty appetite" and "eats everything" they put in front of her. Physical examination findings are consistent with an underweight dog: the patient has a BCS of 3/9. The remainder of the exam is unremarkable. You examine a stool sample that the client brought to the consultation. The feces are acholic. Based upon the history, physical exam findings, and observations about the gross fecal appearance, you prioritize EPI as a differential diagnosis. Hypoadrenocorticism could not be ruled out. Blood was submitted for complete blood count (CBC), serum biochemistry, serum cobalamin, folate, canine trypsin-like immunoreactivity (cTLI), and baseline cortisol. The patient's low cTLI was confirmatory for EPI.

16.9 Add-On Tests That You May Need to Consider and Their Additive Value

Gross observation of a patient's stool sample is merely the first step of fecal analysis. Following gross observation, you should proceed with microscopic assessment. This may include:

- direct smear/fecal cytology/wet mount (see Chapter 17)
- fecal flotation (see Chapter 18)
- fecal culture
- Baermann technique.

Fecal analysis is often paired with bloodwork and urinalysis to screen for occult disease in healthy patients or to further characterize overt clinical illness:

- A CBC is particularly useful in cases that involve apparent hematochezia or melena as a means of quantifying blood loss. In other words, is the patient anemic?
- Many values within a chemistry panel are influenced by the patient's ability to metabolize ingesta. Interpretation of these values in the context of the patient's fecal analysis results guides the diagnostic process. For example, feces that are orange in color point us in the direction of biliary disease or hepatopathy. A serum biochemistry panel will evaluate liver function. For instance, injury to hepatocytes causes the release of cellular enzyme alanine aminotransferase (ALT). Increased ALT is nonspecific; however, this elevation may prompt us to investigate any of the following clinical conditions:
  - infectious disease (e.g. leptospirosis)
  - metabolic disease (e.g. Cushing's disease)

○ neoplasia
○ toxicity (e.g. corticosteroids, phenobarbital, NSAIDs)
• Findings from urinalysis may provide additional clues. For instance, patients with cholestatic liver disease are likely to demonstrate bilirubinuria. This change in urine pigmentation is often concurrent with changes in fecal color.

Puppies and unvaccinated adult dogs that present for acute fever, vomiting, and/or bloody diarrhea should be tested for parvovirus via in-house fecal ELISA antigen testing [12, 52, 80]. This test offers rapid turnaround time and is practical in the clinic setting [12, 52, 80] (see Figures 16.50–16.56).

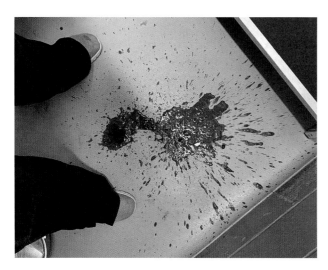

Figure 16.50 Bloody diarrhea from a patient with presumptive parvovirus. *Source:* Courtesy of Rachel Sahrbeck, DVM.

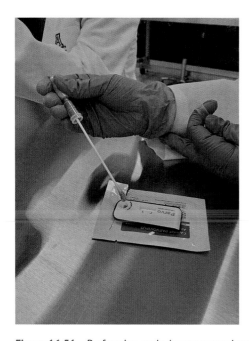

Figure 16.51 Performing an in-house parvovirus fecal ELISA antigen test. *Source:* Courtesy of Simone Conwell.

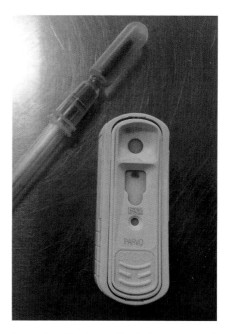

Figure 16.52 A negative in-house parvovirus fecal ELISA antigen test. The blue dot at the top of the display represents the positive control. *Source:* Courtesy of Ryane E. Englar, DVM, DABVP (Canine and Feline Practice).

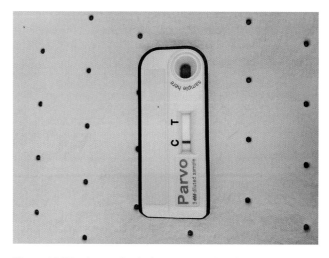

Figure 16.53 A negative in-house parvovirus fecal ELISA antigen test. *Source:* Courtesy of Ryane E. Englar, DVM, DABVP (Canine and Feline Practice). Note the absence of a band at the "T" marker. The "C" marker represents the control.

Canine parvovirus (CPV) is a nonenveloped, DNA virus that replicates within rapidly dividing cells, such as the gut [12, 80]. CPV-2 causes canine parvoviral enteritis [80]. In its original form, it only affected dogs [12, 80]. However, newer strains 2a and 2b are capable of infecting cats [12, 80].

Unvaccinated dogs and pups that have not yet developed protective antibody titers are most are risk [12, 52, 80]. There also appears to be a breed predisposition for CPV-2 among Rottweilers, Doberman Pinschers, Labrador

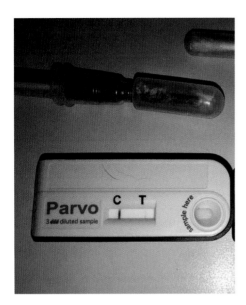

Figure 16.54 A faint-positive in-house parvovirus fecal ELISA antigen test. Note the faint band at the "T" marker. The "C" marker represents the control. *Source:* Courtesy of Ryane E. Englar, DVM, DABVP (Canine and Feline Practice).

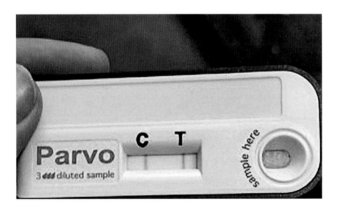

Figure 16.55 A positive in-house parvovirus fecal ELISA antigen test. Note the band at the "T" marker. The "C" marker represents the control. *Source:* Courtesy of Ryane E. Englar, DVM, DABVP (Canine and Feline Practice).

retrievers, German Shepherds, and Staffordshire terriers [12, 52, 80, 82].

At the microscopic level, CPV-2 causes lymphocytolysis and resultant leukopenia, neutropenia, and lymphopenia [12, 52]. Blood loss in stool causes anemia, and malabsorptive syndrome secondary to small intestinal villi destruction leads to hypoproteinemia [12, 52]. Rapid loss of fluid through the gastrointestinal tract leads to life-threatening dehydration [12, 52, 80]. Patients may become septic [12]. Intestinal intussusception is possible [12, 52, 80].

Note that kittens and young adult, nonvaccinated cats may also develop parvovirus [12]. Clinically, this condition is referred to as feline panleukopenia [12, 83]. Feline

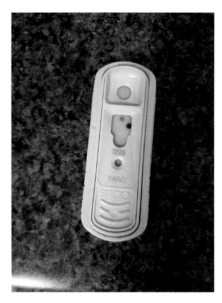

Figure 16.56 A positive in-house parvovirus fecal ELISA antigen test. The blue dot at the top of the display represents the positive control. Note the additional blue dot along the righthand side of the display. This is supportive of a diagnosis of parvovirus. Note, however, that false positives may occur 5–15 days after vaccination with a modified live virus (MLV) [12, 52, 80, 81]. *Source:* Courtesy of Ryane E. Englar, DVM, DABVP (Canine and Feline Practice).

panleukopenia is extraordinarily stable in the environment and is therefore spread most often by indirect contact [12, 83].

Many cases of feline panleukopenia are subclinical [12, 83]. However, clinical disease does occur and preferentially targets the gut [12, 83]. Affected kittens present for evaluation of anorexia, depression, and fever [12, 83]. Vomiting is more likely to be seen than diarrhea; however, diarrheic presentations are possible [12, 83].

On physical examination, patients are markedly dehydrated with palpably thickened loops of intestines [12, 83].

Diagnosis is possible via in-house fecal testing using the ELISA for CPV antigen [52, 80]. This test offers rapid turnaround time and is practical in the clinic setting [52, 80].

16.10 Key Takeaways

- Fecal analysis is incomplete unless observable and olfactory features of patient samples are examined. These include fecal consistency, color, presence/absence of blood and/or mucus, gross parasitism, and odor.
- Observable and olfactory features alone are not pathognomonic for disease; however, they provide clues that guide the diagnostic plan. For instance, black feces should prompt the clinician to consider upper gastrointestinal

bleeds as a differential diagnosis whereas hematochezia should prompt the clinician to consider lower gastrointestinal bleeds.

- To maximize accuracy, fecal samples should be analyzed within two hours of collection. If they cannot be analyzed expediently, then fecal samples should be refrigerated to slow down sample degradation [19, 21]. *in vitro* changes can and will occur in unpreserved feces that are stored at room temperature.
- Refrigerated samples should not be analyzed beyond 24 hours after collection.

16.11 Clinical Pearls

- If your practice sends clients appointment reminders via telephone, text, or email, include instructions to bring in a fresh fecal sample and why doing so is essential.
- Incorporate fecal exams into your annual wellness plan to improve compliance.
- Incorporate year-round, broad-spectrum parasite prevention into your annual wellness plan to protect against endoparasitism (e.g. intestinal parasites) and ectoparasites (e.g. fleas and ticks).
- Do not run a fecal analysis without taking a patient history. History-taking remains one of the most important tools in diagnostic medicine and it is dirt cheap! Approximately two-thirds of diagnoses in human healthcare can be made based upon the patient's history alone [84]. The patient history-taking is likely to play a greater role in veterinary medicine because details about our patient's health must be relayed to us through observant clients. The clients have the answers we need, but it is up to us to actively solicit their perspective and consider what they share.
- Ask owners of diarrheic patients about their appetite.
- Ask owners of diarrheic patients about weight loss. If present, was the weight loss unintended?
- Ask owners of diarrheic patients about fecal volume, mucus, frequency of defecation, urgency to defecate, and whether the patient is exhibiting tenesmus. This should help to localize the diarrhea to either the small or large bowel.
- Confirm vaccination status of diarrheic patients, particularly those presenting with bloody fecal samples.
- Consider in-house fecal antigen testing for canine parvovirus (CPV-2) in diarrheic canine patients, particularly if they are unvaccinated and experiencing bloody stool.
- False positives for in-house fecal antigen testing for CPV-2 may occur 5–15 days after vaccination with a MLV [12, 52, 80, 81].

- Feline patients with the presumptive diagnosis of panleukopenia may be tested using in-house fecal antigen tests for CPV-2.
- Examine the whole patient.
  - ○ Assess the coat for quality and texture. Dry, dull coats often accompany endoparasitism.
  - ○ Assess the coat for evidence of flea dirt (see Figure 16.57). Recall that fleas may be associated with concurrent *Dipylidium caninum* (tapeworm) infestation.
  - ○ Assess the perineum for proglottids (see Figures 16.31 and 16.45).
  - ○ Assess the patient's mucous membranes. Patients are likely to be pale in certain cases of ectoparasite (e.g. flea) and endoparasite (e.g. hookworm) infestation (see Figures 16.58 and 16.59).
  - ○ Perform a rectal examination and examine any residue that adheres to your gloved finger. You may be able to identify streaks of fresh red blood or the dark tar that is associated with melena.
- Physically sift through fecal samples. It is like a treasure hunt! You never know what you may find! (See Figures 16.60 and 16.61.)
- Any amount of fecal material is still worth examining. One drop of liquid feces is still more than you had before.
- Do not get hung up if the fecal sample is older than ideal. Test it anyway.
- Do not get hung up if the fecal sample was not refrigerated overnight. Test it anyway.

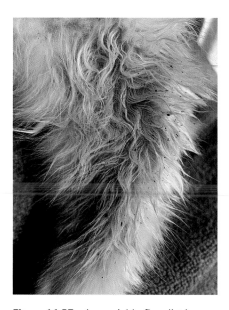

Figure 16.57 Appreciable flea dirt in a seven-month-old kitten. *Source:* Courtesy of Jackie Kucskar, DVM.

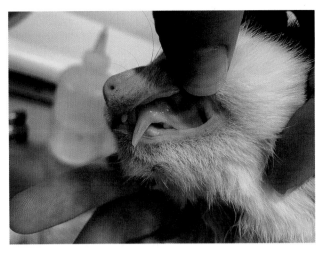

Figure 16.58 Pale oral mucosa in a seven-month-old kitten with severe flea infestation. This kitten had a packed cell volume of 17%. *Source:* Courtesy of Jackie Kucskar, DVM.

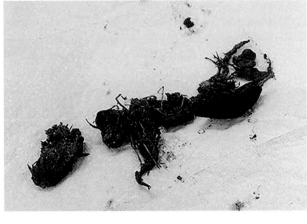

Figure 16.60 Dissected fecal matter. Note that this sample contains an appreciable amount of grass and straw. *Source:* Courtesy of Ryane E. Englar, DVM, DABVP (Canine and Feline Practice).

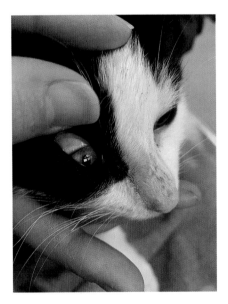

Figure 16.59 Pale conjunctiva in a seven-month-old kitten with severe flea infestation. This kitten had a packed cell volume of 17%. *Source:* Courtesy of Jackie Kucskar, DVM.

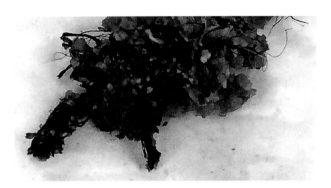

Figure 16.61 This rope toy was extracted from a fecal sample. The presence of this rope toy suggested that this patient had a tendency for pica. Diagnostic imaging confirmed additional foreign bodies that had been ingested, including rocks that required surgical extraction via gastrotomy. *Source:* Courtesy of Ryane E. Englar, DVM, DABVP (Canine and Feline Practice).

- Abnormal fecal color indicates pathology; however, it is nonspecific. In addition, pathology may exist in a fecal sample that is normal in color. Therefore, fecal color is just one of many clues. It is not intended to be used as a stand-alone diagnostic test.
- If fecal color is abnormal, ask questions about:
  - access to toxins (e.g. rodenticide)
  - diet (including snacks)
  - foreign body ingestion (pica)
  - medication (including over-the-counter vitamins and supplements)

References

1 Broussard, J.D. (2003). Optimal fecal assessment. *Clinical Techniques in Small Animal Practice* 18 (4): 218–230.

2 Foreyt, W.J. (1989). Diagnostic parasitology. *The Veterinary Clinics of North America Small Animal Practice* 19 (5): 979–1000.

3 Samples, O.M. (2013(July/August)). Diagnosis of Internal Parasites. *Today's Veterinary Practice* 21–26.

4 Sobotyk, C., Upton, K.E., Lejeune, M. et al. (2021). Retrospective study of canine endoparasites diagnosed by fecal flotation methods analyzed across veterinary

parasitology diagnostic laboratories, United States, 2018. *Parasites & Vectors* 14 (1): 439.

5 Stafford, K., Kollasch, T.M., Duncan, K.T. et al. (2020). Detection of gastrointestinal parasitism at recreational canine sites in the USA: the DOGPARCS study. *Parasites & Vectors* 13 (1): 275.

6 Guidelines for Veterinarians: Prevention of Zoonotic Transmission of Ascarids and Hookworms. https://www. cdc.gov/parasites/zoonotichookworm/resources/ prevention.pdf.

7 Schantz, P.M. (2007). Zoonotic parasitic infections contracted from dogs and cats: How frequent are they? DVM 360 [Internet]. http://veterinarymedicine.dvm360. com/zoonotic-parasitic-infections-contracted-dogs- and-cats-how-frequent-are-they.

8 Bowman, D.D. and Georgi, J.R. (2009). *Georgis' Parasitology for Veterinarians*, 9e. St. Louis, MO: Saunders/Elsevier ix, 451 pp.

9 Schantz, P.M. (2004). Larva migrans syndromes caused by Toxocara species and other helminths. In: *Infectious Diseases* (ed. S.L. Gorbach, J.G. Bartlett and N.R. Blacklow), 1529–1535. Philadelphia: WB Saunders.

10 Glickman, L.T. and Schantz, P.M. (1982). Epidemiology and pathogenesis of zoonotic toxocariasis. *Epidemiologic Reviews* 3: 230–250.

11 Schantz, P.M. (1989). Toxocara larva migrans now. *The American Journal of Tropical Medicine and Hygiene* 41: 21–34.

12 Englar, R.E. (2019). Changes in fecal appearance. In: *Common Clinical Presentations in Dogs and Cats* (ed. R.E. Englar), 647–670. Hoboken, NJ: Wiley-Blackwell.

13 Traversa, D. (2013). Fleas infesting pets in the era of emerging extra-intestinal nematodes. *Parasites & Vectors* 6: 59.

14 Dobler, G. and Pfeffer, M. (2011). Fleas as parasites of the family Canidae. *Parasites & Vectors* 4: 139.

15 Kramer, F. and Mencke, N. (2001). *Flea Biology and Control*. Berlin, Germany: Springer-Verlag Berlin and Heidelberg GmbH & Co.

16 General Guidelines for Dogs and Cats: Companion Animal Parasite Council (CAPC). (2020). https://capcvet. org/guidelines/general-guidelines.

17 Radosta, L. (2015). Coprophagia. NAVC Clinician's Brief [Internet].

18 Englar, R.E. (2019). Abnormal ingestive behaviors. In: *Common Clinical Presentations in Dogs and Cats* (ed. R.E. Englar), 611–616. Hoboken, NJ: Wiley-Blackwell.

19 Hendrix, C.M. and Robinson, E. (2017). Common laboratory procedures for diagnosing parasitism. In: *Diagnostic Parasitology for Veterinary Technicians*, 5e (ed. C.M. Hendrix and E. Robinson), 303–335. St. Louis, Missouri: Elsevier Inc.

20 Greco, D.S. Diagnosis and Dietary Management of Gastrointestinal Disease: Purina Veterinary Diets. https:// www.purinaproplanvets.com/media/1202/gi_quick_ reference_guide.pdf.

21 Foreyt, B. (2001). *Veterinary Parasitology Reference Manual*, 5e. Ames, Iowa: Iowa State University Press viii, 235 pp.

22 Englar, R.E. (2021). The dog that is straining to defecate. In: *The Veterinary Workbook of Small Animal Clinical Cases* (ed. R.E. Englar). Essex, U.K.: 5m Publishing.

23 Englar, R.E. (2021). The adult diarrheic dog. In: *The Veterinary Workbook of Small Animal Clinical Cases* (ed. R.E. Englar). Essex, U.K.: 5m Publishing.

24 Englar, R.E. (2017). *Performing the Small Animal Physical Examination*. Hoboken, NJ: Wiley Pp. 128–131, 353–355.

25 Gaschen, F. (2006). Small intestinal diarrhea - causes and treatment. WSAVA World Congress.

26 Allenspach, K. (2013). Diagnosis of small intestinal disorders in dogs and cats. *The Veterinary Clinics of North America Small Animal Practice* 43 (6): 1227–1240. v.

27 Englar, R.E. (2019). *Common Clinical Presentations in Dogs and Cats*. Hoboken, NJ: Wiley-Blackwell pages cm p.

28 Englar, R.E. (2017). Assessing the big picture: the body, the coat, and the skin of the dog. In: *Performing the Small Animal Physical Examination* (ed. R.E. Englar), 213–260. Hoboken, NJ: Wiley/Blackwell.

29 Burkholder, W.J. (2000). Use of body condition scores in clinical assessment of the provision of optimal nutrition. *Journal of the American Veterinary Medical Association* 217: 650–654.

30 Gant, P., Holden, S.L., Biourge, V., and German, A.J. (2016). Can you estimate body composition in dogs from photographs? *BMC Veterinary Research* 12: 18.

31 Tilley, L.P. and Smith, F.W.K. (2004). *The 5-Minute Veterinary Consult : Canine and Feline*, 3e. Baltimore, MD: Lippincott Williams & Wilkins lviii, 1487 pp.

32 Rothuizen, J., Schrauwen, E., Theyse, L.F.H., and Verhaert, L. (2009). Digestive tract. In: *Medical History and Physical Examination in Companion Animals* (ed. A. Rijnberk and F.J. van Sluijs), 86–100. Philadelphia: Elsevier, Ltd.

33 Trevail, T., Gunn-Moore, D., Carrera, I. et al. (2011). Radiographic diameter of the colon in normal and constipated cats and in cats with megacolon. *Veterinary Radiology & Ultrasound* 52 (5): 516–520.

34 Washabau, R. (2001). Feline Constipation, Obstipation, and Megacolon: Prevention, Diagnosis, and Treatment. World Small Animal Veterinary Association World Congress [Internet]. https://www.vin.com/VINDBPub/ SearchPB/Proceedings/PR05000/PR00118.htm.

35 Washabau, R. (1997). Constipation, obstipation, and megacolon. In: *Consultations in Feline Internal Medicine*, 3e (ed. J.R. August), 104–112. Philadelphia: Saunders.

36 Bredal, W.P., Thoresen, S.I., and Kvellestad, A. (1994). Atresia-coli in a 9-week-old kitten. *The Journal of Small Animal Practice* 35 (12): 643–645.

37 Vandenbroek, A.H.M., Else, R.W., and Hunter, M.S. (1988). Atresia Ani and Urethrorectal Fistula in a Kitten. *The Journal of Small Animal Practice* 29 (2): 91–94.

38 Yam, P. (1997). Decision making in the management of constipation in the cat. *In Practice* 19 (8): 434–440.

39 Hudson, E.B., Farrow, C.S., and Smith, S.L. (1979). Acquired megacolon in a cat. *Modern Veterinary Practice* 60 (8): 625–627.

40 Washabau, R. and Holt, D. (2000). Feline constipation and idiopathic megacolon. In: *Kirk's Current Veterinary Therapy*, 13e (ed. J.D. Bonagura), 648–652. Philadelphia: WB Saunders.

41 Freiche, V., Houston, D., Weese, H. et al. (2011). Uncontrolled study assessing the impact of a psyllium-enriched extruded dry diet on faecal consistency in cats with constipation. *Journal of Feline Medicine and Surgery* 13 (12): 903–911.

42 Jones, B.D. (2000). Constipation, tenesmus, dyschezia, and faecal incontinence. In: *Textbook of Veterinary Internal Medicine* (ed. S.J. Ettinger and E.C. Feldman), 129–135. Philadelphia: Saunders.

43 White, R.N. (2002). Surgical management of constipation. *Journal of Feline Medicine and Surgery* 4 (3): 129–138.

44 Scherk, M. (2003). Feline megacolon. World Small Animal Veterinary Association World Congress [Internet]. https://www.vin.com/apputil/content/defaultadv1.aspx?pId=8768&meta=generic&id=3850188&print=1.

45 Rosin, E., Walshaw, R., Mehlhaff, C. et al. (1988). Subtotal colectomy for treatment of chronic constipation associated with idiopathic megacolon in cats: 38 cases (1979-1985). *Journal of the American Veterinary Medical Association* 193 (7): 850–853.

46 Schiller, L.R. (1999). Secretory diarrhea. *Current Gastroenterology Reports* 1 (5): 389–397.

47 Thiagarajah, J.R., Donowitz, M., and Verkman, A.S. (2015). Secretory diarrhoea: mechanisms and emerging therapies. *Nature Reviews. Gastroenterology & Hepatology* 12 (8): 446–457.

48 Marks, S.L. and Kather, E.J. (2003). Bacterial-associated diarrhea in the dog: a critical appraisal. *The Veterinary Clinics of North America Small Animal Practice* 33 (5): 1029–1060.

49 Greene, C.E. (1998). Enteric bacterial infections. In: *Infectious Diseases of the Dog and Cat* (ed. C.E. Greene), 243–245. St. Louis, MO: Saunders/Elsevier.

50 Cave, N.J., Marks, S.L., Kass, P.H. et al. (2002). Evaluation of a routine diagnostic fecal panel for dogs with diarrhea. *Journal of the American Veterinary Medical Association* 221 (1): 52–59.

51 Guilford, W.G. and Strombeck, D.R. (1996). Gastrointestinal tract infections, parasites, and toxicosis. In: *Stromback's Small Animal Gastroenterology*, 3e (ed. W.G. Guilford and S.A. Center), 411–432. Philadelphia: W.B. Saunders.

52 Magne, M.L. (2006). Selected topics in pediatric gastroenterology. *The Veterinary Clinics of North America. Small Animal Practice* 36 (3): 533–548, vi.

53 Matz, M.E. (2006). Chronic diarrhea in a dog. *NAVC Clinician's Brief* (April): 75–77.

54 Sokolow, S.H., Rand, C., Marks, S.L. et al. (2005). Epidemiologic evaluation of diarrhea in dogs in an animal shelter. *American Journal of Veterinary Research* 66 (6): 1018–1024.

55 Zajac, A.M. (2003). A case of canine diarrhea. *NAVC Clinician's Brief* (April): 13–14.

56 German, A.J. (2006). Large bowel diarrhea. *NAVC Clinician's Brief* (February): 54–55.

57 Lecoindre, P. and Gaschen, F.P. (2011). Chronic idiopathic large bowel diarrhea in the dog. *The Veterinary Clinics of North America. Small Animal Practice* 41 (2): 447–456.

58 Argenzio, R.B. (2004). Digestive and absorptive functions of the intestines. In: *Dukes' Physiology of Domestic Animals*, 12e (ed. H.H. Dukes and W.O. Reece). Ithaca: Comstock Pub. Associates p. xiv, 999 p.

59 Sanada, S., Suzuki, T., Nagata, A. et al. (2020). Intestinal microbial metabolite stercobilin involvement in the chronic inflammation of ob/ob mice. *Scientific Reports* 10 (1): 6479.

60 Morgan, J.A. and Moore, L.E. (2009). A quick review of canine exocrine pancreatic insufficiency. DVM360 [Internet]. http://veterinarymedicine.dvm360.com/quick-review-canine-exocrine-pancreatic-insufficiency.

61 Triolo, A. and Lappin, M.R. (2003). Acute medical diseases of the small intestine. In: *Handbook of Small Animal Gastroenterology*, 2e (ed. T.R. Tams). St. Louis, MO: Saunders.

62 Klaus, J. (2017). Gastrointestinal system motility and integrity. In: *Monitoring and Intervention for the Critically Ill Small Animal: The Rule of 20* (ed. R. Kirby and A.K.J. Linklater). Ames, Iowa, USA: Wiley-Blackwell.

63 Blagburn, B.L. and Dryden, M.W. (2009). Biology, treatment, and control of flea and tick infestations. *The Veterinary Clinics of North America Small Animal Practice* 39 (6): 1173–1200.

64 Dryden, M.W. and Rust, M.K. (1994). The cat flea - biology, ecology and control. *Veterinary Parasitology* 52 (1–2): 1–19.

65 Rust, M.K. and Dryden, M.W. (1997). The biology, ecology, and management of the cat flea. *Annual Review of Entomology* 42: 451–473.

66 Flick, S.C. (1973). Endoparasites in cats: current practice and opinions. *Feline Practice* 4: 21–34.

67 Hitchcock, D.J. (1953). Incidence of gastro-intestinal parasites in some Michigan kittens. *North American Veterinarian* 34: 428–429.

68 Arundel, J.H. (1970). Control of helminth parasites of dogs and cats. *Australian Veterinary Journal* 46 (4): 164–168.

69 Baker, M.K., Lange, L., Verster, A., and van der Plaat, S. (1989). A survey of helminths in domestic cats in the Pretoria area of Transvaal, Republic of South Africa. Part 1: the prevalence and comparison of burdens of helminths in adult and juvenile cats. *Journal of the South African Veterinary Association* 60 (3): 139–142.

70 Boreham, R.E. and Boreham, P.F.L. (1990). Dipylidium-Caninum - life-cycle, epizootiology, and control. *Compendium on Continuing Education for The Practicing Veterinarian* 12 (5): 667–671.

71 Collins, G.H. (1973). A limited survey of gastro-intestinal helminths of dogs and cats. *New Zealand Veterinary Journal* 21 (8): 175–176.

72 Coman, B.J. (1972). A survey of the gastro-intestinal parasites of the feral cat in Victoria. *Australian Veterinary Journal* 48 (4): 133–136.

73 Coman, B.J. (1972). Helminth parasites of the dingo and feral dog in Victoria with some notes on the diet of the host. *Australian Veterinary Journal* 48 (8): 456–461.

74 Coman, B.J., Jones, E.H., and Driesen, M.A. (1981). Helminth parasites and arthropods of feral cats. *Australian Veterinary Journal* 57 (7): 324–327.

75 Engbaek, K., Madsen, H., and Larsen, S.O. (1984). A survey of helminths in stray cats from Copenhagen with ecological aspects. *Zeitschrift für Parasitenkunde* 70 (1): 87–94.

76 Griffiths, H.J. (1978). *Handbook of Veterinary Parasitology*. Minnesota: University of Minnesota.

77 Hall, E.J. and German, A.J. (2005). Diseases of the small intestine. In: *Textbook of Veterinary Internal Medicine*, 6e (ed. S.J. Ettinger and E.C. Feldman), 1332–1378. Philadelphia: WB Saunders.

78 Hussein, H. and Sunvold, G. (2000). Dietary strategies to decrease dog and cat faecal odour components. In: *Recent Advances in Canine and Feline Nutrition* (ed. D.P. Carey, G.A. Reinhart and Iams Company), 153–168. Wilmington, Ohio: Orange Frazer Press.

79 Miyazaki, M., Miyazaki, T., and Nishimura, T. (2018). The chemical basis of species, sex, and individual recognition using feces in the domestic cat. *Journal of Chemical Ecology* 44: 364–373.

80 McCaw, D.L. and Hoskins, J.D. (2006). Canine viral enteritis. In: *Infectious Diseases of the Dog and Cat*, 3e (ed. C.E. Greene), 63–73. St. Louis, MO: Saunders/Elsevier.

81 Rewerts, J.M. and Cohn, L.A. (2000). CVT update: diagnosis and treatment of parvovirus. In: *Kirk's Current Veterinary Therapy XIII* (ed. J.D. Bonagura), 629–632. Philadelphia: WB Saunders.

82 Glickman, L.T., Domanski, L.M., Patronek, G.J., and Visintainer, F. (1985). Breed-related risk factors for canine parvovirus enteritis. *Journal of the American Veterinary Medical Association* 187 (6): 589–594.

83 Greene, C.E. and Addie, D.D. (2006). Feline parvovirus infections. In: *Infectious Diseases of the Dog and Cat*, 3e (ed. C.E. Greene), 78–88. St. Louis, MO: Saunders/Elsevier.

84 Lichstein, P.R. (1990). The medical interview. In: *Clinical Methods: The History, Physical, and Laboratory Examinations* (ed. H.K. Walker, W.D. Hall and J.W. Hurst). Boston: Butterworths.

17

Direct Smears
Ryane E. Englar

17.1 Procedural Definition: What Is This Test About?

Direct "wet mount" smears are add-on diagnostic tests that screen fecal samples for motile organisms, including trophozoites, that may not survive the hypertonic solutions that are involved in the flotation aspect of fecal analysis [1–4]. Trophozoites represent one of many stages in the life cycle of certain protozoa.

Recall from basic biology that protozoa are unicellular eukaryotes. Some are flagellated for the purpose of enhancing movement, feeding, and/or attachment to substrates. Two flagellate protozoans in particular, *Giardia* spp. and *Tritrichomonas foetus*, have been implicated as causative agents of gastrointestinal disease of companion animals. These organisms can be identified on wet mounts, contingent upon the examiner's experience and skill [1, 3].

Direct smears are also an effective tool for the identification of amoebae (e.g. *Entamoeba histolytica*), nematode larvae (e.g. *Strongyloides* spp.), spores of *Clostridium* spp., and motile bacteria, such as *Campylobacter* [2, 3, 5].

17.2 Procedural Purpose: Why Should I Perform This Test?

Diarrhea is a common clinical presentation among companion animal patients. Protozoal and enteric bacterial pathogens are capable of inducing both acute and chronic disease.

Routine fecal analysis typically includes macroscopic assessment of the sample as well as fecal flotation to identify helminth ova (e.g. those from roundworms, hookworms, and whipworms) and digested skin mites (e.g. *Demodex* spp. and *Cheyletiella*) [6] (see Figure 17.1).

However, protozoal cysts, oocysts, and trophozoites from *Giardia* spp. and *Tritrichomonas foetus* are notoriously difficult to identify using routine methods. In fact, the solutions that are routinely used for fecal flotation are hypertonic, which tends to distort, if not kill, motile trophozoites. Because of this, trophozoites tend to be misdiagnosed or underdiagnosed, particularly *Giardia* spp., which are shed intermittently. Cysts from *Giardia* spp. may be mistaken as yeast because they are sized and shaped similarly.

It is critical that we broaden our diagnostic toolbox to include a combination of methods particularly in diarrheic patients so that we are more likely to diagnose accurately. Expedient diagnosis is vital so that active infections in symptomatic patients do not persist.

17.2.1 The Rationale for Employing Wet Mounts to Diagnose Giardiasis

Giardiasis is a clinical condition that causes intermittent intestinal disease in humans, companion animals, livestock, and wild animals [7–15]. Both symptomatic patients and asymptomatic carriers shed cysts intermittently for indefinite periods. This life cycle promotes recurrent infection and persistence of *Giardia* spp. within the environment [7].

Infection of dogs with *Giardia duodenalis* is common [16]. Although prevalence of giardiasis varies regionally within the United States, 15.6% of dogs with diarrhea are infected with *Giardia*, and prevalence increases among dogs that frequent dog parks [16].

Patients typically become infected through ingestion of cysts found in contaminated food or water [17–21]. Cysts are resistant to cold temperatures and damp environments [18, 19, 21]. Cysts release trophozoites within the small bowel [19, 21]. Trophozoites can be free-floating throughout

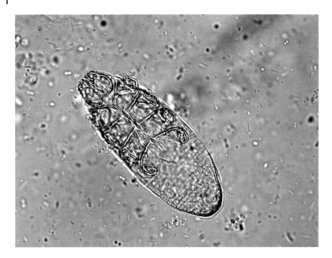

Figure 17.1 *Demodex gatoi*, 40x, as observed on routine fecal analysis from a feline patient. *Source:* Courtesy of Dr. Araceli Lucio-Forster, Cornell University College of Veterinary Medicine.

the lumen, or they may attach to intestinal mucosa via a ventral sucking disc [19, 21]. As these parasites move toward the colon, they undergo encystation [19, 21].

Patients that are symptomatic exhibit small bowel diarrhea and potentially weight loss, stunted growth, and lack of thriftiness [18, 21–24]. Pediatric patients are more likely to be symptomatic [18, 20–23, 25]. Adult infections may be clinical or subclinical [18, 21, 23, 24]. Diarrhea may become chronic if the patient remains untreated [21, 24].

Cats can also become infected with *Giardia*.

Diagnosis can be achieved by identification of cysts via zinc sulfate fecal flotation [11, 18, 21, 24, 26] (see Figure 17.2).

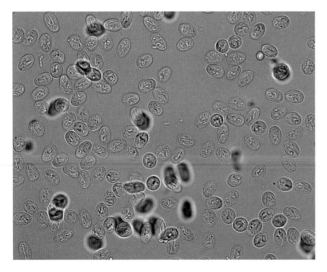

Figure 17.2 *Giardia* cysts in a feline patient, 40x. Concentrated from feces by zinc sulfate centrifugal flotation. *Source:* Courtesy of Araceli Lucio-Forster, PhD.

However, sensitivity of microscopic identification is low [11, 17, 21, 23, 27, 28]. *Giardia* cysts are small and are frequently mistaken for yeast [11]. Cysts are also shed intermittently, which means that serial fecal testing may be necessary to increase the sensitivity of detection in this manner [7, 11].

The trophozoite stage of *Giardia* is better suited for visualization via direct smear. The concave underside of the trophozoite's tear-shaped body makes it appear cupped or spoon-like as it moves through space in a pattern that resembles a falling leaf [18, 20, 21].

Although zoonotic transmission is possible in human patients that are immunocompromised, for instance, those with human immunodeficiency virus (HIV), genotypes of *Giardia* that commonly infect dogs and cats are not typically the same as those that infect people [9, 17, 21, 29].

17.2.2 The Rationale for Employing Wet Mounts to Diagnose Trichomoniasis

Trichomoniasis was first described in cattle as a venereal disease that caused infertility, abortion, and endometriosis [30–32]. In the late 1990s and early 2000s, *Tritrichomonas foetus* was linked to chronic diarrhea in cats [30, 33–36]. Cats become infected via the fecal–oral route [30].

Young cats are at increased risk for infection [30, 35, 37]. Prevalence is also increased amidst crowded populations [30].

Because many cats that are affected with *Tritrichomonas foetus* have concurrent coinfections, it is unclear if *Tritrichomonas foetus* alone causes diarrhea or if clinical signs are precipitated by other enteropathogens [30, 32, 33, 38–40].

Affected cats exhibit intermittent or chronic large bowel diarrhea [21, 30, 41]. Large bowel diarrhea is suggestive of colitis and is characterized by the presence of fresh blood and/or fecal mucus in samples that range from semi-solid to liquid consistency [21, 30]. Patients may be flatulent and/or fecal incontinent [30]. Defecation often involves tenesmus [30]. If tenesmus is severe, patients may experience perianal irritation, inflammation, and/or rectal prolapse [30] (see Figures 17.3 and 17.4).

Affected cats do not typically exhibit weight loss because diarrhea is localized to the large bowel, meaning that nutrient absorption across the small bowel is not impaired [30]. However, during diarrheic bouts, patients may demonstrate depression, anorexia, and fever [30]. Affected cats may also vomit [30].

Tritrichomonas foetus cannot be identified via routine fecal analysis through flotation because its trophozoite

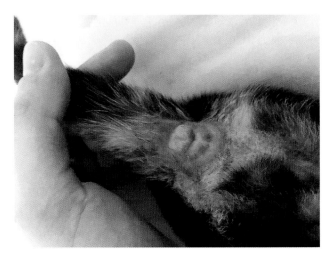

Figure 17.3 Perianal irritation. *Source:* Courtesy of Dr. Jule Schweighoefer.

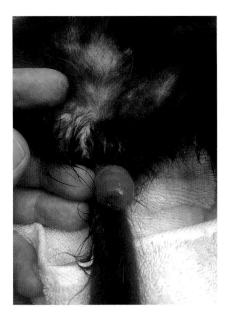

Figure 17.4 Rectal prolapse in a cat. *Source:* Courtesy of Frank Isom, DVM.

phase is destroyed during fecal flotation due to hypertonic solutions [30]. Therefore, direct examination via wet mount is indicated as a first pass attempt to detect *Tritrichomonas foetus* [30, 42]. The progressive movement of *Tritrichomonas foetus* is distinct from that of *Giardia* spp. because trichomonads propel forward in an erratic fashion [41, 42].

The use of direct smears to diagnose *Tritrichomonas foetus* is clinically challenging because of the low specificity and sensitivity that are attributed to this test [30, 41]. In spite of these challenges, wet mounts offer a simple and inexpensive starting point [30, 42].

17.2.3 The Rationale for Employing Wet Mounts to Diagnose *Campylobacter* spp.

Campylobacter spp. are transmitted through the fecal–oral route [43]. Sources of transmission include [43]:

- undercooked or raw food
- unpasteurized milk
- water that has become contaminated with infected feces
- ingestion of infected feces
- indirect contact with other animals, as through the environment, vectors, and fomites.

Campylobacter spp. have been implicated as causative agents of bacterial diarrhea among companion animal patients in addition to the following pathogens [21, 22, 44, 45]:

- *Clostridium* spp.
- *Escherichia coli*
- *Salmonella* spp.
- *Yersinia enterocolitica.*

The primary challenge associated with isolating bacteria in cases involving acute or chronic diarrhea is determining whether the bacteria are in fact causing pathology or are simply present within the gastrointestinal tract [21, 22]. Colonization of the gut with *Campylobacter* spp. can be normal [21, 46].

As an added complication, many bacteria are opportunistic: they will not cause disease in and of themselves, but they may cause disease if the intestinal milieu is disrupted [21, 22, 44].

Both healthy and diarrheic patients may produce feces that contain *Campylobacter* spp. [21, 46–51] *Campylobacter* spp. are particularly abundant in stool samples from young patients and those patients that are stressed [21, 43, 46]. *Campylobacter* spp. are also more prevalent among those housed in groups, as is true of shelter or kennel settings [43].

Microscopically, *Campylobacter* spp. are Gram-negative, curved bacteria. When viewed under light microscopy, *Campylobacter* spp. take on a seagull wing S-shape [21]. This shape is not pathognomonic for *Campylobacter* spp. [21, 46]. Other bacteria with this characteristic shape include *Helicobacter, Arcobacter,* and *Anaerobiospirillum* [21, 46].

Fecal culture can confirm the presence of *Campylobacter* spp., but this diagnostic test requires additional time and the ability to ship samples to outside diagnostic laboratories [22]. Therefore, a direct smear is an appropriate first step.

Campylobacter spp. are zoonotic [46, 52–57]. Therefore, diagnosis is essential to protect those who are living in close contact with affected patients, particularly those who may be immunocompromised [43].

17.3 Equipment

Performing a direct smear via wet mount requires minimal supplies [2, 3, 5, 20, 30]:

- exam gloves for handling biosamples
- a microscope with the ability to adjust the condenser diaphragm
- microscope slides
- newsprint
- 0.9% (physiologic) saline (NaCl) at room temperature or slightly warmed
- wooden applicator stick or comparable tool for mixing feces and saline
- cover slip
- Lugol's iodine
- a fresh sample of feces.

Fecal samples should be fresh, ideally five minutes old or less [2, 36, 58].

Samples are typically taken directly from the rectum via gloved finger during rectal examination. Mucous and/or diarrheic samples are appropriate specimen because sample size is small – roughly the size of the head of a match (1–2 mm^3) [5].

Direct smears can also be made from fecal matter that clings to a rectal thermometer following its insertion into the rectum [4, 59].

An alternate means of sample collection is via rectal saline lavage [3]. In this method, 6–12 ml of 0.9% saline is inserted into the rectum through a soft rubber catheter to which a water-based lubricant has been applied [3]. The saline is aspirated and delivery into the rectum is repeated several times [3].

17.4 Procedural Steps [1–5, 20, 30, 60–62]

1) Gather supplies (see Figure 17.5).
2) Apply fecal sample to a microscope slide (see Figures 17.6 and 17.7).
3) Apply one drop of 0.9% saline to the same microscope slide unless the sample was obtained by rectal lavage, in which case you can skip ahead to the next step (see Figure 17.8).
4) Mix the fecal sample and the saline with a wooden applicator stick or comparable tool to form a slurry that spans approximately 1×1 centimeter (see Figures 17.9 and 17.10).
5) Check the "thickness" of the slurry against newsprint. You should be able to read newsprint through the wet mount. If you cannot, then the mixture is too dense and will need to be thinned out by removing some of the fecal sample, adding more saline, or both (see Figure 17.11).

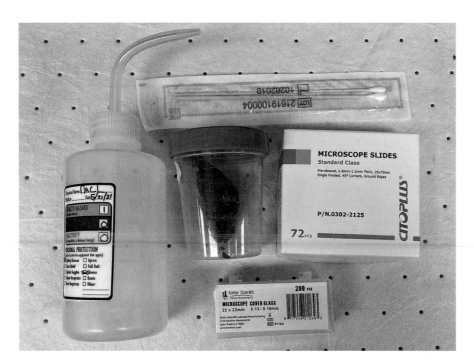

Figure 17.5 Supplies for direct smear. *Source:* Courtesy of Jeremy Bessett, Inaugural Class of 2023, University of Arizona College of Veterinary Medicine.

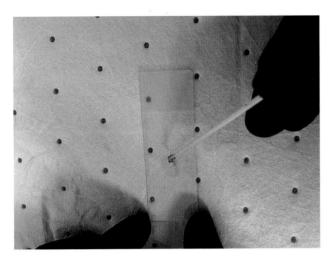

Figure 17.6 Using a wooden applicator stick to apply the patient's fecal sample to a microscope slide. *Source:* Courtesy of Jeremy Bessett, Inaugural Class of 2023, University of Arizona College of Veterinary Medicine.

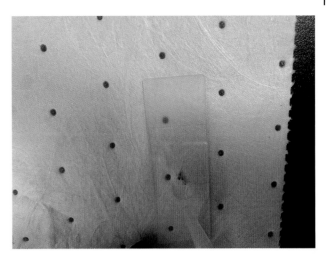

Figure 17.8 Adding one drop of 0.9% saline to the slide that contains the fecal sample. *Source:* Courtesy of Jeremy Bessett, Inaugural Class of 2023, University of Arizona College of Veterinary Medicine.

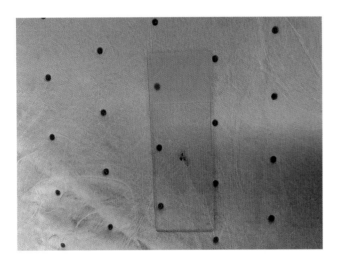

Figure 17.7 The patient's sample has been added to a microscope slide. *Source:* Courtesy of Jeremy Bessett, Inaugural Class of 2023, University of Arizona College of Veterinary Medicine.

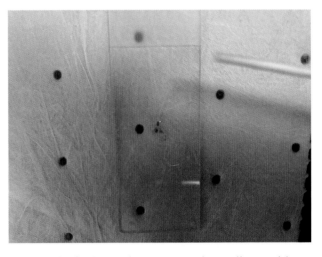

Figure 17.9 Getting ready to use a wooden applicator stick to mix the saline and fecal sample. *Source:* Courtesy of Jeremy Bessett, Inaugural Class of 2023, University of Arizona College of Veterinary Medicine.

6) Place a coverslip over the slurry (see Figure 17.12).
7) Place the microscope slide on the stage of the microscope.
8) Look through the microscope oculars.
9) Adjust the position of the oculars so that you can look through both oculars at the same time to view a single image.
10) Adjust the condenser diaphragm so that it is not opened too wide. You do not want illumination to be too bright.
11) Scan the slide for eggs, cysts, and larvae at low magnification (10×).

12) Increase the magnification to 20×, then 40×, and scan the slide with each adjustment to magnifying power, evaluating for motile trophozoites.
13) Increase the magnification to 100× under oil immersion and scan the slide to search for motile bacteria.
14) Following thorough scans for motile trophozoites and bacteria, apply iodine to the edge of the cover glass to assist in the identification of organisms. Note that iodine will kill motile organisms; however, it will make them more visible and therefore more readily identified.

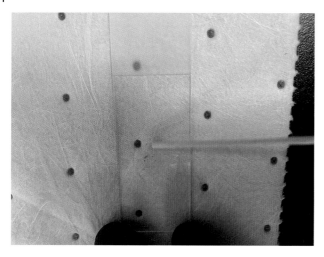

Figure 17.10 Using a wooden applicator stick to mix the saline and fecal sample. *Source:* Courtesy of Jeremy Bessett, Inaugural Class of 2023, University of Arizona College of Veterinary Medicine.

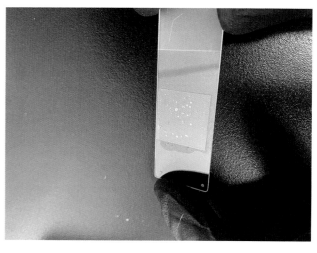

Figure 17.12 Placing a coverslip over the slurry in preparation for viewing via light microscopy. *Source:* Courtesy of Jeremy Bessett, Inaugural Class of 2023, University of Arizona College of Veterinary Medicine.

17.5 Time Estimate to Perform Test

Less than five minutes.

17.6 Procedural Tips and Troubleshooting

- This technique is not intended to analyze thick samples. When samples are solid rather than diarrheic, you must dilute the sample with sufficient 0.9% saline. Otherwise, the opacity of the fecal slurry will block detection of motile organisms [1, 2, 4, 60, 61].
- Trophozoites are transparent. Adjust the condenser diaphragm so that it is not opened too wide [20]. If the illumination is too bright, you will be challenged to see trophozoites [20]. You are watching for their movement and require contrast to be successful.
- The addition of iodine to the slide will aid the identification of organisms by staining internal features; however, iodine kills the organisms of interest [2, 20, 62]. Therefore, do not apply iodine to the slide until after you have fully scanned the slide at 10, 20, 40, and 100× magnification to detect motile organisms. After the addition of iodine, organisms will no longer be motile.
- If this diagnostic test is unsuccessful at identifying organisms, do *not* send wet mount slides to outside diagnostic laboratories [2]. The slides will dry out in transit and results will be inconclusive [2]. A better approach would be to perform dry mounts on additional fecal samples and send these to pathologists with a clear description of what you found on the wet mounts in-house [2].

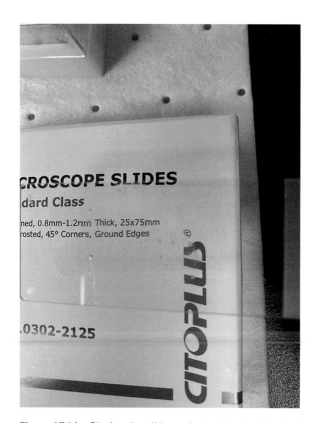

Figure 17.11 Placing the slide against written text to check the slurry's thickness. You can read words through the slurry, which means that this sample is of the appropriate thickness. *Source:* Courtesy of Jeremy Bessett, Inaugural Class of 2023, University of Arizona College of Veterinary Medicine.

17.7 Interpreting Test Results

The advantage of the direct smear is that it provides an opportunity to scan the slide for visible movement.

It is in fact the movement of the motile organisms that assists most with identification. After all, trophozoites of *Tritrichomonas foetus* and *Giardia* spp. are similar in size but differ in how they move [30].

- The concave underside of *Giardia*'s tear-shaped body makes it appear cupped or spoon-like as it moves through space in a pattern that resembles a falling leaf [18, 20, 21, 30].
- By contrast, the trophozoite of *Tritrichomonas foetus* has a progressive forward movement [30, 41, 42].

Movement is *not* something that can be captured in text form. Movement is something that must be witnessed either in person or via videography.

What we can appreciate in this text is how both *Giardia* spp. and *Tritrichomonas foetus* appear in still-frames (see Figures 17.13–17.25).

In addition to visualizing motile trophozoites, you should examine direct smears for motile bacteria. Again, the advantage of the direct smear is that it provides an opportunity to scan the slide for visible movement.

What was stated previously concerning trophozoites also applies to bacteria. Movement of motile bacteria is *not* something that can be captured in text form.

What we can appreciate in this text is how bacteria may appear in still-frames (see Figures 17.26–17.29).

Recall that we scan the slide for motile bacteria at 100× using oil immersion [2]. *Campylobacter*-like organisms

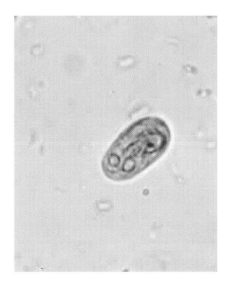

Figure 17.14 *Giardia* cyst magnified and stained with iodine, direct smear. *Source:* Courtesy of Ryane E. Englar, DVM, DABVP (Canine and Feline Practice).

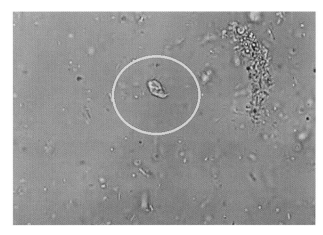

Figure 17.15 *Giardia* trophozoite as seen on direct smear. *Source:* Courtesy of Ryane E. Englar, DVM, DABVP (Canine and Feline Practice).

exhibit a rapid darting motion due to long-sheathed polar flagella. Motility of these organisms is not long-lasting because of sensitivity to oxygen.

Additional diagnostic tools are often indicated to differentiate bacterial morphology. For instance, we may consider adding on a Gram stain [2] (see Figure 17.30).

Alternate stains may be indicated depending upon your index of suspicion [2]. For instance, if you suspect *Cryptosporidium*, then you should consider utilizing an acid-fast stain [2].

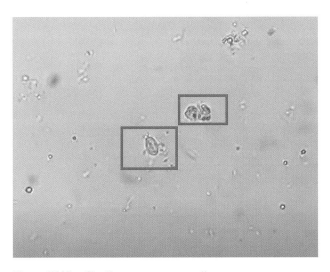

Figure 17.13 *Giardia* cysts as seen on direct smear. *Source:* Courtesy of Ryane E. Englar, DVM, DABVP (Canine and Feline Practice).

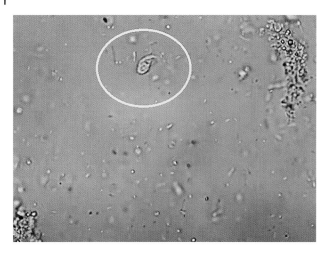

Figure 17.16 *Giardia* trophozoite as seen on direct smear. *Source:* Courtesy of Ryane E. Englar, DVM, DABVP (Canine and Feline Practice).

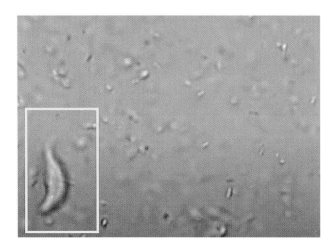

Figure 17.17 Sideview of *Giardia* trophozoite, magnified, as seen on direct smear. *Source:* Courtesy of Ryane E. Englar, DVM, DABVP (Canine and Feline Practice).

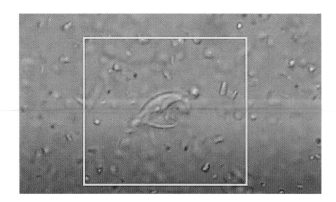

Figure 17.18 *Giardia* trophozoite, magnified, as seen on direct smear. *Source:* Courtesy of Ryane E. Englar, DVM, DABVP (Canine and Feline Practice).

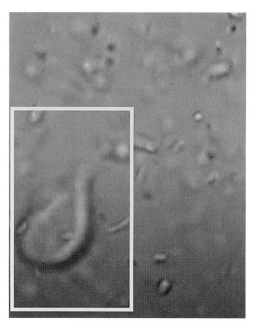

Figure 17.19 Tear-drop shape of *Giardia* trophozoite, magnified, as seen on direct smear. *Source:* Courtesy of Ryane E. Englar, DVM, DABVP (Canine and Feline Practice).

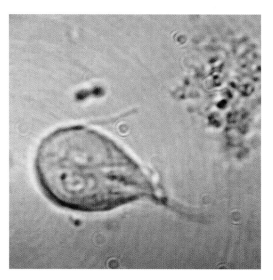

Figure 17.20 *Giardia* trophozoite, magnified and stained with iodine, as seen on direct smear. Note that the *Giardia* trophozoite is said by some to resemble a clown's face. You can appreciate what appear to be two cartoony eyes staring out at you in this photograph. These "eyes" are formed by two nuclei. *Source:* Courtesy of Ryane E. Englar, DVM, DABVP (Canine and Feline Practice).

17.8 Clinical Case Example(s)

A young adult intact female domestic short-haired (DSH) stray cat was recently adopted by your client from a local shelter. The client presents the cat to you for evaluation of chronic, watery, foul-smelling diarrhea. At times, the feces

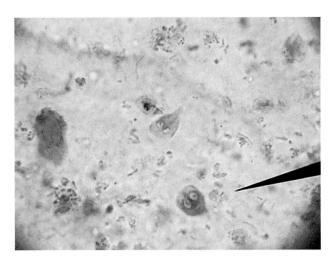

Figure 17.21 *Giardia* trophozoite, magnified and stained with Giemsa, as seen on direct smear. Note that the *Giardia* trophozoite is said by some to resemble a clown's face. You can appreciate what appear to be two cartoony eyes staring out at you in this photograph. These "eyes" are formed by two nuclei. *Source:* Courtesy of Dr. Robert Eisemann.

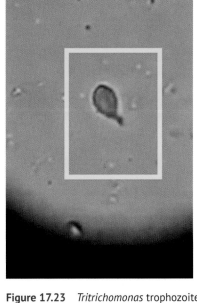

Figure 17.23 *Tritrichomonas* trophozoite as seen on direct smear. *Source:* Courtesy of Ryane E. Englar, DVM, DABVP (Canine and Feline Practice).

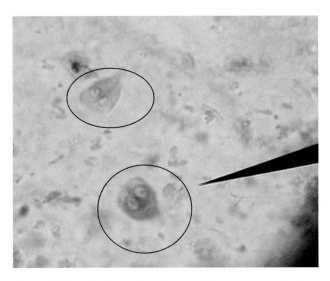

Figure 17.22 *Giardia* trophozoite, magnified and stained with Giemsa, as seen on direct smear. Note that the *Giardia* trophozoite is said by some to resemble a clown's face. You can appreciate what appear to be two cartoony eyes staring out at you in this photograph. These "eyes" are formed by two nuclei. *Source:* Courtesy of Dr. Robert Eisemann.

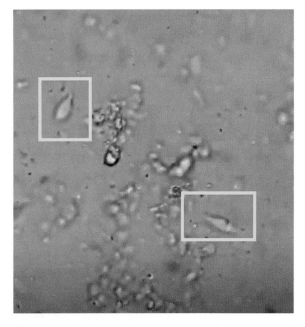

Figure 17.24 Two *Tritrichomonas* trophozoites as seen on direct smear. *Source:* Courtesy of Ryane E. Englar, DVM, DABVP (Canine and Feline Practice).

appear to dribble from the cat's rectum as if the cat is fecally incontinent. When the client contacted the shelter for medical records, the shelter disclosed that the cat had produced pudding-like feces while under their care, but that the cat had been recently dewormed with fenbendazole. The shelter had presumptively diagnosed the cat with stress colitis. Fecal flotation performed at that time was reportedly negative for ova. The shelter anticipated that the feces

would firm up after the cat was placed in a stable home environment. Unfortunately, that does not seem to be the case and the client is frustrated. On physical examination today, the cat is thin with a body condition score of 3/9. The patient's perianal fur is wet and the patient dribbles brown-tinged watery diarrhea from the anus during abdominal palpation. A wet mount is performed and discloses motile

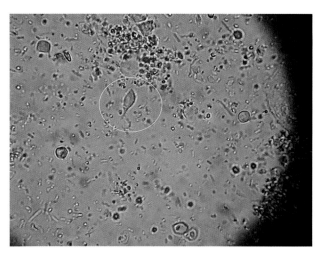

Figure 17.25 *Tritrichomonas* trophozoite as seen on direct smear. *Source:* Courtesy of Ryane E. Englar, DVM, DABVP (Canine and Feline Practice).

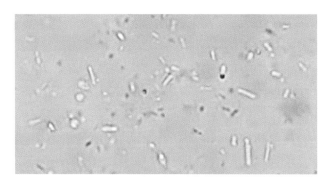

Figure 17.26 Scanning slide for bacteria, as seen on direct smear. *Source:* Courtesy of Ryane E. Englar, DVM, DABVP (Canine and Feline Practice).

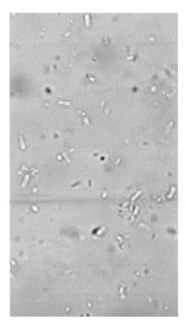

Figure 17.27 Scanning slide for bacteria, as seen on direct smear. *Source:* Courtesy of Ryane E. Englar, DVM, DABVP (Canine and Feline Practice).

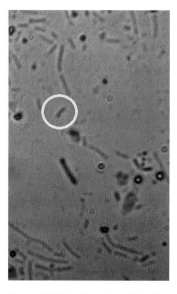

Figure 17.28 Scanning slide for bacteria, as seen on direct smear. Iodine has been added for contrast. A rod-shaped bacterium has been circled in yellow. This was motile when viewed via light microscopy. *Source:* Courtesy of Ryane E. Englar, DVM, DABVP (Canine and Feline Practice).

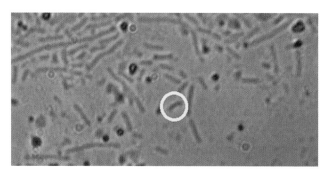

Figure 17.29 Scanning slide for bacteria, as seen on direct smear. Iodine has been added for contrast. A rod-shaped bacterium has been circled in yellow. This was motile when viewed via light microscopy. *Source:* Courtesy of Ryane E. Englar, DVM, DABVP (Canine and Feline Practice).

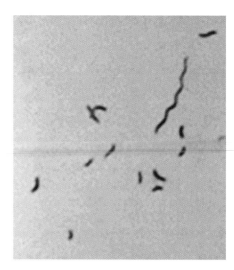

Figure 17.30 *Campylobacter*-like organisms on fecal examination. Note the characteristic gull wing or S-shape. Some refer to this as a comma shape. *Source:* Courtesy of Ryane E. Englar, DVM, DABVP (Canine and Feline Practice).

flagellated organisms that exhibit a forward progressive movement. Based upon morphology and the motility pattern, trichomonads were prioritized as the diagnosis. A stained dry mount subsequently confirmed that the patient was infected with *Tritrichomonas foetus:* three anterior flagella, one posterior flagellum, one nucleus, and an undulating membrane.

17.9 Add-On Tests That You May Need to Consider and Their Additive Value

Direct smears are just one of many diagnostic tools that may collectively be involved in performing fecal analysis.

Although direct smears are a means by which to microscopically assess feces, false negatives are common because of the small sample size used for this procedure and because many of the organisms that we are searching for shed intermittently [1, 4, 5].

Therefore, the following additional modalities may be of benefit, particularly in chronic cases that have escaped diagnosis:

- fecal flotation (see Chapter 18)
- *Giardia* antigen detection test
- fecal culture using In Pouch ™ TF Feline
- polymerase chain reaction (PCR) testing for *Tritrichomonas foetus*
- dry mount fecal cytology.

17.9.1 The Rationale for Fecal Flotation as an Add-On Diagnostic Test

Fecal flotation will be discussed in detail in Chapter 18. Because fecal flotation is a method that concentrates parasitic ova and cysts based upon differences in density, it has a greater chance of detecting *Giardia* cysts, provided that the solution employed is zinc sulfate [2, 20]. Hypertonic solutions such as sucrose, sodium chloride, and sodium nitrate are more likely to shrivel the cysts beyond recognition [20, 63, 64].

17.9.2 The Rationale for Giardia Antigen Detection Tests an Add-on Diagnostic Tool

Giardia antigen detection tests may also be employed to detect dogs and cats that have clinical disease. These tests offer an in-house enzyme-linked immunosorbent assay (ELISA) that detects *Giardia* cyst antigen [1]. There are several different commercially available products by which a rapid detection of *Giardia* cyst antigen is possible (see Figures 17.31–17.34).

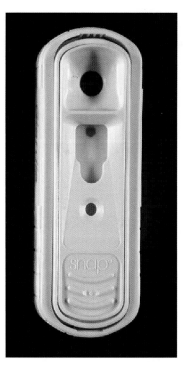

Figure 17.31 A negative in-house *Giardia* ELISA antigen test. The blue dot at the top of the display represents the positive control. *Source:* Courtesy of Ryane E. Englar, DVM, DABVP (Canine and Feline Practice).

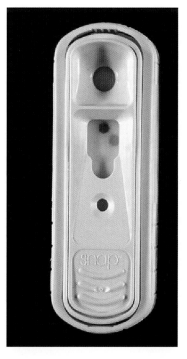

Figure 17.32 A positive in-house *Giardia* ELISA antigen test. The blue dot at the top of the display represents the positive control. Note the additional blue dot along the righthand side of the display. *Source:* Courtesy of Ryane E. Englar, DVM, DABVP (Canine and Feline Practice).

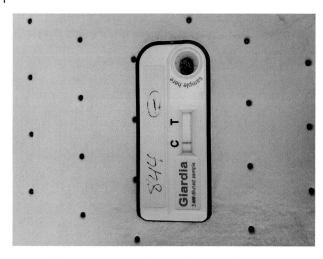

Figure 17.33 A negative in-house *Giardia* ELISA antigen test. *Source:* Courtesy of Ryane E. Englar, DVM, DABVP (Canine and Feline Practice). Note the absence of a band at the "T" marker. The "C" marker represents the control. *Source:* Courtesy of Ryane E. Englar, DVM, DABVP (Canine and Feline Practice).

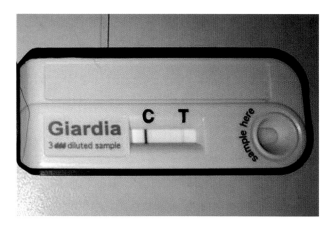

Figure 17.34 A faint-positive in-house *Giardia* ELISA antigen test. Note the faint band at the "T" marker. The "C" marker represents the control. *Source:* Courtesy of Ryane E. Englar, DVM, DABVP (Canine and Feline Practice). Courtesy of Ryane E. Englar, DVM, DABVP (Canine and Feline Practice).

Advantages of *Giardia* antigen detection tests include convenience and expedience. However, because cysts are shed intermittently, false negatives are possible [1].

Interpretation of *Giardia* antigen detection tests may also prove challenging if used in asymptomatic dogs and cats that subsequently test positive. In these situations, it is unclear whether the patients are chronic carriers or whether environmental contamination is to blame [1]. In clinical practice, this is a frequent occurrence when stool is sent to outside diagnostic labs that routinely pair *Giardia* antigen detection tests with fecal flotation. What do you do with a patient that tests positive, but is exhibiting no clinical signs?

17.9.3 The Rationale for Add-On Diagnostic Tests for Detection of *Tritrichomonas Foetus*

It is difficult to diagnose *T. foetus* because trichomonads are shed intermittently [21, 65]. The fact that they are the same size as *Giardia* adds an additional layer of complexity to their diagnosis because they may be mistaken for *Giardia* by inexperienced examiners [21]. In addition, *Tritrichomonas foetus* is less hardy than *Giardia* because there is no cyst stage [21, 23]. Therefore, *Tritrichomonas foetus* trophozoites do not survive refrigeration or fecal flotation [21, 23, 65].

Performing a fecal culture by inoculating the In Pouch™ TF Feline may increase yield of trophozoites, thereby increasing the likelihood of a true positive diagnosis [21, 23, 41, 65] (see Figure 17.35).

Stool must be freshly collected, either from a voided sample, via rectal loop-collection, or via rectal lavage [21, 41, 65]. Pouches are inoculated with a sample of feces that approximates the size of a peppercorn [21, 65]. Pouch contents are examined every other day in-house for 12 days [21, 65].

The gold standard for diagnosis of *Tritrichomonas foetus* is to perform PCR on fecal matter [41]. However, this requires contracting with outside diagnostic laboratories.

17.9.4 The Rationale for Dry Mount Fecal Cytology as an Add-On Diagnostic Tool

Dry mount cytology allows you to evaluate fecal flora [3]. This test requires the examiner to understand what constitutes normal fecal cytology [3]. Rod-shaped bacteria are typically the predominant fecal flora with the occasional yeast and rare coccoid bacteria [3]. Mucus and debris may be present in, but you should not observe erythrocytes or many (if any) epithelial cells if fecal samples were collected without rectal scraping [3].

Dry mounts are prepared using very little feces [2]. As was true of wet mounts, thick dry mount slides are difficult to interpret. They are also difficult to process. Thick slides do not stain well [2]. Furthermore, large pieces of fecal matter may become dislodged in the processing stage [2].

Once fecal matter has been smeared onto the slide, the slide should be allowed to air dry to preserve cellular morphology [2]. The slide is then typically stained using either Wright–Giemsa or Diff-Quik [2].

The slide should be first scanned at low magnification so that the examiner broadly surveys the sample before they dive in to assess cellular morphology and bacteria at 100× using oil immersion [2].

Gram staining may highlight different populations of bacteria [2].

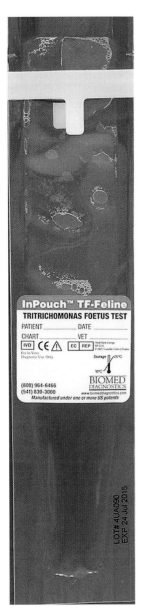

Figure 17.35 In Pouch ™ TF Feline in-house test for *Tritrichomonas foetus,* prior to inoculation with feces. *Source:* Courtesy of Ryane E. Englar, DVM, DABVP (Canine and Feline Practice).

Alternate stains, such as acid-fast, may be indicated depending upon your index of suspicion (e.g. if you suspect *Cryptosporidium*) [2].

Fecal cytology can detect bacterial and fungal overgrowth as well as inflammatory infiltrates [3]. Neither erythrocytes nor leukocytes are present on dry mounts of healthy canine patients [3]. The presence of increased numbers of neutrophils on dry mounts is consistent with bacterial enteritis, colitis, whipworm infestation, chronic primary inflammatory disease, and neoplasia [3]. Incidentally, puppies that are diagnosed with parvovirus do not have fecal neutrophils despite hemorrhagic diarrhea and peripheral blood neutropenia [3].

Fecal eosinophils may be present in cases of eosinophilic enteritis or nematode infestation [3].

17.10 Key Takeaways

- Wet mounts require a very small amount of feces and analysis can be performed immediately with limited equipment [1, 4].
- Prep slides with only a thin layer of feces [59]! Fecal organisms may be obscured if the slide prep is too thick, causing an abundance of fecal debris [4].

  You still should be able to read newsprint through the slide of a direct smear [60]. If you cannot do so, then the smear is too thick [60].

  If the smear is too thick, add one or more drops of 0.9% (physiologic) saline until the appropriate dilution has been attained [61].
- If the sample tests negative, then the direct smear is inconclusive [59].
- The diagnostic capacity for wet mounts is contingent upon the examiner's experience and skill [1]. The examiner must be able to differentiate pathogenic from nonpathogenic organisms [1]. For example, it is not uncommon to observe nonpathogenic *Pentatrichomonas hominis* in canine feces [2, 5]. The examiner may also identify a significant number of treponeme-like spirochetes on wet mounts, particularly those of diarrheic samples [2, 3]. These are considered to be nonpathogenic yet could be mistaken for pathogenic organisms if the examiner is inexperienced [2, 3].
- Because wet mounts only require a small sample, they are not an appropriate measure of parasite load and false negatives are common [1, 4, 5]. Serial fecal sampling can be helpful in terms of increasing the number of samples that are positive and test positive [7].
- Unlike fecal flotation, wet mounts do not concentrate ova. Therefore, you will underdiagnose helminths that produce few eggs using this diagnostic test [60].
- Do not get discouraged by the low specificity and low sensitivity of this test [30, 66]. To test positive, fresh fecal samples must contain many viable trophozoites [66]. Most samples contain few, if any, even though they are derived from affected patients [30]. This accounts for the test's low sensitivity [30]. The test's low specificity is attributed to the examiner's ability to identify and differentiate trophozoites [30]. To assist the examiner with differentiation:
  - *Tritrichomonas foetus* is characterized by pear-shaped trophozoites with three anterior flagella, one nucleus, and an undulating membrane [30].

- *Giardia* spp. are characterized by trophozoites that lack an undulating membrane. They have two nuclei and one ventral disc [30].
- Trophozoites from both *Tritrichomonas foetus* and *Giardia* spp. are similar in terms of size, but different in terms of movement [30].
- The concave underside of *Giardia's* tear-shaped body makes it appear cupped or spoon-like as it moves through space in a pattern that resembles a falling leaf [18, 20, 21, 30].
- By contrast, the trophozoite of *Tritrichomonas foetus* has a progressive forward movement [30, 41, 42].

17.11   Clinical Pearls

- The reason why we choose saline instead of water to mix with the fecal sample is because water lyses trophozoites and/or distorts them through osmosis [59].
- On the wet mount, look for the clown face that is characteristic of the *Giardia* trophozoite.
  The two "eyes" are formed by two nuclei.
  The "mouth" is formed by the dark median bodies.
- You can apply the same procedural technique of direct smear to oropharyngeal swabs from birds to evaluate avian patients for *Giardia* or *Trichomonas*.

References

1   Dryden, M.W. and Payne, P.A. (2010). *Fecal Examination Techniques*, –13, 6. NAVC Clinician's Brief.

2   Broussard, J.D. (2003). Optimal fecal assessment. *Clin. Tech. Small Anim. Pract.* 18 (4): 218–230.

3   Trumel, C. and Dossin, O. (2020). Fecal cytology. In: *Veterinary Cytology* (ed. L.C. Sharkey, M.J. Radin and D. Seelig), 407–410. Hoboken, NJ: Wiley-Blackwell.

4   Hendrix, C.M. and Robinson, E. (2017). Common laboratory procedures for diagnosing parasitism. In: *Diagnostic Parasitology for Veterinary Technicians*, 6e (ed. C.M. Hendrix and E. Robinson), 303–335. St. Louis, Missouri: Elsevier Inc.

5   Foreyt, W.J. (1989). Diagnostic parasitology. *Vet. Clin. North Am. Small Anim. Pract.* 19 (5): 979–1000.

6   Haller, J. (2021). The Veterinary Nurse's Guide to Fecal Flotation Techniques. *Today's Veterinary Nurse* [Internet] Fall.

7   Uchoa, F.F.M., Sudre, A.P., Macieira, D.B., and Almosny, N.R.P. (2017). The influence of serial fecal sampling on the diagnosis of giardiasis in humans, dogs, and cats. *Rev. Inst. Med. Trop. Sao Paulo* 59: e61.

8   Esch, K.J. and Petersen, C.A. (2013). Transmission and epidemiology of zoonotic protozoal diseases of companion animals. *Clin. Microbiol. Rev.* 26 (1): 58–85.

9   Thompson, R.C. (2004). The zoonotic significance and molecular epidemiology of Giardia and giardiasis. *Vet. Parasitol.* 126 (1–2): 15–35.

10   Thompson, R.C., Palmer, C.S., and O'Handley, R. (2008). The public health and clinical significance of Giardia and Cryptosporidium in domestic animals. *Vet. J.* 177 (1): 18–25.

11   Olson, M.E., Leonard, N.J., and Strout, J. (2010). Prevalence and diagnosis of Giardia infection in dogs and cats using a fecal antigen test and fecal smear. *Can. Vet. J.* 51 (6): 640–642.

12   Swan, J.M. and Thompson, R.C. (1986). The prevalence of Giardia in dogs and cats in Perth, Western Australia. *Aust. Vet. J.* 63 (4): 110–112.

13   Shukla, R., Giraldo, P., Kraliz, A. et al. (2006). Cryptosporidium spp. and other zoonotic enteric parasites in a sample of domestic dogs and cats in the Niagara region of Ontario. *Can. Vet. J.* 47 (12): 1179–1184.

14   Papini, R., Gorini, G., Spaziani, A., and Cardini, G. (2005). Survey on giardiosis in shelter dog populations. *Vet. Parasitol.* 128 (3–4): 333–339.

15   Jacobs, S.R., Forrester, C.P., and Yang, J. (2001). A survey of the prevalence of Giardia in dogs presented to Canadian veterinary practices. *Can. Vet. J.* 42 (1): 45–46.

16   Giardia: Companion Animal Parasite Council (CAPC) (2019). https://capcvet.org/guidelines/giardia.

17   Schantz, P.M. (2007). Zoonotic parasitic infections contracted from dogs and cats: How frequent are they? DVM 360 [Internet]. http://veterinarymedicine.dvm360.com/zoonotic-parasitic-infections-contracted-dogs-and-cats-how-frequent-are-they.

18   Giardiasis, S.V. (2013). NAVC Clinician's Brief. (February):71–86.

19   Barr, S.C. (2006). Enteric protozoal infections. In: *Infectious Diseases of the Dog and Cat* (ed. C.E. Greene), 736–742. St. Louis, MO: Elsevier, Inc.

20   Kirkpatrick, C.E. (1987). Giardiasis. *Vet. Clin. North Am. Small Anim. Pract.* 17 (6): 1377–1387.

21   Englar, R.E. (2019). Changes in fecal appearance. In: *Common Clinical Presentations in Dogs and Cats* (ed. R.E. Englar), 647–670. Hoboken, NJ: Wiley-Blackwell.

22   Magne, M.L. (2006). Selected topics in pediatric gastroenterology. *Vet. Clin. North Am. Small Anim. Pract.* 36 (3): 533–548, vi.

23 Little, S. (ed.) (2011). Diarrhea in kittens and young cats. In: *WSAVA World Congress*. Jeju, Korea.

24 Bowman, D. (2009). Canine and feline cryptosporidiosis and giardiasis DVM 360 [Internet]. http://veterinarycalendar.dvm360.com/canine-and-feline-cryptosporidiosis-and-giardiasis-proceedings.

25 Tangtrongsup, S. and Scorza, V. (2010). Update on the diagnosis and management of Giardia spp infections in dogs and cats. *Top. Companion Anim. Med.* 25 (3): 155–162.

26 Steiner, J.M. (2010). Workup of dogs with chronic diarrhea. DVM 360.

27 Dryden, M.W., Payne, P.A., and Smith, V. (2006). Accurate diagnosis of Giardia spp and proper fecal examination procedures. *Vet. Ther.* 7 (1): 4–14.

28 Hackett, T. and Lappin, M.R. (2003). Prevalence of enteric pathogens in dogs of north-Central Colorado. *J. Am. Anim. Hosp. Assoc.* 39 (1): 52–56.

29 Slifko, T.R., Smith, H.V., and Rose, J.B. (2000). Emerging parasite zoonoses associated with water and food. *Int. J. Parasitol.* 30 (12–13): 1379–1393.

30 Bastos, B.F., Almeida, F.M., and Brener, B. (2019). What is known about Tritrichomonas foetus infection in cats? *Rev. Bras. Parasitol. Vet.* 28 (1): 1–11.

31 Felleisen, R.S. (1999). Host-parasite interaction in bovine infection with Tritrichomonas foetus. *Microbes Infect.* 1 (10): 807–816.

32 Bissett, S.A., Gowan, R.A., O'Brien, C.R. et al. (2008). Feline diarrhoea associated with Tritrichomonas cf. foetus and Giardia co-infection in an Australian cattery. *Aust. Vet. J.* 86 (11): 440–443.

33 Gookin, J.L., Stebbins, M.E., Hunt, E. et al. (2004). Prevalence of and risk factors for feline Tritrichomonas foetus and giardia infection. *J. Clin. Microbiol.* 42 (6): 2707–2710.

34 Romatowski, J. (2000). Pentatrichomonas hominis infection in four kittens. *J. Am. Vet. Med. Assoc.* 216 (8): 1270–1272.

35 Gookin, J.L., Breitschwerdt, E.B., Levy, M.G. et al. (1999). Diarrhea associated with trichomonosis in cats. *J. Am. Vet. Med. Assoc.* 215 (10): 1450–1454.

36 Levy, M.G., Gookin, J.L., Poore, M. et al. (2003). Tritrichomonas foetus and not Pentatrichomonas hominis is the etiologic agent of feline trichomonal diarrhea. *J. Parasitol.* 89 (1): 99–104.

37 Yaeger, M.J. and Gookin, J.L. (2005). Histologic features associated with tritrichomonas foetus-induced colitis in domestic cats. *Vet. Pathol.* 42 (6): 797–804.

38 Stockdale, H.D., Givens, M.D., Dykstra, C.C., and Blagburn, B.L. (2009). Tritrichomonas foetus infections in surveyed pet cats. *Vet. Parasitol.* 160 (1–2): 13–17.

39 Gookin, J.L., Levy, M.G., Law, J.M. et al. (2001). Experimental infection of cats with Tritrichomonas foetus. *Am. J. Vet. Res.* 62 (11): 1690–1697.

40 Gookin, J.L., Birkenheuer, A.J., St John, V. et al. (2005). Molecular characterization of trichomonads from feces of dogs with diarrhea. *J. Parasitol.* 91 (4): 939–943.

41 Gould, E. and Tolbert, M.K. (2017). *Tritrichomonas Foetus Infection in Cats*, 29–31. NAVC Clinician's Brief.

42 Maki, E. and Pohlman, L.M. (2021). *Watery Diarrhea and Frequent Fecal Dribbling in a Cat*. NAVC Clinician's Brief [Internet].

43 Acke, E. (2018). Campylobacteriosis in dogs and cats: a review. *N. Z. Vet. J.* 66 (5): 221–228.

44 Hall, E.J. and German, A.J. (2005). Diseases of the small intestine. In: *Textbook of Veterinary Internal Medicine*, 6e (ed. S.J. Ettinger and E.C. Feldman), 1332–1378. Philadelphia: WB Saunders.

45 Hoskins, J.D. and Dimski, D. (1990). The digestive system. In: *Veterinary Pediatrics* (ed. J.D. Hoskins), 133–187. Philadelphia: WB Saunders.

46 Weese, J.S. (2011). Bacterial enteritis in dogs and cats: diagnosis, therapy, and zoonotic potential. *Vet. Clin. North Am. Small Anim. Pract.* 41 (2): 287–309.

47 Burnens, A.P., Angeloz-Wick, B., and Nicolet, J. (1992). Comparison of Campylobacter carriage rates in diarrheic and healthy pet animals. *Zentralbl. Veterinarmed. B* 39 (3): 175–180.

48 Fox, J.G., Hering, A.M., Ackerman, J.I., and Taylor, N.S. (1983). The pet hamster as a potential reservoir of human campylobacteriosis. *J. Infect. Dis.* 147 (4): 784.

49 Acke, E., Whyte, P., Jones, B.R. et al. (2006). Prevalence of thermophilic Campylobacter species in cats and dogs in two animal shelters in Ireland. *Vet. Rec.* 158 (2): 51–54.

50 Rossi, M., Hanninen, M.L., Revez, J. et al. (2008). Occurrence and species level diagnostics of Campylobacter spp., enteric Helicobacter spp. and Anaerobiospirillum spp. in healthy and diarrheic dogs and cats. *Vet. Microbiol.* 129 (3–4): 304–314.

51 Sandberg, M., Bergsjo, B., Hofshagen, M. et al. (2002). Risk factors for Campylobacter infection in Norwegian cats and dogs. *Prev. Vet. Med.* 55 (4): 241–253.

52 Adak, G.K., Cowden, J.M., Nicholas, S., and Evans, H.S. (1995). The public health laboratory service national case-control study of primary indigenous sporadic cases of campylobacter infection. *Epidemiol. Infect.* 115 (1): 15–22.

53 Damborg, P., Olsen, K.E., Moller Nielsen, E., and Guardabassi, L. (2004). Occurrence of Campylobacter jejuni in pets living with human patients infected with C. jejuni. *J. Clin. Microbiol.* 42 (3): 1363–1364.

54 Fullerton, K.E., Ingram, L.A., Jones, T.F. et al. (2007). Sporadic campylobacter infection in infants: a population-based surveillance case-control study. *Pediatr. Infect. Dis. J.* 26 (1): 19–24.

55 Gillespie, I.A., O'Brien, S.J., Adak, G.K. et al. (2003). Point source outbreaks of Campylobacter jejuni infection-are they more common than we think and what might cause them? *Epidemiol. Infect.* 130 (3): 367–375.

56 Tam, C.C., Higgins, C.D., Neal, K.R. et al. (2009). Chicken consumption and use of acid-suppressing medications as risk factors for Campylobacter enteritis. *England. Emerg. Infect. Dis.* 15 (9): 1402–1408.

57 Tenkate, T.D. and Stafford, R.J. (2001). Risk factors for campylobacter infection in infants and young children: a matched case-control study. *Epidemiol. Infect.* 127 (3): 399–404.

58 Willard, M.D. and Twedt, D.C. (1991). Gastrointestinal, pancreatic, and hepatic disorders. In: *Small Animal Clinical Diagnosis by Laboratory Methods* (ed. M.D. Willard, D.C. Twedt and H. Turnwald), 172–207. Philadelphia, PA: Saunders.

59 Bowman, D.D. and Georgi, J.R. (2003). Diagnostic Parasitology. In: *Georgis' Parasitology for Veterinarians*, 8e (ed. D.D. Bowman and J.R. Georgi), 287–358. Saunders/Elsevier: St. Louis, Mo.

60 Greiner, E.C. (1989). Parasite diagnosis by fecal examination. *J. Assoc. Avian Vet.* 3 (Summer): 69–72.

61 Sellon, R.K. (2008). Gastrointestinal cytology (Proceedings). DVM360.

62 Samples, O.M. (2013). Diagnosis of internal parasites. Today's veterinary. *Practice* 21–26.

63 Kirkpatrick, C.E. (1982). Techniques for the diagnosis of intestinal parasites. *Anim. Health Technol.* 3: 324–331.

64 Kirkpatrick, C.E. (1984). Enteric protozoal infections. In: *Clinical Microbiology and Infectious Diseases of the Dog and Cat* (ed. C.E. Greene), 806–823. Philadelphia: WB Saunders Co.

65 Gookin, J.L. (2006). Trichomoniasis. In: *Infectious Diseases of the Dog and Cat* (ed. C.E. Greene), 745–750. St. Louis, MO: Elsevier, Inc.

66 Hale, S., Norris, J.M., and Slapeta, J. (2009). Prolonged resilience of Tritrichomonas foetus in cat faeces at ambient temperature. *Vet. Parasitol.* 166 (1–2): 60–65.

18

Fecal Flotation

Ryane E. Englar and Jeremy Bessett

18.1 Procedural Definition: What is This Test About?

Fecal flotation is a routine diagnostic test that screens concentrated fecal samples for evidence of parasitic infection. This test can recover cysts, oocysts, and eggs of mature parasites that live inside the body and reproduce [1, 2]. To perform this test, the diagnostician bathes macerated feces in hypertonic solutions of concentrated sugar or salts [1, 2]. These solutions force parasitic components, which are less dense, to float to the top, where they can be retrieved for microscopic examination [1–5]. This requires an understanding of specific gravity.

Specific gravity was first introduced in Chapter 13 with regard to urinalysis. Recall that when we measure specific gravity, we are making an assessment about density [6]. Density is a measure of the mass of an object relative to the space that it occupies [6]. When we consider density of a solution, then what we are really investigating is the mass of solute per volume of solution.

Fresh water is said to have a specific gravity of 1.000 at 4°C at sea level [6].

Tap water is said to have a specific gravity that is just above 1.000 [1].

Solutions that have a specific gravity less than 1.000 are less dense than water and will float. These include gasoline, automotive oil, kerosene, jet fuel, lard oil, and corn oil (see Figure 18.1).

Objects that are less dense than water will also float. Consider, for instance, ice cubes, and corks (see Figure 18.2).

Solutions that have a specific gravity greater than 1.000 are denser than water and will sink. These include whole milk, 5% sodium chloride, and propylene glycol.

Objects that are denser than water will also sink. Consider, for instance, parasite eggs. Regardless of which parasite they come from, ova have a specific gravity that exceeds 1.000 [1]. This means that if we tried to separate

ova from tap water through centrifugation in an attempt to get them to rise to the surface, we would be unsuccessful. The eggs would be too heavy. They would sink to the bottom instead [1].

The specific gravity of most parasite ova falls between 1.05 and 1.203 [1, 7]:

- Ascarid eggs have a specific gravity of 1.0900 [2].
- Hookworm eggs have a specific gravity of 1.0559 [2].
- Whipworm eggs have a specific gravity of 1.1453 [2].

To float ova, we must suspend them in a solution that exceeds their specific gravity [1, 2, 5, 7]. We achieve this by creating hypertonic flotation solutions that heavily concentrate sugar or salts [2].

Hypertonicity of flotation solutions is essential. However, there is such a thing as too much. If the flotation solution's specific gravity is too high, then we run the risk of rupturing ova or protozoal cysts, or at the very least, distorting them as they lose water via osmosis to the solution in which they are being bathed [5, 7].

We also want to discourage larger particulate matter that is suspended within fecal samples from also rising to the top when placed in solution [1, 5]. This would make it challenging to discern parasites from fecal debris. We must therefore keep in mind the specific gravity of feces when selecting an ideal flotation solution. Fecal matter has a specific gravity that exceeds 1.3 [1]. Therefore, our ideal fecal flotation solution should have a specific gravity that exceeds 1.2 but is less than 1.3. This provides an efficient means by which to separate out most parasitic life stages from fecal matter [1]. Because feces are heavier than the flotation solution, they will sink along with any particulate matter contained within [1, 4].

Because eggs, larvae, and cysts are less dense than most flotation solutions, they will rise to the top for sampling by the diagnostician [1, 4]. This is achieved by positioning a glass microscope slide over top of the solution. Anything

Low-Cost Veterinary Clinical Diagnostics, First Edition. Ryane E. Englar and Sharon M. Dial.
©2023 John Wiley & Sons, Inc. Published 2023 by John Wiley & Sons, Inc.

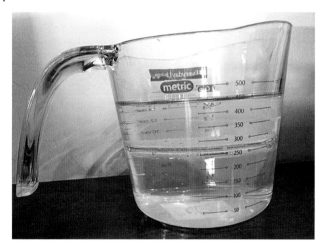

Figure 18.1 Oil mixed with water. Note that the oil is less dense than water, so the oil floats to the top, supported by the water beneath. *Source:* Courtesy of Ryane E. Englar, DVM, DABVP (Canine and Feline Practice).

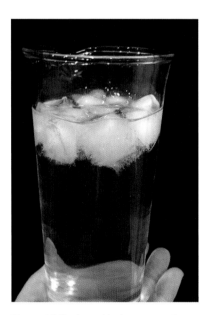

Figure 18.2 Ice added to a cup of water. The ice is less dense than water, so the ice floats to the top, supported by the water beneath. *Source:* Courtesy of Ryane E. Englar, DVM, DABVP (Canine and Feline Practice).

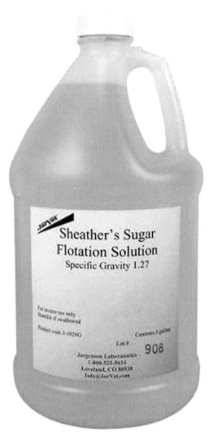

Figure 18.3 One commercially available brand of Sheather's sugar solution. *Source:* Courtesy of Ryane E. Englar, DVM, DABVP (Canine and Feline Practice).

that rises to the surface of the solution will adhere to the slide. The slide can then be examined under a microscope to facilitate identification of parasites.

Common fecal flotation solutions that are used in veterinary practice include [1, 2, 5, 7–10]:

- Sheather's sugar solution (see Figure 18.3)
  - recipe:
    - 454 g granulated sugar
    - 355 ml tap water
    - 6 ml formaldehyde
  - specific gravity: 1.27–1.33
  - advantages:
    - readily available
    - inexpensive
    - can be made in-house
    - has the highest specific gravity among the other flotation solutions that are listed here, which means that it floats most parasite eggs, including *Taenia* and *Physaloptera* species.
      - *Taenia* spp. (tapeworm) – specific gravity: 1.2251 [2]
      - *Physaloptera* (stomach worm) – specific gravity: 1.2376 [2]
    - capable of floating coccidian oocysts
    - capable of floating the eggs of the salmon poisoning fluke, *Nanophyetus salmincola,* more so than salt solutions.
    - causes less distortion of eggs than salt solutions.
  - disadvantages:
    - contains formaldehyde, which is a concern if team members have formaldehyde hypersensitivity
    - stickiness may attract arthropods, especially flies, if not kept sealed

- stickiness complicates clean-up
- viscous; takes approximately 15–20 minutes for eggs to float to the surface, as compared with sodium nitrate, which takes 10 [11]
- floats fewer eggs than sodium nitrate solution
- saturated sodium chloride (NaCl)
  - recipe:
    - 350 g–400 ml NaCl
    - 1000 ml tap water
  - specific gravity: 1.18–1.20
  - advantages:
    - inexpensive
    - easy to prepare in-house
    - readily available for purchase
  - disadvantages:
    - corrodes compound microscopes and centrifuges
    - slides dry out very quickly
    - forms crystals on the microscope slides; crystals challenge the ability of the examiner to identify parasites
    - causes distortion of fecal eggs within a few hours of preparation
    - does not float some of the heavier eggs because the specific gravity of this solution is 1.18–1.2
      - *Taenia* spp. (tapeworm) – specific gravity: 1.2251 [2]
      - *Physaloptera* (stomach worm) – specific gravity: 1.2376 [2]
- magnesium sulfate (Epsom salt; $MgSO_4$)
  - recipe:
    - 400–450 g $MgSO_4$
    - 1000 ml tap water
  - specific gravity: 1.20
  - advantages:
    - inexpensive
    - easy to prepare in-house
    - readily available for purchase
  - disadvantages:
    - crystallizes on the microscope slide
    - does not float some of the heavier eggs because the specific gravity of this solution is 1.18–1.2.
      - *Taenia* spp. (tapeworm) – specific gravity: 1.2251 [2]
      - *Physaloptera* (stomach worm) – specific gravity: 1.2376 [2]
- zinc sulfate ($ZnSO_4$) (see Figure 18.4)
  - recipe
    - 331–371 g $ZnSO_4$
    - 1000 ml warm tap water
  - specific gravity: 1.18–1.20
  - advantages:
    - comparable to sugar solution in terms of efficiency of use
    - readily available for purchase
    - preferred method for concentrating *Giardia* cysts.

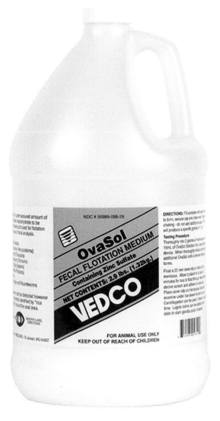

Figure 18.4 One commercially available brand of zinc sulfate solution. *Source:* Courtesy of Ryane E. Englar, DVM, DABVP (Canine and Feline Practice).

The specific gravity of Sheather's sugar solution is too high and may cause the eggs or protozoal cysts to rupture.
  - disadvantages:
    - does not float some of the heavier eggs because the specific gravity of this solution is 1.18–1.2
      - *Taenia* spp. (tapeworm) – specific gravity: 1.2251 [2]
      - *Physaloptera* (stomach worm) – specific gravity: 1.2376 [2]
- sodium nitrate ($NaNO_3$) (see Figure 18.5)
  - recipe:
    - 338–400 g $NaNO_3$
    - 1000 ml tap water
  - specific gravity: 1.18–1.20
  - advantages:
    - less viscous than Sheather's sugar solution; therefore, sodium nitrate requires only 10 minutes for the sample to be prepped for microscopic examination [11]
  - disadvantages:
    - purchased commercially and can be difficult to acquire
    - tends to be more expensive

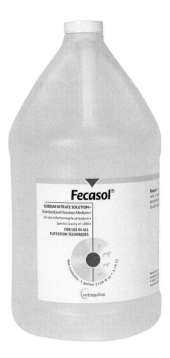

Figure 18.5 One commercially available brand of sodium nitrate solution. *Source:* Courtesy of Ryane E. Englar, DVM, DABVP (Canine and Feline Practice).

- forms crystals on slides
- does not float some of the heavier eggs because the specific gravity of this solution is 1.18–1.2
  - *Taenia* spp. (tapeworm) – specific gravity: 1.2251 [2]
  - *Physaloptera* (stomach worm) – specific gravity: 1.2376 [2]

Specific gravity of flotation solutions should be confirmed at least monthly via hydrometers [2, 7]. This is particularly important if the solution is being prepared in-house. Evaporation of the stock solution will unintentionally raise the solution's specific gravity [7]. This may be undesirable, particularly if the evaporating solution's specific gravity becomes high enough to cause rupture of cysts or ova [7].

18.2 Procedural Purpose: Why Should I Perform This Test?

Although the direct smear technique that was outlined in the preceding chapter (see Chapter 17) is a valuable diagnostic tool, its small sample size significantly reduces the likelihood that parasite eggs, larvae, or protozoal cysts will be identified [1]. Alternate methods that concentrate fecal matter provide additional value by increasing the chance that one or more developmental stages of parasites will be observed [1].

Fecal-borne parasites are prevalent among companion animals. Given the zoonotic potential of many of these parasites, fecal egg shedding represents a significant public health issue [8, 12]. Zoonotic species include, but are not limited to, *Toxocara canis, Toxocara cati, Ancylostoma caninum, Giardia* spp., *Cryptosporidium parvum*, and *Toxoplasma gondii* [8].

Although many people associate parasitic infections with tropical regions of the world, Americans are also at risk of contracting parasitic disease [13]. In 2020, the Center for Disease Control (CDC) named five parasitic infections as priorities for increasing public awareness [13]. Based upon the sheer numbers of those infected and the severity of disease, the CDC prioritized Chagas disease, neurocysticercosis, toxocariasis, toxoplasmosis, and trichomoniasis [13]. Human exposure to toxocariasis is climbing. The CDC reported exposure of 14% of the US population in 2020 with an estimated 70 people annually becoming blind because of infection [13].

A 2016 study by Lucio-Forster evaluated a cumulative data set from 2011 to 2014 that was compiled by the Companion Animal Parasite Council (CAPC). The goal of the study was to determine prevalence of *Toxocara* egg shedding from more than 500,000 feline and 2.5 million canine fecal samples [14]. Shedding of *Toxocara* by companion animals ranged from 0% to 18.2% in cats and from 0% to 5.3% in dogs depending upon the state of residence [14]. However, most states demonstrated a prevalence between 1% and 8% in cats and between 1% and 3% in dogs [14]. What this means is that for every 20 cats across the nation, 1 is shedding *Toxocara* eggs, and one out of every 60 dogs is doing the same, except for in the southwestern United States, where prevalence is higher among canine patients [14].

What is most concerning about this is that fecal samples from cats are examined less often than samples from dogs [14]. From 2011 to 2014, nearly five times as many fecal tests were submitted for canine patients as compared with feline patients, yet cats are a major source of environmental contamination when it comes to shedding of ova, particularly roundworms [14].

Lucio-Forster and Bowman examined fecal samples from 1,322 cats from shelters and affiliated foster homes in upstate New York over a 3.5-year period [15]. Eighteen different parasites were identified by the research team, and at least one parasite was detected in 50.9% of all samples [15]. The feline roundworm, *Toxocara cati*, and *Cystoisospora* spp. were most prevalent [15]. Twenty-one percent of all samples contained *Toxocara cati* [15]. Twenty-one percent of all samples contained *Cystoisospora* spp. [15]. Additional parasites and their associated percentages include: *Giardia* spp. (8.9%), the lungworm, *Aelurostrongylus abstrusus* (6.2%), ova from *Taenia* spp. (3.9%), *Cryptosporidium* spp. (3.8%), *Aonchotheca* spp. (3.7%), *Eucoleus* spp. (2.3%), *Ancylostoma* spp. (2.2%), *Cheyletiella* spp. (2.0%), *Dipylidium caninum* (1.1%), *Otodectes* spp., *Toxoplasma*-like oocysts and *Sarcocystis* spp. (0.8% each), *Demodex* and *Spirometra* spp. (0.4% each), and *Alaria* spp. and *Felicola subrostratus* (0.2% each) [15].

Regional differences in parasite distribution have been reported. For instance, a 2019 report by Hoggard et al. documented the prevalence of parasites from shelter cats in northeastern Georgia. Flotation of 103 samples using a sugar solution disclosed eggs of *Toxocara cati* (17.5%), oocysts of *Cystoisospora felis* (16.5%), *Ancylostoma* sp. (11.7%), oocysts of *Cystoisospora rivolta* (8.7%), ova from *Taenia* spp. (3.9%), *Spirometra mansonoides* (2.9%), *Mesocestoides* sp. (1%), *Dipylidium caninum* (1%), and *Eucoleus aerophilus* (1%) [16].

Over one-third of cats euthanized by animal control agencies in Northwestern Georgia (39.6%) tested positive for gastrointestinal helminths [17]. Coinfection with two helminths was present in 6.1% of the sampled population [17]. Coinfection with three or more helminths was identified in 1.1% of the sampled population [17].

These are just a handful of studies in the growing veterinary medical literature concerning gastrointestinal parasitism. These and others demonstrate that risk of feline patients acquiring intestinal parasites is real despite years of being overlooked by pet owners and veterinarians alike.

For the benefit and well-being of our patients and their caretakers, it is essential for veterinary professionals to emphasize the importance of fecal screens within the context of preventative care. We need to accurately diagnose affected patients irrespective of whether they are clinical for disease so that we can effectively implement parasite control strategies. We also need to catch and curb asymptomatic patients that contribute to environmental contamination through fecal shedding of ova.

Fecal flotation is a critical diagnostic test that identifies most gastrointestinal parasites, including roundworm, hookworm, and whipworm ova as well as protozoal oocysts, such as *Coccidia* and *Toxoplasma* [4]. In addition, fecal flotation can recover digested skin mites like *Demodex* spp. or *Cheyletiella* spp., thereby contributing to dermatologic diagnosis [4].

According to the 2020 guidelines from the CAPC, fecal analysis should take place at least four times during the first year of life for puppies and kittens [18]. Thereafter, canine and feline patients should be subject to fecal examinations at least twice per year throughout adulthood [18]. Recognize that patient health and lifestyle as well as parasite prevalence within the geographical residence of the patient may further influence frequency of fecal examination [18].

In addition to routine screening, fecal analysis must be considered an essential part of the diagnostic workup for those patients that present with aberrant defecation histories and/or clinical presentations, including, but not limited to [19]:

- constipation – prolonged retention of feces within the colon, resulting in infrequent or difficult evacuation of the feces
- coprophagia – ingestion of fecal matter [20]
- diarrhea – loose, liquid bowel movements
- dyschezia – difficult or painful defecation
- hematochezia – the presence of fresh (red) blood in the stool from lower gastrointestinal bleeds
- melena – dark-colored (often black) tarry feces containing digested blood from upper gastrointestinal bleeds
- obstipation – inability to evacuate accumulated, dry, hard feces due to diminished or absent function of the large bowel, causing impaction that may extend the entire length of the colon
- pica – the intentional consumption of nonfood items [21]
- tenesmus – straining to defecate.

18.3 Options Available for Fecal Flotation

There is more than one way to perform fecal flotation. In veterinary practice, two methodologies are commonly employed [4]:

- passive (gravitational) flotation
- centrifugal flotation
  (see Figures 18.6 and 18.7).

Passive flotation is predominant among veterinary clinics because it is efficient, expedient, and economical: disposable kits are available for purchase commercially and you do not require a centrifuge [4]. All you need is a sample, a disposable kit, flotation solution, and a microscope. Greater detail concerning equipment and procedural steps will be provided below.

Centrifugal flotation relies upon a centrifuge to separate particulate material based upon differential densities so that less dense ova or cysts float to the surface of the solution [22]. There are two types of centrifuges that you might choose to support fecal analysis in private practice:

- swinging bucket
- fixed-angle rotor
  (see Figures 18.8 and 18.9).

Regardless of which model you purchase, centrifugal flotation is considered the gold standard both in the clinic setting and at reference laboratories [4, 7, 8, 22–26]. Centrifugal flotation offers greater recovery of ova [8] as well as greater reliability in the diagnosis of *Trichuris vulpis* and *Giardia*

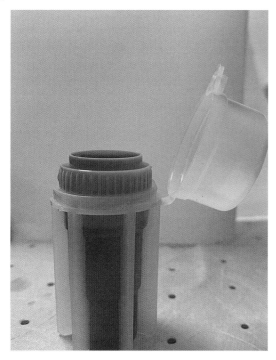

Figure 18.6 Passive (gravitational) fecal flotation. *Source: Courtesy of Jeremy Bessett, Inaugural Class of 2023, University of Arizona College of Veterinary Medicine.*

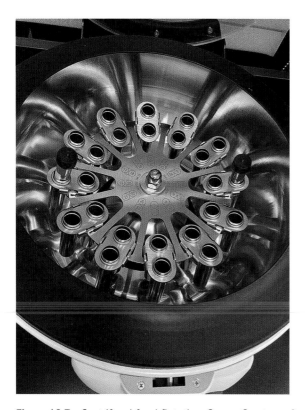

Figure 18.7 Centrifugal fecal flotation. *Source: Courtesy of Jeremy Bessett, Inaugural Class of 2023, University of Arizona College of Veterinary Medicine.*

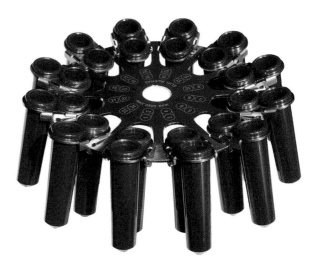

Figure 18.8 Centrifuge model that reflects the swinging bucket style. This style of centrifuge allows you to place the prepared sample into a bucket in the centrifuge, add flotation solution to form a rounded meniscus at the top of the tube, and place a coverslip on the tube. This coverslip will stay in place for the duration of centrifugation. *Source: Courtesy of Ryane E. Englar, DVM, DABVP (Canine and Feline Practice).*

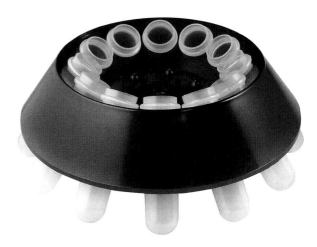

Figure 18.9 Centrifuge model that reflects the fixed-angle rotor style. Note that because the sample is placed within the centrifuge at an angle, you cannot place a coverslip on the tube during centrifugation. You also cannot form a meniscus at the top of the sample tube with flotation solution or else you risk that the sample will overflow into the centrifuge. *Source: Courtesy of Ryane E. Englar, DVM, DABVP (Canine and Feline Practice).*

lamblia [25], whereas passive fecal flotation may miss as many as 50.5% of infected dogs [27].

For ease of chapter flow, we will review centrifugal flotation first, followed by passive fecal flotation.

Note that when performing centrifugal flotation, you can choose to use either a swinging bucket centrifuge or a fixed-angle centrifuge. We have chosen to outline the procedure for a fixed-angle centrifuge below.

18.4 Equipment

Equipment that is required for fecal flotation with fixed-angle centrifuge includes:

- gloves
- fecal sample
- two 15-ml conical centrifuge tubes
  - Tubes with caps are *preferred.*
- fecal flotation solution
  - Sheather's sugar solution or zinc sulfate is *preferred.*
- two cups/containers to mix feces and flotation solution
- tongue depressor to assist with the maceration of feces
- tea strainer or woven gauze (4″ × 4″)
- microscope
- microscope slide(s)
- 22 × 22 mm glass coverslip
- centrifuge with adjustable speed
  - The centrifuge needs to be able to decrease rpm to ~1000–1200 rpm.
- laboratory tube rack.

18.5 Procedural Steps: Fecal Flotation with Fixed-Angle Centrifuge [1–4, 8, 11, 22, 23, 28]

1) After donning appropriate personal protective equipment (PPE) (at minimum, gloves, but ideally protective eyewear, too), place 2–5 g of your patient's sample into a disposable cup/ container (see Figure 18.10).

    Smaller wax paper cups work best in the authors' experience, rather than plastic cups. The flexibility of the wax paper will ultimately facilitate pouring the solution into the conical tubes. Plastic cups are more difficult to manipulate during this critical step in the process.

    Larger sample volumes of feces (e.g., 6–10 g) are acceptable provided that you use a larger volume of flotation solution (e.g., 35 ml).

2) Add ~20–35 ml of fecal flotation solution to the sample cup (see Figure 18.11). Use the larger volume (e.g., 35 ml) if you have enough feces. This is advantageous because you will then have a sufficient volume of fecal slurry to fill two conical tubes. This will yield two samples for you to examine, which increases the likelihood that you will recover eggs, cysts, or oocysts, if present.

    Having two tubes handy also automatically gives you a means by which to balance out the centrifuge.

    If you only have sufficient sample to fill one tube, then you will have to create a balancer for the

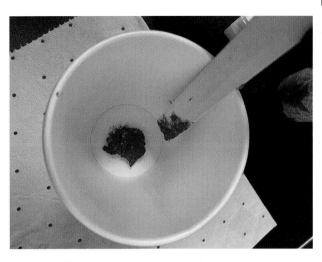

Figure 18.10 Appropriate sample size for centrifugal fecal flotation. For reference, one Hershey's Kiss weighs roughly 4.6 g. This amount is less than the size of an adult's thumb and is roughly the size of a quarter's surface. *Source:* Courtesy of Jeremy Bessett, Inaugural Class of 2023, University of Arizona College of Veterinary Medicine.

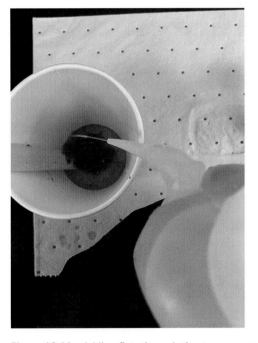

Figure 18.11 Adding flotation solution to cup containing fecal sample. *Source:* Courtesy of Jeremy Bessett, Inaugural Class of 2023, University of Arizona College of Veterinary Medicine.

centrifuge. You do this by filling another conical tube to the same volume with flotation solution.

3) Thoroughly macerate the fecal sample by mixing it with the flotation solution using the tongue depressor to break down whole feces into a slurry (see Figure 18.12).

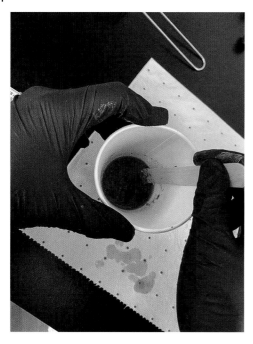

Figure 18.12 Mixing fecal sample and flotation solution. *Source:* Courtesy of Jeremy Bessett, Inaugural Class of 2023, University of Arizona College of Veterinary Medicine.

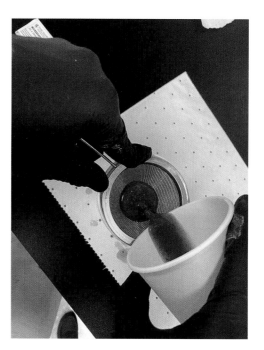

Figure 18.13 Filtering the mixture of feces and fecal flotation solution through a strainer. *Source:* Courtesy of Jeremy Bessett, Inaugural Class of 2023, University of Arizona College of Veterinary Medicine.

Strain the slurry by pouring it through a tea strainer into a clean cup or other suitable container. Use a tongue depressor to agitate the slurry to facilitate its passage through the strainer (see Figures 18.13 and 18.14).

If you are using woven gauze in lieu of a strainer, unfold the gauze so that you are straining the slurry through a single layer.

As the slurry filters through the gauze, apply pressure to the solid matter in the center of the gauze to facilitate the material squishing through. This is very helpful, especially if Sheather's sugar solution is used. Sheather's sugar solution is viscous with a high surface tension. As a result, the solution has a propensity to stick to the gauze. A significant portion of your slurry can get "stuck" within the gauze, meaning that you will lose a good amount of your sample to the gauze if you do not gently squeeze the solid matter to help dislodge excess solution.

4) Once you have successfully filtered the slurry through the strainer or woven gauze, you are left with a suspension of sample in one cup and solid matter in the other. Discard the cup with solid matter.

5) Pour the remaining suspension into conical centrifuge tubes, filling the tube approximately 0.5 to 1 cm from the top. Secure the cap on the conical tube (see Figures 18.15 and 18.16).

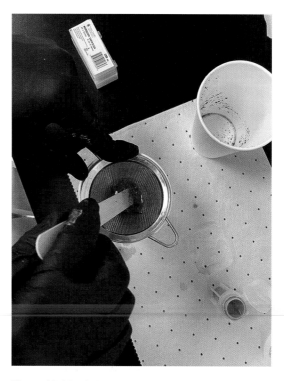

Figure 18.14 Agitating the mixture of feces and fecal flotation solution as it is strained through a filter. *Source:* Courtesy of Jeremy Bessett, Inaugural Class of 2023, University of Arizona College of Veterinary Medicine.

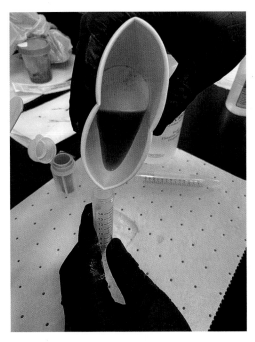

Figure 18.15 Pouring filtrate into a conical tube. *Source: Courtesy of Jeremy Bessett, Inaugural Class of 2023, University of Arizona College of Veterinary Medicine.*

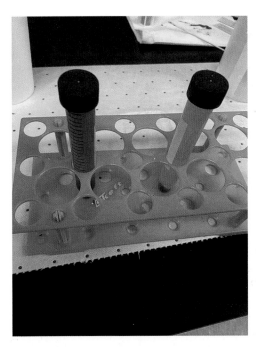

Figure 18.16 Capping the conical tube and placing it in the tube rack prior to centrifugation. *Source:* Courtesy of Jeremy Bessett, Inaugural Class of 2023, University of Arizona College of Veterinary Medicine.

6) Place the sample tube(s) in the fixed-angle centrifuge. If you had sufficient sample to fill two tubes, then there is no need for an additional balancer. Place both sample tubes opposite each other in the centrifuge and they will effectively balance each other out.

   If you only had sufficient sample to fill one tube, you need to create a balancer. To do so, fill another conical tube with flotation solution to the same volume as the sample tube and place the balancer tube opposite the sample tube in the centrifuge (see Figure 18.17).

7) You are now ready to begin the centrifugation process. Centrifuge sample(s) at approximately 1000–1200 rpm for five minutes.

8) Remove sample tubes from the centrifuge (see Figure 18.18).

9) Remove caps from sample tubes and place tubes in tube rack oriented vertically.

   Fill the sample tubes with fresh flotation solution to form a *slight* meniscus (see Figure 18.19).

10) Place a coverslip on top of the meniscus. When you do so, little to no solution should spill over. Note that a

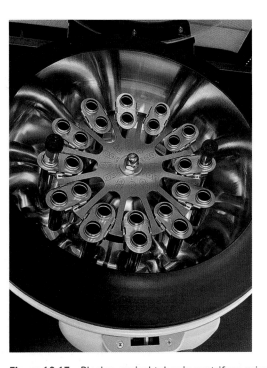

Figure 18.17 Placing conical tubes in centrifuge prior to centrifugation. Note that there are two tubes and that these tubes have been placed opposite each other in the centrifuge to balance each other out. The centrifuge that is pictured here is a swinging bucket type. The authors did not have a comparable picture using the fixed-angle rotor. *Source:* Courtesy of Jeremy Bessett, Inaugural Class of 2023, University of Arizona College of Veterinary Medicine.

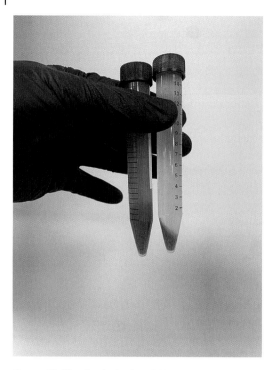

Figure 18.18 Conical tubes following centrifugation. Note the supernatant and pellet, which are both particularly prominent in the sample on the right. *Source:* Courtesy of Jeremy Bessett, Inaugural Class of 2023, University of Arizona College of Veterinary Medicine.

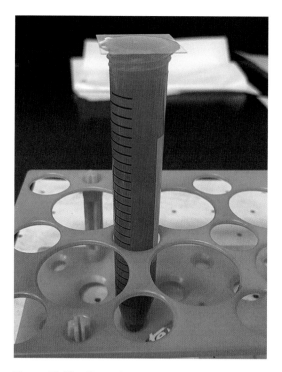

Figure 18.20 Coverslip placed on top of meniscus. *Source:* Courtesy of Jeremy Bessett, Inaugural Class of 2023, University of Arizona College of Veterinary Medicine.

small air bubble under the coverslip is acceptable (see Figure 18.20).

The amount of time for the coverslip to rest upon the meniscus is variable. It depends upon the flotation solution that you used:

- When you choose sodium nitrate as a flotation solution, 10 minutes is sufficient to allow the eggs to float to the coverslip.
- When you choose zinc sulfate as a flotation solution, 10–12 minutes is sufficient.
- When you choose Sheather's sugar solution, 15 minutes is ideal. The high viscosity of the Sheather's solution causes the ova to rise more slowly.

11) Remove the coverslip and place it directly on a glass slide with the wet side down (e.g., the side that had been in contact with the fecal suspension) (see Figures 18.21 and 18.22).

12) Scan the *entire* glass slide first at 10×.

13) Further evaluate the slide at 40× to assist with identification of ova.

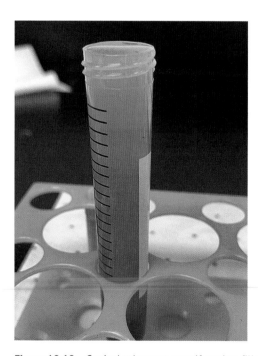

Figure 18.19 Conical tube post-centrifugation, filled with fresh flotation solution to achieve meniscus. *Source:* Courtesy of Jeremy Bessett, Inaugural Class of 2023, University of Arizona College of Veterinary Medicine.

18.6 Time Estimate to Perform Fecal Flotation with Fixed-Angle Centrifuge

Twenty to thirty minutes.

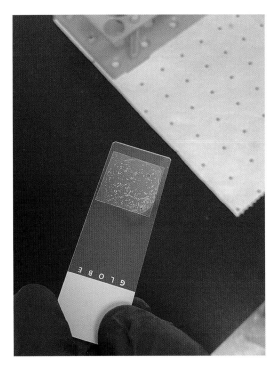

Figure 18.21 Creating one slide from a single sample.
Source: Courtesy of Jeremy Bessett, Inaugural Class of 2023, University of Arizona College of Veterinary Medicine.

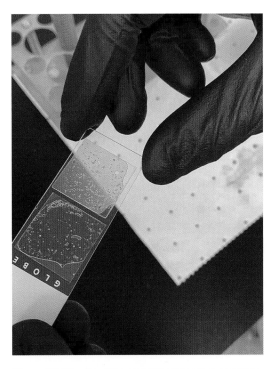

Figure 18.22 Creating one slide from two samples.
Source: Courtesy of Jeremy Bessett, Inaugural Class of 2023, University of Arizona College of Veterinary Medicine.

18.7 Brief Consideration of the Procedural Steps in the Event a Swinging Bucket Centrifuge Is Used

The swinging bucket style of centrifuge allows you to add flotation solution directly to the sample as it sits in the tube holder within the centrifuge so that you can place a coverslip over the slight meniscus prior to centrifugation. The coverslip will stay in place for the duration of centrifugation if you gradually increase the speed of the rotor during centrifugation to *no more than* 800 rpm. This step is critical because it allows the centrifuge bucket to move slowly into a horizontal position. If you ignore this step and attempt to go from 0 to 800 rpm rapidly, then the coverslip is likely to be dislodged from the sample tube. This defeats the purpose of fecal flotation using a swinging bucket centrifuge.

18.8 Equipment

In Section 18.5, we reviewed the procedural steps for fecal flotation with a fixed-angle centrifuge, as is considered to be the gold standard. Let us now shift our attention to a method that predominates in many veterinary clinics due to its perceived efficiency: passive (gravitational) flotation. One advantage of passive (gravitational) flotation is that disposable kits are available for purchase commercially and you do not require a centrifuge [4].

All that you require is:

- gloves
- fecal sample
- fecal flotation solution
- disposable fecal diagnostic kit
- microscope slide(s)
- 22 mm × 22 mm glass coverslip
- microscope
  (see Figure 18.23).

18.9 Procedural Steps

For passive fecal flotation,

1) After donning appropriate PPE (at minimum, gloves, but ideally protective eyewear, too), gather supplies, including the patient sample (e.g., 2–5 g of feces).
2) Lift the cap of the disposable fecal diagnostic kit (e.g. Fecalyzer® or Ovassay®) (see Figures 18.24 and 18.25).

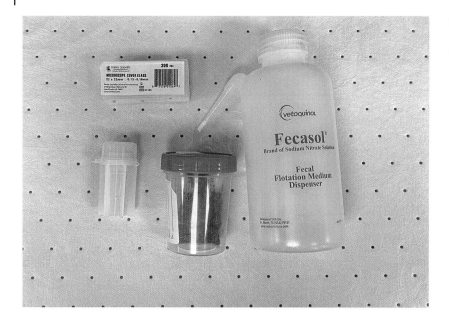

Figure 18.23 Materials needed for passive fecal flotation. *Source:* Courtesy of Jeremy Bessett, Inaugural Class of 2023, University of Arizona College of Veterinary Medicine.

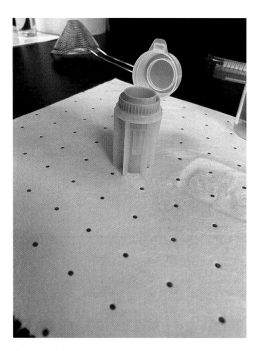

Figure 18.24 Profile view of disposable fecal diagnostic kit, ready to be filled. *Source:* Courtesy of Jeremy Bessett, Inaugural Class of 2023, University of Arizona College of Veterinary Medicine.

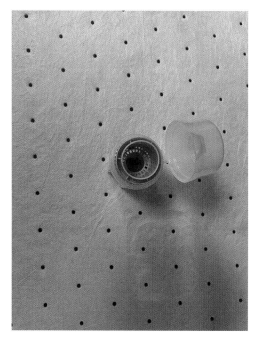

Figure 18.25 Aerial view of disposable fecal diagnostic kit, ready to be filled. *Source:* Courtesy of Jeremy Bessett, Inaugural Class of 2023, University of Arizona College of Veterinary Medicine.

3) Remove the green insert.
   Press the small end of the insert into the fecal sample. You may need to scoop or pour diarrheic feces into the small end of the insert (see Figure 18.26).
   Replace the green insert into the device (see Figure 18.27).

4) With the sample-loaded insert in place, add the flotation solution until the fluid level reaches about halfway up the device (see Figures 18.28 and 18.29).

5) Mix the fecal sample and flotation solution by rotating the insert to macerate the feces (see Figures 18.30 and 18.31).

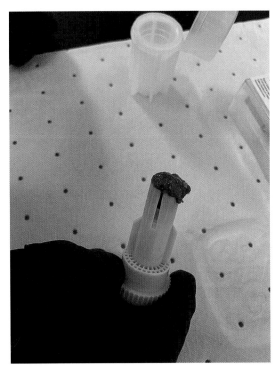

Figure 18.26 Appropriate sample size for passive fecal flotation. *Source:* Courtesy of Jeremy Bessett, Inaugural Class of 2023, University of Arizona College of Veterinary Medicine.

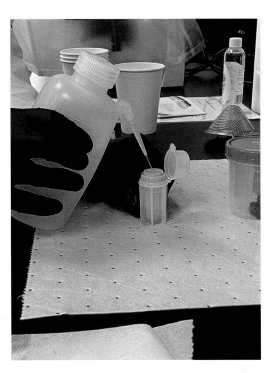

Figure 18.28 Profile view of adding flotation solution to the disposable fecal diagnostic kit. *Source:* Courtesy of Jeremy Bessett, Inaugural Class of 2023, University of Arizona College of Veterinary Medicine.

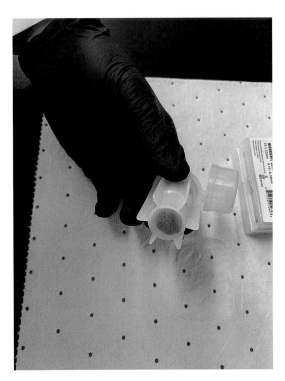

Figure 18.27 Disposable fecal diagnostic kit, to which feces have been added. *Source:* Courtesy of Jeremy Bessett, Inaugural Class of 2023, University of Arizona College of Veterinary Medicine.

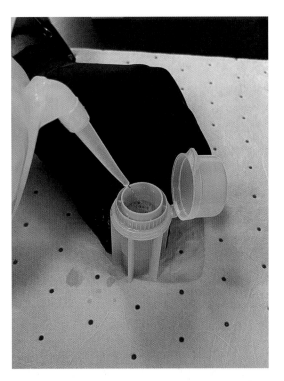

Figure 18.29 Close-up view of adding flotation solution to the disposable fecal diagnostic kit. *Source:* Courtesy of Jeremy Bessett, Inaugural Class of 2023, University of Arizona College of Veterinary Medicine.

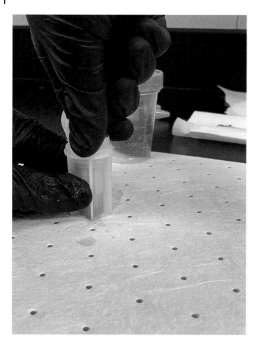

Figure 18.30 Mixing the sample of feces and flotation solution by rotating the insert. *Source:* Courtesy of Jeremy Bessett, Inaugural Class of 2023, University of Arizona College of Veterinary Medicine.

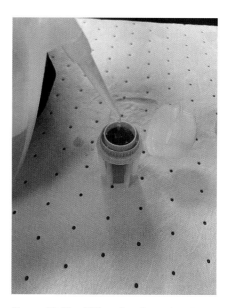

Figure 18.32 Filling the disposable fecal diagnostic kit to achieve a slight meniscus. *Source:* Courtesy of Jeremy Bessett, Inaugural Class of 2023, University of Arizona College of Veterinary Medicine.

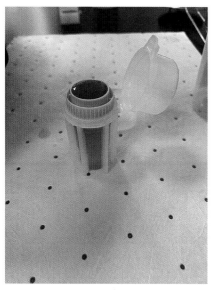

Figure 18.33 Slight meniscus has been achieved. *Source:* Courtesy of Jeremy Bessett, Inaugural Class of 2023, University of Arizona College of Veterinary Medicine.

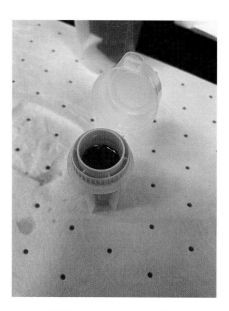

Figure 18.31 Close-up view of the appropriately mixed slurry. *Source:* Courtesy of Jeremy Bessett, Inaugural Class of 2023, University of Arizona College of Veterinary Medicine.

6) With the bottom edge of the cap, push on the insert until it is firmly seated in the device.
7) Fill the device with flotation solution to form a slight meniscus (see Figures 18.32–18.34).
8) Place cover slip on the meniscus for the prescribed number of minutes. Follow the instructions that have been provided by the manufacturer of the disposable fecal

diagnostic kits that you have purchased as the number of minutes that you will wait will be determined by the type of flotation solution that the kits require.

For instance, the package insert for Ovassay®, which uses zinc sulfate as a flotation solution, reports that there is a five-minute wait time.

The package insert for Fecalyzer®, which makes use of Fecasol® (sodium nitrate) as a flotation solution, reports that there is a 15–20 minute wait time (see Figures 18.35 and 18.36).

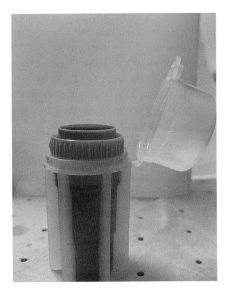

Figure 18.34 Profile view of slight meniscus. *Source:* Courtesy of Jeremy Bessett, Inaugural Class of 2023, University of Arizona College of Veterinary Medicine.

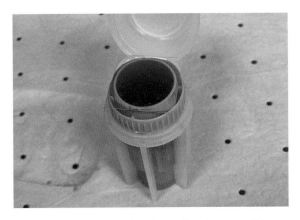

Figure 18.35 Coverslip has been placed on top of the meniscus. *Source:* Courtesy of Jeremy Bessett, Inaugural Class of 2023, University of Arizona College of Veterinary Medicine.

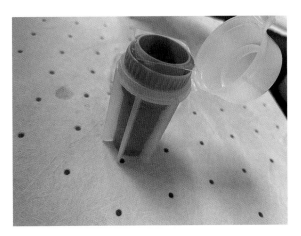

Figure 18.36 Alternate view of coverslip in place over meniscus. *Source:* Courtesy of Jeremy Bessett, Inaugural Class of 2023, University of Arizona College of Veterinary Medicine.

9) Transfer the cover slip to a microscope for examination.
10) Close the cap tightly for easy disposal.

18.10   Time Estimate to Perform Passive Fecal Flotation

Ten to twenty-five minutes, depending upon test kit manufacturer instructions.

18.11   Procedural Tips and Troubleshooting for Fecal Flotation

- Check your equipment before you begin. If you are performing centrifugal flotation, invest in a centrifuge that is smooth-running and both accelerates and decelerates slowly [3].
- Fresh samples are essential. Older samples make it more likely that parasites will have developed to a stage that is not typically identified in the feces [10]. For instance, hookworm eggs will expediently hatch out to first-stage larvae [10].
- If clients cannot bring in a fresh sample, then encourage refrigeration of the sample unless you suspect giardiasis [10].
- *Giardia* cysts are unlikely to survive refrigeration. If you suspect that your patient has giardiasis, then wait until you are able to test a fresh sample [7].
- When samples are diarrheic, the number of parasite eggs or cysts that can be recovered is reduced because parasites are diluted out by the water content of the sample [10]. In this instance, increase the volume of feces that you will examine to compensate for the dilution effect [10].
- Allow the sample to stand for the specified amount of time before examining it under the microscope [8]. Prep time is essential because it allows the parasite eggs to rise to the surface of the flotation solution. If you rush the process, then you are likely to miss out on identifying parasitic life stages that would have floated to the top, had you just allowed them the time to do so.
- At the same time, you do not want to delay microscopic review of the prepped sample indefinitely. In this case, more time is not always better. Unnecessary delays in microscopic examination increase the chance that crystals will precipitate out of salt solutions (see Figure 18.37). Crystals obscure the examiner's view and contribute to false negative results.

18.12   Interpreting Test Results

The goal of fecal flotation is to recover cysts, oocysts, and eggs of mature parasites that live inside the body and reproduce [1, 2].

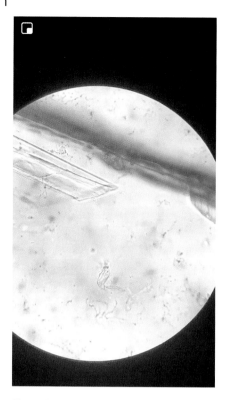

Figure 18.37 Crystal artifact as seen under the microscope after delaying review of a prepped sample. *Source:* Courtesy of Ryane Englar, DVM, DABVP (Canine and Feline Practice).

The primary purpose of this chapter is to provide the reader with the tools to perform this procedure efficiently in a manner that can be repeated successfully to improve the yield and accuracy of test results.

This chapter is *not* intended to be an atlas of all parasites and their associated life stages. Only the most common fecal parasites in cats and dogs will be shown here. *For additional information, please refer to a veterinary parasitology text.*

18.12.1 Ascarids (Roundworms)

Ascarids (roundworms) are zoonotic helminths that are ubiquitous in soil and cause infection when dogs and cats ingest ova by eating dirt and/or drinking infected milk [19, 29–31]. Transplacental infection is also possible [19]. Because of vertical transmission, puppies and kittens are assumed to have roundworm infections at birth or shortly thereafter [19]. Therefore, prophylactic deworming is standard practice in companion animal medicine [19, 29–32].

Clinically important roundworms in dogs and cats include [19, 29–31]:

- *Toxocara canis*
- *Toxocara cati*
- *Toxocara leonina.*

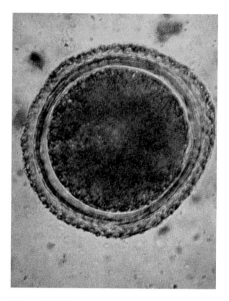

Figure 18.38 *Toxocara canis* egg on fecal examination, using light microscopy. *Source:* Courtesy of Dr. Araceli Lucio-Forster, Cornell University College of Veterinary Medicine.

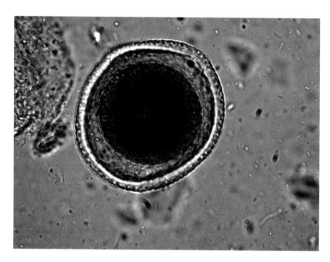

Figure 18.39 *Toxocara cati* egg on fecal examination, using light microscopy. *Source:* Courtesy of Dr. Araceli Lucio-Forster, Cornell University College of Veterinary Medicine.

Affected patients may present with a rounded belly, dry or dull coat, poor weight gain, and/or stunted growth, diarrhea, and/or vomiting [19].

Diagnosis of ascariasis is via detection of ova by fecal flotation or gross observation of roundworms in the feces or vomitus [19] (see Figures 18.38–18.41).

18.12.2 Hookworms

Hookworms are also zoonotic helminths [19]. They are acquired by dogs and cats primarily through nursing; however, larvae may also penetrate the vertebrate host's skin [19, 29–31, 33].

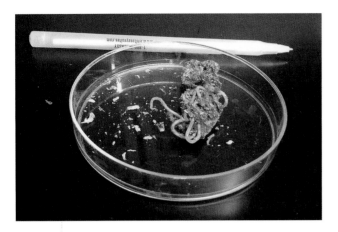

Figure 18.40 Adult *Toxocara cati* in a stool sample.
Source: Courtesy of Dr. Araceli Lucio-Forster, Cornell University College of Veterinary Medicine.

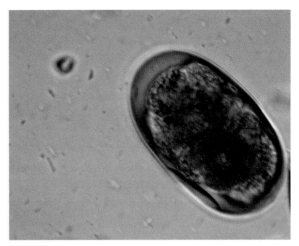

Figure 18.42 *Uncinaria* egg on fecal examination, using light microscopy. *Source:* Courtesy of Dr. Araceli Lucio-Forster, Cornell University College of Veterinary Medicine.

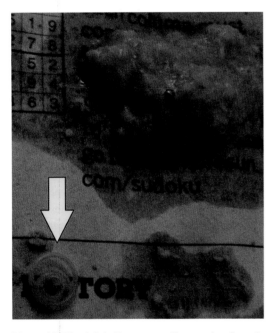

Figure 18.41 Adult *Toxocara cati* in sample of vomitus.
Source: Courtesy of Sigma and Cassandra Filloramo.

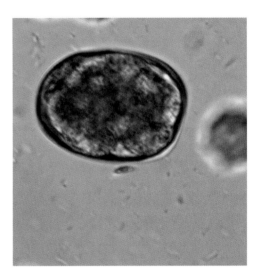

Figure 18.43 *Ancylostoma* egg on fecal examination, using light microscopy. *Source:* Courtesy of Dr. Araceli Lucio-Forster, Cornell University College of Veterinary Medicine.

Clinically important hookworms in dogs and cats include [19, 34]:

- *Ancylostoma caninum*
- *Ancylostoma tubaeforme*
- *Uncinaria stenocephala.*

Because hookworms ingest a large amount of blood from their hosts, patients may present with varying degrees of anemia in addition to diarrhea and/or dark, tarry stool [19, 29].

Diagnosis of hookworms is via detection of hookworm eggs via fecal flotation [19] (see Figures 18.42 and 18.43).

Unlike adult roundworms, hookworms cannot be seen by the naked eye.

18.12.3 Tapeworms

Tapeworms are zoonotic cestodes, that is, parasitic flatworms [19, 31].

Commonly diagnosed tapeworms in dogs and cats include [19, 34]:

- *Dipylidium caninum*
- *Taenia* spp.

Let us begin with *Dipylidium caninum*. Fleas are vectors of *Dipylidium caninum* [19, 35–48]. Vertebrate hosts become infected with *Dipylidium caninum* when they ingest fleas that contain tapeworm larvae. Within the small intestine of the vertebrate host, the tapeworm larvae mature into adults. This process takes, on average, a month. The adult tapeworms attach themselves to the small intestinal walls of their host [19]. As they mature, they produce eggs that are stored within terminal segments called proglottids [19].

Once a proglottid is full of eggs, it detaches from the host's intestinal wall and is shed in the host's feces [19]. Proglottids are visible to the naked eye and may resemble grains of white rice or cucumber seeds [19, 31, 49] (see Figures 18.44 and 18.45). Affected dogs and cats may

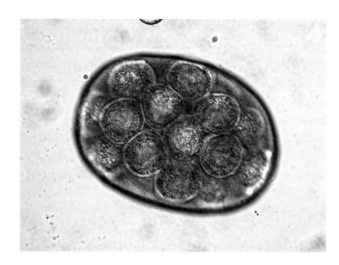

Figure 18.46 *Dipylidium caninum* egg packet, 20×.
Source: Courtesy of Dr. Araceli Lucio-Forster, Cornell University College of Veterinary Medicine.

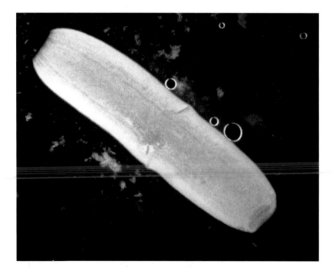

Figure 18.44 *Dipylidium caninum* proglottid. *Source:* Courtesy of Sarah Bashaw, DVM.

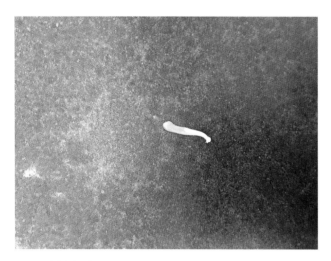

Figure 18.45 Magnified *Dipylidium* segment. *Source:* Courtesy of Dr. Araceli Lucio-Forster, Cornell University College of Veterinary Medicine.

exhibit perianal pruritus and/or scooting as proglottids emerge from the rectum [19].

Each proglottid contains egg capsules or packets, each containing 5–30 hexacanth ova [19, 31]. These eggs are released into the environment when each proglottid breaks open [19] (see Figure 18.46).

Now let us shift gears to consider *Taenia* spp. as another type of cestode. *Taenia taeniaeformis* is found in both canine and feline patients, whereas *Taenia pisiformis* is found primarily in domestic and wild canids [19]. These species cause disease in cats and dogs when they ingest intermediate hosts [19]. Intermediate hosts for *Taenia* spp. are infected rodents or hares [19, 31].

When cats or dogs ingest infected rodents or hares, they inadvertently consume larvae of *Taenia* spp. [19]. These larvae migrate to the small intestine where they mature [19]. As they mature, they produce eggs that are stored within proglottids, just like *Dipylidium caninum* [19]. Once a proglottid is full of eggs, it detaches and is shed in the host's feces [19]. The *Taenia* proglottid can be distinguished from the *Dipylidium caninum* proglottid based upon its shape when viewed microscopically (see Figure 18.47).

Diagnosis of *Taenia* spp. more typically occurs through detection of eggs during fecal flotation (see Figure 18.48).

18.12.4 Whipworms

Whipworms are large intestinal parasites that are named because their shape resembles a whip: they have a wider head that tapers to a narrow tail [19, 31]. They are most often acquired through vertical transmission; however, adult dogs may also acquire whipworms by ingesting infected wildlife, feces, soil, or water [19, 50].

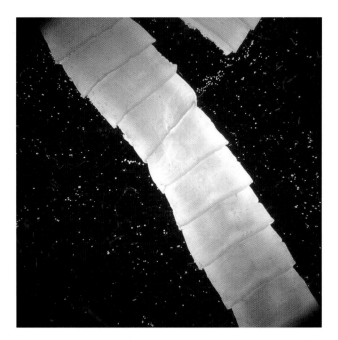

Figure 18.47 Magnified *Taenia* segment. *Source:* Courtesy of Dr. Araceli Lucio-Forster, Cornell University College of Veterinary Medicine.

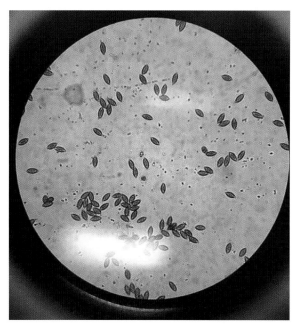

Figure 18.49 Whipworm eggs, low magnification. *Source:* Courtesy of Dr. Laura Nelson.

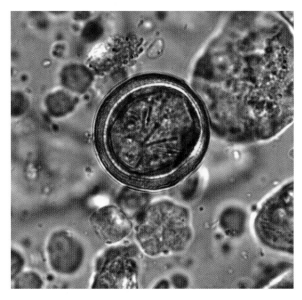

Figure 18.48 *Taenia* egg, 40×. *Source:* Courtesy of Dr. Araceli Lucio-Forster, Cornell University College of Veterinary Medicine.

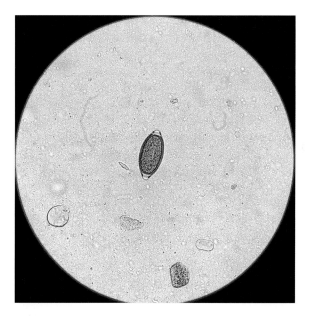

Figure 18.50 Whipworm egg, higher magnification. *Source:* Courtesy of Ryane E. Englar, DVM, DABVP (Canine and Feline Practice).

Trichuris vulpes is a clinically important canine whipworm [34]. Affected dogs typically present for diarrhea, weight loss, anemia, and/or hematochezia [50].

Diagnosis is via detection of eggs via fecal flotation [50]. Eggs are football-shaped with polar plugs at both ends [50] (see Figures 18.49 and 18.50).

The football shape is easy to identify; however, it is not pathognomonic for whipworms [19, 50]. Ova from respiratory parasites, such as the capillarids *Eucoleus (Capillaria) aerophila* and *Eucoleus (Capillaria) boehmi* share the same shape [19, 50]. However, the capillarid eggs tend to be smaller in size than those of *Trichuris vulpes* [19, 50].

18.12.5 Protozoa

Helminths and cestodes are not the only clinically relevant intestinal parasites in companion animals.

Clinically important protozoa in dogs and cats include [34]:

- Coccidia
- *Cryptosporidium* spp.
- *Giardia* spp. (see Chapter 17)
- *Tritrichomonas foetus* (see Chapter 17).

Coccidiosis is caused by a number of species, including *Hammondia, Isospora,* and *Sarcocystis* spp. [19, 31]. In addition, cats may become infected with *Besnoitia* spp. [19, 31]. Of these, *Isospora* spp. are most often identified in dogs and cats with clinical disease [19].

Isospora spp. tend to be host-specific [19].

- Feline coccidiosis is most often caused by *I. felis* and *I. rivolta* [19].
- Canine coccidiosis is most often caused by *I. canis, I. ohioensis, I. burrowsi,* and *I. neorivolta* [19].

The diagnosis of coccidiosis is made by detecting eggs via fecal flotation (see Figures 18.51–18.54).

Cryptosporidiosis is another cause of protozoal diarrhea in dogs and cats [19, 34, 51]. *Cryptosporidium canis* and *Cryptosporidium felis* infect dogs and cats respectively [19, 51]. Both are zoonotic [19, 51]. Oocysts are detected on fecal examination; however, false negatives are common due to intermittent shedding as well as the fact that oocysts are very small and easy to miss [52]. Please refer to a textbook of veterinary parasitology for a visual of how these oocysts appear via light microscopy.

For addition information about *Giardia* spp. or *Tritrichomonas foetus*, please refer to Chapter 17. Although *Giardia* cysts can be seen through fecal flotation, the trophozoite stage is better suited for visualization via direct smear (refer to Figures 17.7 and 17.8). The concave underside of the trophozoite's tear-shaped body makes it appear cupped or spoon-like as it moves through space in a pattern that resembles a falling leaf [19, 53, 54].

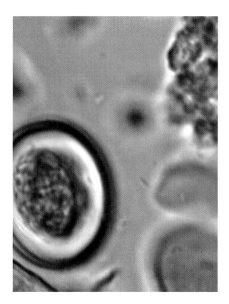

Figure 18.52 *Isospora rivolta. Source:* Courtesy of Dr. Araceli Lucio-Forster, Cornell University College of Veterinary Medicine.

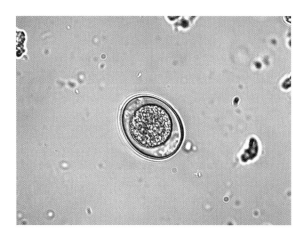

Figure 18.53 *Isospora canis. Source:* Courtesy of Dr. Araceli Lucio-Forster, Cornell University College of Veterinary Medicine.

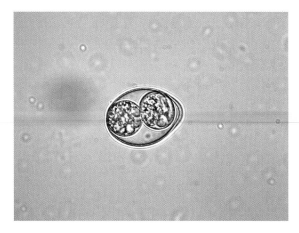

Figure 18.54 *Isospora ohioensis. Source:* Courtesy of Dr. Araceli Lucio-Forster, Cornell University College of Veterinary Medicine.

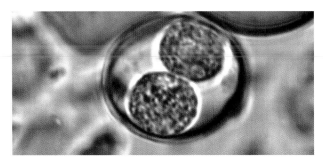

Figure 18.51 *Isospora felis. Source:* Courtesy of Dr. Araceli Lucio-Forster, Cornell University College of Veterinary Medicine.

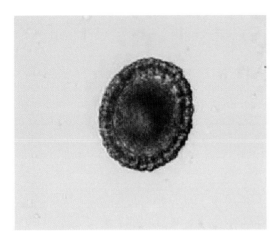

Figure 18.55 *Baylisascaris procyonis* ovum. *Source:* Courtesy of Ryane E. Englar, DVM, DABVP (Canine and Feline Practice).

18.13 Clinical Case Example(s)

A four-year-old female intact Coonhound from Maryland is presented for routine wellness examination. The client shares that their land backs up to a reservoir and that the patient is allowed to freely roam throughout acres of forest because hunting is illegal throughout the preserved land. The client's only concern is that the patient scavenges and bring back parts of carcasses. Examination discloses that the patient is apparently healthy with a body condition score of 4/9. A sample of feces is submitted for centrifugal flotation as part of a routine preventative screen. The sample tests positive for an unusual egg that is smaller in size than *Toxocara canis* and darker (see Figure 18.55).

You research the mystery egg and discover that the patient is shedding ova from *Baylisascaris procyonis*. *Baylisascaris procyonis* is a relatively common parasite of raccoons and is seen most typically in the northeastern and midwestern United States [55].

If untreated, this patient may remain aclinical. However, the infection may develop into progressive neurologic disease [55]. In addition, *Baylisascaris procyonis* is known to cause ocular and/or visceral larval migrans in people [55].

18.14 Add-On Tests That You May Need to Consider and Their Additive Value

Flotation is just one of many diagnostic tools that is routinely involved in performing fecal analysis. Although it is one of the best tools to recover cysts, oocysts, and eggs of mature internal parasites, false negatives do occur, and the procedure is not ideal for identification of motile trophozoites.

Therefore, additional modalities may be of benefit, particularly in chronic cases that have eluded diagnosis. These include:

- history-taking
- direct smear (see Chapter 17)
- *Giardia* antigen detection test (see Chapter 17)
- complete blood count (CBC) and chemistry profile
- Baermann test.

18.14.1 The Rationale for History-Taking as an Add-On Diagnostic Tool

The successful practice of veterinary medicine requires attentive history-taking, which contributes to diagnostic accuracy through clinical reasoning [56, 57]. Traditionally, the value of observation and touch has been prioritized by clinicians. Veterinarians are trained to use their eyes and hands to identify key structures and to differentiate normal from abnormal physical exam findings. However, clinicians gather significant data before the exam even begins, by asking the client a combination of open-ended and closed-ended questions.

History-taking is especially important when investigating cases involving diarrheic patients. The answers that we obtain during history-taking allow us to localize disease within the gastrointestinal tract. Disease localization facilitates diagnosis. For instance, consider the canine whipworm, *Trichuris vulpis*. This parasite resides in the cecum or ascending colon. Although infections may be subclinical, patients that experience heavy worm burdens are symptomatic and often present for evaluation of large bowel diarrhea [50]. We can discover whether the patient has large bowel diarrhea by asking the right questions during history-taking. We know, for example, that large bowel diarrhea is characterized by [19, 58]:

- gelatinous semi-formed stool
- high volume of mucus
- increased frequency of defecation
- increased urgency of defecation
- tenesmus
- +/− hematochezia.

So, if we ask the client questions about frequency and urgency of defecation, whether the patient is exhibiting straining, and what the diarrhea looks (and feels!) like, then we are likely to narrow down our list of differentials. If we discover through the process of history-taking that our patient does indeed have large bowel diarrhea, then we must add whipworms to our growing list of differential diagnoses.

18.14.2 The Rationale for the Direct Smear as an Add-On Diagnostic Tool

Direct "wet mount" smears are add-on diagnostic tests that screen fecal samples for motile organisms, including trophozoites, that may not survive the hypertonic solutions that are involved in fecal flotation [1, 26, 59, 60]. Trophozoites represent one of many stages in the life cycle of certain protozoa. The two flagellate protozoans that we prioritize in companion animal medicine are *Giardia* spp. and *Tritrichomonas foetus*. Both have been implicated as causative agents of gastrointestinal disease of companion animals. These organisms can be identified on wet mounts, contingent upon the examiner's experience and skill [59, 60]. Direct smears are also an effective tool for the identification of amoebae (e.g. *Entamoeba histolytica*), nematode larvae (e.g. *Strongyloides* spp.), spores of *Clostridium* spp., and motile bacteria, such as *Campylobacter* [26, 60, 61].

Please refer to Chapter 17 for additional information.

18.14.3 The Rationale for Giardia Antigen Detection Tests as an Add-On Diagnostic Tool

Centrifugal fecal flotation with zinc sulfate is the preferred method for concentrating *Giardia* cysts [2]. However, this statement presumes that veterinary practices have adequately trained personnel [2, 62–64].

In the words of Drs. Dryden, Payne, Ridley, and Smith, "*Giardia* is one of the most commonly misdiagnosed, underdiagnosed, and overdiagnosed parasites." [2] Patients that are infected with *Giardia* spp. shed small, fragile cysts intermittently [2]. Although centrifugation using zinc sulfate is the preferred method for concentrating *Giardia* cysts, cyst misidentification is common [2]. This led to the development of fecal antigen tests with high sensitivity in human healthcare [2]. The goal was to reduce the number of false negatives, meaning that fewer cases of disease were missed.

Giardia antigen detection tests have also been developed for use in veterinary practice to facilitate diagnosis of dogs and cats with clinical disease. These tests are convenient and augment the chance of recording a positive finding if used in combination with fecal flotation [2].

Please refer to Chapter 17 for additional information – in particular, Figures 17.23–17.26.

18.14.4 The Rationale for CBC and Blood Chemistry Profile Tests as Add-On Diagnostic Tools

Although fecal analysis should be routinely performed as a screening test in asymptomatic patients, it is typically run more often as part of a gastrointestinal workup [26].

A structured approach to the gastrointestinal workup expedites diagnosis, which allows us to initiate treatment sooner.

When a patient presents with gastrointestinal signs, such as vomiting, diarrhea, regurgitation, weight loss, altered appetite, abdominal distension, and/or abdominal pain, we need to first determine whether disease is localized or systemic (e.g. metabolic).

Fecal analysis plays an essential role; however, parasitism is not the only cause of gastrointestinal distress. For example, renal and hepatic disease may contribute to gastrointestinal signs. So, too, can endocrinopathies such as Addison's disease.

Even if a parasite is to blame, depending upon the parasite load and fecal shedding, we may or may not be able to identify the offending organism(s). Therefore, it helps for us to maintain a broad rather than narrow scope in trying to gather a complete portrait of disease. This includes expanding the diagnostic workup to include other laboratory tests such as a CBC and chemistry profile.

To appreciate how an expanded diagnostic profile facilitates case management, let us reconsider the canine whipworm, *Trichuris vulpis*. Infection with *Trichuris vulpis* is often associated with the following changes on the patient's CBC:

- anemia
- eosinophilia
- hypoproteinemia.

The following changes on the patient's serum biochemistry profile are also consistent with infection with *Trichuris vulpis* [65–69]:

- hyponatremia
- hyperkalemia
- decreased sodium to potassium (Na : K) ratio (normal: 27–40).

These changes in electrolytes cause clinical signs of weakness that mimic Addison's disease [65–69]. For this reason, whipworm infection is often referred to as Pseudo-Addison Disease [65–69]. However, the results of basal and post-ACTH stimulation cortisolemia for a dog with whipworm infection will be within normal limits [65–69].

18.14.5 The Rationale for the Baermann Test as an Add-On Diagnostic Tool

If you suspect nematode larvae, such as *Aelurostrongylus* spp., the Baermann test is the preferred diagnostic tool [7, 70].

Aelurostrongylus spp. are lungworms [70–74]. Additional species of lungworms that infect cats include [70, 71, 74–78]:

- *Capillaria aerophila* or *Eucoleus aerophilus*
- *Paragonimus kellicotti*
- *Troglostrongylus brevior.*

Lungworms of the following species infect dogs [70, 72, 75, 79–81]:

- *Angiostrongylus vasorum*
- *Capillaria aerophila* or *Eucoleus aerophilus*
- *Crenosoma vulpis*
- *Eucoleus boehmi*
- *Filaroides hirthi*
- *Filaroides milksi*
- *Oslerus osleri*
- *P. kellicotti.*

Lungworm infection mirrors asthma and other bronchial diseases [70, 71, 76]. Coughing and wheezing are commonly reported in cases of *Aelurostrongylus abstrusus* infection [70, 71, 76, 82, 83]. Sneezing and nasal discharge are also frequent [70, 71, 76, 82, 83]. Young, debilitated, or immunosuppressed patients may present with tachypnea, dyspnea, or open-mouth breathing that leads to respiratory distress and potentially sudden death [70, 71, 84].

Diagnosis of lungworm infection is challenging because the radiographic appearance of lungworm-associated respiratory pathology is identical to feline asthma [70, 71, 85, 86].

Thankfully, the first-stage larvae (L1s) of lungworms hop aboard the cat's mucociliary clearance mechanism [70, 87]. In so doing, they travel from the feline lung to the pharynx, where they are swallowed [70, 87]. Following digestion, they appear microscopically in feces [87].

Unfortunately, the yield from fecal flotation is low [70, 71]. The hypertonicity of fecal flotation solutions often damages lungworm larvae beyond our ability to recognize them [70, 71, 82, 88].

Larval identification is made possible by the Baermann migration method [70, 71, 76, 88, 89]. Results are not immediate. Samples may not test positive until 12–48 hours after set-up [70, 71, 76, 88, 89].

18.15 Key Takeaways

- There is a misconception among veterinarians and the public that well cared for pets do not get exposed to parasites; however, companion animal shedding of intestinal parasites, including their ova, is common among shelter patients as well as owned pets [14–17].

- Environmental contamination with shed parasites and their ova contributes to new infections as well as reinfection among repeat offenders.
- Fecal shedding of parasites and their ova is a significant public health issue, given that many gastrointestinal parasites are zoonotic [8, 12, 90].
- Accurate and frequent fecal analysis is key to maintaining preventative health care of our patients and their caretakers alike [90].
- Flotation is one component of fecal analysis that can recover cysts, oocysts, and eggs of mature parasites that live inside the body and reproduce [1, 2].
- Fecal flotation involves macerating feces in hypertonic solutions of concentrated sugar or salts, followed by centrifugation to separate particles based upon differential densities [1, 2, 22]. Ova and cysts are less dense, so they float to the top of the solution.
- There are two types of fecal flotation: passive (gravitational) and centrifugal.
- Centrifugation recovers more eggs than passive flotation [7, 8, 26] and is more likely to detect those parasites with low numbers of dense eggs, for instance, *Trichuris* spp. [7, 10].
- Passive (gravitational) fecal flotation is readily performed in clinical practice due to ease and convenience [27], but often misses the diagnosis of giardiasis [8, 27].
- Regardless of whether you use passive or centrifugal flotation and regardless of which flotation solution you use, adhere to the guidelines with respect to timing when you should examine your fecal preps.
- A negative result does not guarantee that the patient is free of intestinal parasites. A true negative signifies that no parasites or ova were seen today.
- Examiner error and methodology also impact the sensitivity of fecal examination methods [27].
- False negatives may occur when an infected animal is tested during asymptomatic pre-patent periods [27].
- False negatives also may occur if the parasite infection is light, meaning that few ova or cysts are being shed at any given time in the feces [27].

18.16 Clinical Pearls

- There is often a mentality in practice that "it's *just* a fecal test." This attitude is in many respects what leads practices to delegate fecal analysis to the least trained member of the veterinary team. The reality is that it is not *just* a fecal test. A fecal analysis is as important as any other diagnostic test. Furthermore, because some internal parasites are zoonotic, we owe it to our clients and our team as much as our patients to evaluate samples methodically and with accuracy [2].

- Dwight Bowman said it best: "Feces puddling is by no means an exact science. The actual procedure followed is less important than a show of respect for the basic principles involved" [11].
- If samples are collected from the ground, then there is the potential that the sample will be contaminated with free-living organisms [10].
- Fecal samples that are contaminated with urine may also contain eggs of the bladder worm, *Pearsonema (Capillaria) plica* [50].
- You can also freeze prepared slides for months or even years [5].
- Alternatively, apply fingernail polish or quick-drying glue around the coverslip to increase the shelf life of a fecal flotation slide [5].

- *Trichuris* eggs are football-shaped eggs with polar plugs and a clear-brown unstriated shell [50].
- The football shape is easy to identify; however, it is not pathognomonic for whipworms. The same shape is seen among ova from capillarids of the respiratory tree – *Eucoleus (Capillaria) aerophilia* and *Eucoleus (Capillaria) boehmi* [50]
- *Capillarid* eggs have a striated shell and are yellower in color, with polar plugs that are not directly opposite one another [50].
- The eggs of *Baylisascaris* are slightly smaller and darker than the eggs of *Toxocara canis*, and lack a pitted surface [55].

References

1 Hendrix, C.M. and Robinson, E. (2017). Common laboratory procedures for diagnosing parasitism. In: *Diagnostic Parasitology for Veterinary Technicians*, 5e (ed. C.M. Hendrix and E. Robinson), 303–335. St. Louis, Missouri: Elsevier Inc.

2 Dryden, M.W., Payne, P.A., Ridley, R.K., and Smith, V.E. (2006). *Gastrointestinal Parasites: The Practice Guide to Accurate Diagnosis and Treatment*, vol. 28. Compendium: Continuing Education for Veterinarians (8(A)).

3 Ballweber, L.R., Beugnet, F., Marchiondo, A.A., and Payne, P.A. (2014). American Association of Veterinary Parasitologists' review of veterinary fecal flotation methods and factors influencing their accuracy and use--is there really one best technique? *Veterinary Parasitology* 204 (1–2): 73–80.

4 Haller, J. (2021). The Veterinary Nurse's Guide to Fecal Flotation Techniques. Today's Veterinary Nurse [Internet]. (Fall).

5 Foreyt, B. (2001). *Veterinary Parasitology Reference Manual*, 5e, vol. viii, 235 p. Ames, Iowa: Iowa State University Press.

6 Polzin, D.J. and Osborne, C.A. (2012). Urinalysis in acutely and critically ill dogs and cats. In: *Advanced Monitoring and Procedures for Small Animal Emergency and Critical Care* (ed. J.M. Burkitt Creedon and H. Davis), 409–420. Chichester, West Sussex: Wiley-Blackwell.

7 Knoll, J.S. (2010). An Egg Hunt for Parasites. DVM360 [Internet]. https://www.dvm360.com/view/egg-hunt-parasites.

8 Dryden, M.W., Payne, P.A., Ridley, R., and Smith, V. (2005). Comparison of common fecal flotation techniques for the recovery of parasite eggs and oocysts. *Veterinary Therapeutics* 6 (1): 15–28.

9 Samples, O.M. (2013(July/August)). Diagnosis of internal parasites. Today's veterinary. *Practice* 21–26.

10 Blagburn, B.L. (2003). Diagnosing Internal Parasites in Cats. DVM360 [Internet]. https://www.dvm360.com/view/diagnosing-internal-parasites-cats.

11 Bowman, D.D. and Georgi, J.R. (2003). Diagnostic Parasitology. In: *Georgis' Parasitology for Veterinarians*, 8e (ed. D.D. Bowman and J.R. Georgi), 287–358. Saunders/Elsevier: St. Louis, Mo.

12 Jones, J.L., Kruszon-Moran, D., Won, K. et al. (2008). Toxoplasma gondii and Toxocara spp. co-infection. *The American Journal of Tropical Medicine and Hygiene* 78 (1): 35–39.

13 Parasites - Parasitic Infections in the United States: Center for Disease Control. (2020) https://www.cdc.gov/parasites/npi/index.html.

14 Lucio-Forster, A., Mizhquiri Barbecho, J.S., Mohammed, H.O. et al. (2016). Comparison of the prevalence of Toxocara egg shedding by pet cats and dogs in the U.S.A., 2011–2014. *Veterinary Parasitology: Regional Studies and Reports* 5: 1–13.

15 Lucio-Forster, A. and Bowman, D.D. (2011). Prevalence of fecal-borne parasites detected by centrifugal flotation in feline samples from two shelters in upstate New York. *Journal of Feline Medicine and Surgery* 13 (4): 300–303.

16 Hoggard, K.R., Jarriel, D.M., Bevelock, T.J., and Verocai, G.G. (2019). Prevalence survey of gastrointestinal and respiratory parasites of shelter cats in northeastern Georgia, USA. *Veterinary Parasitology: Regional Studies and Reports* 16: 100270.

17 Carleton, R.E. and Tolbert, M.K. (2004). Prevalence of Dirofilaria immitis and gastrointestinal helminths in cats euthanized at animal control agencies in Northwest Georgia. *Veterinary Parasitology* 119 (4): 319–326.

18 General Guidelines for Dogs and Cats: Companion Animal Parasite Council (CAPC). (2020) https://capcvet.org/guidelines/general-guidelines.

19 Englar, R.E. (2019). Changes in fecal appearance. In: *Common Clinical Presentations in Dogs and Cats* (ed. R.E. Englar), 647–670. Hoboken, NJ: Wiley-Blackwell.

20 Coprophagia, R.L. (2015). NAVC Clinician's Brief [Internet]. (July).

21 Englar, R.E. (2019). Abnormal Ingestive behaviors. In: *Common Clinical Presentations in Dogs and Cats* (ed. R.E. Englar), 611–616. Hoboken, NJ: Wiley-Blackwell.

22 B. B. Why fecal centrifugation is better: Companion Animal Parasite Council (CAPC). (2022) https://capcvet.org/articles/why-fecal-centrifugation-is-better.

23 Blagburn, B.L. and Butler, J.M. (2006). Optimize intestinal parasite detection with centrifugal fecal flotation. *Veterinary Medicine* 101 (7): 455–464.

24 Dryden, M.W., Payne, P.A., and Smith, V. (2006). Accurate diagnosis of Giardia spp and proper fecal examination procedures. *Veterinary Therapeutics* 7 (1): 4–14.

25 Zajac, A.M., Johnson, J., and King, S.E. (2002). Evaluation of the importance of centrifugation as a component of zinc sulfate fecal flotation examinations. *Journal of the American Animal Hospital Association* 38 (3): 221–224.

26 Broussard, J.D. (2003). Optimal fecal assessment. *Clinical Techniques in Small Animal Practice* 18 (4): 218–230.

27 Gates, M.C. and Nolan, T.J. (2009). Comparison of passive fecal flotation run by veterinary students to zinc-sulfate centrifugation flotation run in a diagnostic parasitology laboratory. *The Journal of Parasitology* 95 (5): 1213–1214.

28 Knoll, J.S. (2010). Procedure for centrifugal fecal flotation. DVM360 [Internet]. https://www.dvm360.com/view/procedure-centrifugal-fecal-flotation.

29 Guidelines for Veterinarians: Prevention of Zoonotic Transmission of Ascarids and Hookworms. https://www.cdc.gov/parasites/zoonotichookworm/resources/prevention.pdf.

30 Schantz, P.M. (2007). Zoonotic parasitic infections contracted from dogs and cats: How frequent are they? DVM 360 [Internet]. http://veterinarymedicine.dvm360.com/zoonotic-parasitic-infections-contracted-dogs-and-cats-how-frequent-are-they.

31 Bowman, D.D. and Georgi, J.R. (2009). *Georgis' Parasitology for Veterinarians*, 9e, vol. ix. St. Louis, Mo: Saunders/Elsevier 451 p.

32 Hall, E.J. and German, A.J. (2005). Diseases of the small intestine. In: *Textbook of Veterinary Internal Medicine*, 6e (ed. S.J. Ettinger and E.C. Feldman), 1332–1378. Philadelphia: WB Saunders.

33 Burke, T.M. and Roberson, E.L. (1985). Prenatal and lactational transmission of Toxocara canis and Ancylostoma caninum: experimental infection of the bitch at midpregnancy and at parturition. *International Journal for Parasitology* 15 (5): 485–490.

34 Magne, M.L. (2006). Selected topics in pediatric gastroenterology. *The Veterinary Clinics of North America. Small Animal Practice* 36 (3): 533–548, vi.

35 Blagburn, B.L. and Dryden, M.W. (2009). Biology, treatment, and control of flea and tick infestations. *The Veterinary Clinics of North America. Small* 39 (6): 1173-+.

36 Dryden, M.W. and Rust, M.K. (1994). The cat flea - biology, ecology and control. *Veterinary Parasitology* 52 (1–2): 1–19.

37 Rust, M.K. and Dryden, M.W. (1997). The biology, ecology, and management of the cat flea. *Annual Review of Entomology* 42: 451–473.

38 Traversa, D. (2013). Fleas infesting pets in the era of emerging extra-intestinal nematodes. *Parasites & Vectors* 6: 59.

39 Flick, S.C. (1973). Endoparasites in cats: current practice and opinions. *Feline Practice* 4: 21–34.

40 Hitchcock, D.J. (1953). Incidence of gastro-intestinal parasites in some Michigan kittens. *North America Veterinary* 34: 428–429.

41 Arundel, J.H. (1970). Control of helminth parasites of dogs and cats. *Australian Veterinary Journal* 46 (4): 164–168.

42 Baker, M.K., Lange, L., Verster, A., and van der Plaat, S. (1989). A survey of helminths in domestic cats in the Pretoria area of Transvaal, Republic of South Africa. Part 1: the prevalence and comparison of burdens of helminths in adult and juvenile cats. *Journal of the South African Veterinary Association* 60 (3): 139–142.

43 Boreham, R.E. and Boreham, P.F.L. (1990). Dipylidium-caninum - life-cycle, epizootiology, and control. *Compendium on Continuing Education for the Practising* 12 (5): 667-&.

44 Collins, G.H. (1973). A limited survey of gastro-intestinal helminths of dogs and cats. *New Zealand Veterinary Journal* 21 (8): 175–176.

45 Coman, B.J. (1972). A survey of the gastro-intestinal parasites of the feral cat in Victoria. *Australian Veterinary Journal* 48 (4): 133–136.

46 Coman, B.J. (1972). Helminth parasites of the dingo and feral dog in Victoria with some notes on the diet of the host. *Australian Veterinary Journal* 48 (8): 456–461.

47 Coman, B.J., Jones, E.H., and Driesen, M.A. (1981). Helminth parasites and arthropods of feral cats. *Australian Veterinary Journal* 57 (7): 324–327.

48 Engbaek, K., Madsen, H., and Larsen, S.O. (1984). A survey of helminths in stray cats from Copenhagen with ecological aspects. *Zeitschrift für Parasitenkunde* 70 (1): 87–94.

49 Griffiths, H.J. (1978). *Handbook of Veterinary Parasitology*. Minnesota: University of Minnesota.

50 Zajac, A.M. (2003(April)). A Case of Canine Diarrhea. *NAVC Clinician's Brief* 13. 4.

51 Bowman, D. (2009). Canine and feline cryptosporidiosis and giardiasis DVM 360 [Internet]. http://veterinarycalendar.dvm360.com/canine-and-feline-cryptosporidiosis-and-giardiasis-proceedings.

52 Little, S. (ed.) (2011). *Diarrhea in Kittens and Young Cats. WSAVA World Congress*. Jeju, Korea.

53 Giardiasis, S.V. (2013). NAVC Clinician's Brief. (February):71–86.

54 Kirkpatrick, C.E. (1987). Giardiasis. *The Veterinary Clinics of North America. Small Animal Practice* 17 (6): 1377–1387.

55 Kazacos, K.R. (2006(June)). Unusual Fecal Parasite in a Dog. *NAVC Clinician's Brief* 37–39.

56 Englar, R. (2019). The problem-oriented approach to clinical medicine. In: *Common Clinical Presentations in Dogs and Cats*, 3–10. Hoboken, NJ: Wiley.

57 Englar, R. (2019). The role of the comprehensive patient history in the problem-oriented approach. In: *Common Clinical Presentations in Dogs and Cats*, 11–18. Hoboken, NJ: Wiley.

58 Englar, R.E. (2021). The adult diarrheic dog. In: *The Veterinary Workbook of Small Animal Clinical Cases* (ed. R.E. Englar). Essex, U.K: 5m Publishing.

59 Dryden, M.W. and Payne, P.A. (2010(April)). Fecal Examination Techniques. *NAVC Clinician's Brief* 13–16.

60 Trumel, C. and Dossin, O. (2020). Fecal cytology. In: *Veterinary Cytology* (ed. L.C. Sharkey, M.J. Radin and D. Seelig), 407–410. Hoboken, NJ: Wiley-Blackwell.

61 Foreyt, W.J. (1989). Diagnostic parasitology. *The Veterinary Clinics of North America. Small Animal Practice* 19 (5): 979–1000.

62 Zimmer, J.F. and Burrington, D.B. (1986). Comparison of four techniques of fecal examination for detecting canine giardiasis. *Journal of the American Animal Hospital Association (JAAHA).* 22: 161–167.

63 Payne, P.A., Dryden, M.W., and Ridley, R. (2002). Evaluation of the efficacy of Drontal plus and GiardiaVax to eliminate cyst shedding in dogs naturally infected with Giardia spp. *Journal of the American Veterinary Medical Association (JAVMA).* 220 (3): 330–333.

64 Barr, S.C., Bowman, D.D., and Erb, H.N. (1992). Evaluation of two test procedures for diagnosis of giardiasis in dogs. *American Journal of Veterinary Research* 53 (11): 2028–2031.

65 Venco, L., Valenti, V., Genchi, M., and Grandi, G. (2011). A dog with Pseudo-Addison disease associated with Trichuris vulpis infection. *Journal of Parasitology Research* 2011: 682039.

66 DiBartola, S.P., Johnson, S.E., Davenport, D.J. et al. (1985). Clinicopathologic findings resembling hypoadrenocorticism in dogs with primary gastrointestinal disease. *Journal of the American Veterinary Medical Association* 187 (1): 60–63.

67 Graves, T.K., Schall, W.D., Refsal, K., and Nachreiner, R.F. (1994). Basal and ACTH-stimulated plasma aldosterone concentrations are normal or increased in dogs with trichuriasis-associated pseudohypoadrenocorticism. *Journal of Veterinary Internal Medicine* 8 (4): 287–289.

68 Car, S., Croton, C., and Haworth, M. (2019). Pseudohypoadrenocorticism in a Siberian husky with Trichuris vulpis infection. *Case Reports in Veterinary Medicine* 2019: 3759683.

69 DiBartola, S.P. and De Morais, H.A. (2000). Clinical Cases. In: *Fluid Therapy in Small Animal Practice*, 2e (ed. S.P. DiBartola), 548–597. Philadelphia, PA: WB Saunders.

70 Englar, R.E. (2019). Sneezing and coughing. In: *Common Clinical Presentations in Dogs and Cats* (ed. R.E. Englar). Hoboken, NJ: Wiley-Blackwell.

71 Traversa, D. and Di Cesare, A. (2016). Diagnosis and management of lungworm infections in cats: cornerstones, dilemmas and new avenues. *Journal of Feline Medicine and Surgery* 18 (1): 7–20.

72 Palma, D. (2016(October)). Common Pulmonary Diseases in Dogs. *NAVC Clinician's Brief* 77–109.

73 Palma D. Common pulmonary diseases in cats. NAVC Clinician's Brief. 2017(March):107–15.

74 Conboy, G. (2009). Helminth parasites of the canine and feline respiratory tract. *The Veterinary Clinics of North America. Small Animal Practice* 39 (6): 1109–1126. vii.

75 Pechman, R.D. (1994). Respiratory parasites. In: *The Cat: Diseases and Clinical Management* (ed. R.G. Sherding), 613–622. New York: Churchill Livingstone.

76 Traversa, D. and Di Cesare, A. (2013). Feline lungworms: what a dilemma. *Trends in Parasitology* 29 (9): 423–430.

77 Brianti, E., Giannetto, S., Dantas-Torres, F., and Otranto, D. (2014). Lungworms of the genus Troglostrongylus (Strongylida: Crenosomatidae): neglected parasites for domestic cats. *Veterinary Parasitology* 202 (3–4): 104–112.

78 Bowman, D.D., Hendrix, C.M., and Lindsay, D.S. (2002). *Feline Clinical Parasitology*, 262–272. Ames, IA: Iowa State University Press; 338–350 p.

79 Herman, L.H. and Helland, D.R. (1966). Paragonimiasis in a cat. *Journal of the American Veterinary Medical Association* 149 (6): 753-&.

80 Pechman, R.D. (1976). Radiographic features of pulmonary paragonimiasis in dog and cat. *Journal of the American Veterinary Radiology Society* 17 (5): 182–191.

81 Pechman, R.D. (1980). Pulmonary paragonimiasis in dogs and cats - review. *The Journal of Small Animal Practice* 21 (2): 87–95.

82 Traversa, D., Di Cesare, A., Milillo, P. et al. (2008). Aelurostrongylus abstrusus in a feline colony from Central Italy: clinical features, diagnostic procedures and molecular characterization. *Parasitology Research* 103 (5): 1191–1196.

83 Traversa, D., Lia, R.P., Iorio, R. et al. (2008). Diagnosis and risk factors of Aelurostrongylus abstrusus (Nematoda, Strongylida) infection in cats from Italy. *Veterinary Parasitology* 153 (1–2): 182–186.

84 Pechman, R.D. Jr. (1984). Newer knowledge of feline bronchopulmonary disease. *The Veterinary Clinics of North America. Small Animal Practice* 14 (5): 1007–1019.

85 Losonsky, J.M., Thrall, D.E., and Prestwood, A.K. (1983). Radiographic evaluation of pulmonary abnormalities after Aelurostrongylus abstrusus inoculation in cats. *American Journal of Veterinary Research* 44 (3): 478–482.

86 Mahaffey, M.B. (1979). Radiographic-pathologic findings in experimental Aelurostrongylus-Abstrusus infection in cats. *Journal of the American Veterinary Radiology Society* 20 (2): 81-.

87 Carruth, A.J., Buch, J.S., Braff, J.C. et al. (2019). Distribution of the feline lungworm Aelurostrongylus abstrusus in the USA based on fecal testing. *JFMS Open Reports* 5 (2): 2055116919869053.

88 Traversa, D., Di Cesare, A., and Conboy, G. (2010). Canine and feline cardiopulmonary parasitic nematodes in Europe: emerging and underestimated. *Parasites & Vectors* 3: 62.

89 Lacorcia, L., Gasser, R.B., Anderson, G.A., and Beveridge, I. (2009). Comparison of bronchoalveolar lavage fluid examination and other diagnostic techniques with the Baermann technique for detection of naturally occurring Aelurostrongylus abstrusus infection in cats. *Journal of the American Veterinary Medical Association* 235 (1): 43–49.

90 Blagburn, B.L. (2006). A strategic approach to diagnosing and treating gastrointestinal parasites. *Compendium: Continuing Education for Veterinarians.* 28 (8(A)).

Part 5

Quick Assessment of Body Cavity Fluids

19

Body Cavity Fluid Analysis

Sharon M. Dial

19.1 Procedural Definition: What Is This Test About?

The analysis of the fluid from the thorax, pericardium, and abdomen provides information necessary in determining the type of fluid (effusion) and will assist in determining the cause of the fluid accumulation, choosing additional diagnostic tests, and developing an appropriate treatment plan. The complete body cavity fluid analysis provides a nucleated cell count, total protein, and cytologic evaluation of the nucleated cells seen in the sample.

19.2 Procedural Purpose: Why Should I Perform This Test?

Accumulation of any fluid within a body cavity compartment warrants analysis of the fluid to determine the protein and cellular constituents of the fluid. The character of the fluid within a body cavity assists in determining the underlying mechanism that caused the fluid accumulation and, in turn, will assist in developing an appropriate differential diagnosis list for the patient. Fluid accumulates within body cavities by the following mechanisms:

- alterations in intravascular hydrostatic pressure
  - venous hypertension
  - arteriolar hypertension
  - lymphatic obstruction
- alterations in vascular permeability
  - inflammation/vasculitis
- alterations in intravascular oncotic pressure
  - hypoproteinemia – most often hypoalbuminemia
- hemorrhage or lymphatic rupture
- loss of fluid from gall bladder (bile peritonitis), urinary bladder (uroabdomen), gastrointestinal perforation.

The concentration of protein, nucleated cell count, and types of cells within the fluid are used to characterize fluid accumulation into several types of effusions:

- transudate – fluids with low total protein and low cellularity
- exudate – fluids with high total protein and high cellularity
- high-protein (protein-rich) transudate – high-protein and low to moderate cellularity.

The last category was previously called "modified transudates". However, the term modified transudate is insufficiently informative to be useful. It is even more useful to categorize some effusions by mechanism and cellular components:

- hemorrhagic effusion
- chylous effusion/lymphocytic effusion
- inflammatory effusions
  - suppurative exudate ± sepsis
  - pyogranulomatous exudate ± sepsis
  - bile peritonitis
  - uroabdomen
- neoplastic effusion.

The abdominal and pleural cavities of the healthy dog and cat do not contain sufficient fluid to allow collection and determination of reference intervals. As a result, the total protein and cell counts provided for interpretation are based on the values found in patients known to have a specific disease process and mechanism for fluid accumulation or from necropsy of dogs and cats without evidence of disease.

The differential diagnoses for body cavity effusions include:

- transudate – fluids with low total protein and low cellularity

- ○ venous obstruction due to mass occupying lesions
  - ▪ heart-based masses
  - ▪ mediastinal masses
  - ▪ acute lung torsion
  - ○ severe hypoalbuminemia (serum albumin < 1.5)
    - ▪ protein-losing nephropathy
    - ▪ protein-losing enteropathy
    - ▪ end-stage liver disease
- high-protein (protein-rich) transudate – high-protein low to moderate cellularity
  - ○ venous hypertension
    - ▪ cardiac disease
    - ▪ portal hypertension (pre- and posthepatic portal hypertension)
    - ▪ mass occupying lesions
    - ▪ vasculitis (including feline infectious peritonitis)
    - ▪ bile peritonitis
    - ▪ uroabdomen
- exudate – fluids with high total protein and high cellularity
  - ○ suppurative exudate with sepsis
    - ▪ penetrating wounds of the thorax or abdomen
    - ▪ gastrointestinal rupture or perforation
      - • esophageal perforation – thorax
      - • intestinal perforation – abdomen
    - ▪ compromised gastrointestinal wall without perforation
  - ○ suppurative exudate without sepsis
    - ▪ pancreatitis
    - ▪ uroabdomen
    - ▪ bile peritonitis
  - ○ pyogranulomatous (mixed inflammation) exudate with sepsis
    - ▪ fungal disease
    - ▪ parasitic disease (mesocestoides)
    - ▪ chronic bacterial disease
    - ▪ feline infectious peritonitis
  - ○ pyogranulomatous (mixed inflammation) without sepsis
    - ▪ chronic fluid accumulation from transudative processes
    - ▪ vasculitis
    - ▪ neoplasia
- hemorrhagic effusion
  - ○ rupture or trauma to abdominal viscera (spleen and liver)
  - ○ vascular neoplasia (atrial and splenic hemangiosarcoma)
  - ○ mass lesions eroding into major vessels (neoplasia, granuloma)
  - ○ inherited or acquired coagulopathies
- chylous effusion/lymphocytic effusion
  - ○ lymphatic vessel rupture (thoracic duct most common)
  - ○ lymphatic obstruction
  - ○ lymphoid neoplasia
- neoplastic effusion.

19.3 Equipment

Equipment used for this test includes:

- Body cavity fluid collected in Ethylenediaminetetraacetic acid (EDTA) anticoagulant
- refractometer
- glass slides
- Romanowski stain set
- pipette or microhematocrit tube
- conical centrifuge tubes
- centrifuge.

19.4 Procedural Steps: How Do I Perform This Test?

Common procedures for all fluids, no cavity specified.

- Collect all equipment and supplies for the procedure (see Figure 19.1).

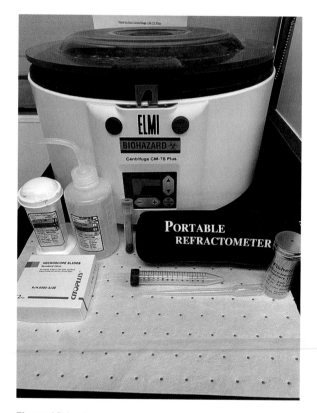

Figure 19.1 Equipment and supplies needed for performing a body cavity fluid analysis include: fluid collected in ethylenediaminetetraacetic acid anticoagulant, refractometer, glass slides, Romanowsky stain set, pipette, or microhematocrit tube, and conical centrifuge tubes. *Source:* Jeremy Bessett (Contributor).

- Collect fluid samples for fluid analysis into a blood collection tube with ethylenediaminetetraacetic acid (EDTA) anticoagulant.
  - The collection tube should be filled at least half way to avoid an artifactual increase in fluid total protein by refractometer.
  - If there is suspicion for a possible septic process, collect additional fluid in a sterile tube without anticoagulant. EDTA can inhibit bacterial cell growth. Do not use this sample for any of the in-house procedures. It is reserved for culture if needed.
- Record the color and clarity of the fluid (see Figure 19.2a–c).
- Perform a fluid total protein by following the procedure outlined in Chapter 4 to determine total plasma protein using the refractometer.
  - If the fluid appears to be highly cellular (cloudy), a small portion of the fluid can be centrifuged and the total protein can be performed on the supernatant. Cloudy fluids can make it difficult to read the total protein.
  - The sediment from the centrifuged sample can be used for making a sediment preparation for cytology.
- If the fluid is red and cloudy, consistent with a hemorrhagic effusion, perform a PCV to compare with a peripheral blood PCV of the patient.

Note: Always reserve a portion of the fluid sample to be submitted to a reference laboratory before performing any of the in-house procedures that require centrifugation.

- While a full fluid analysis includes a total nucleated cell count, this procedure does not include a nucleated cell count because the WBC counting systems used for manual nucleated cell counts are difficult to find.
  - Some in-house hematology instruments can provide a nucleated cell count. However, most do not recommend running fluid samples in these instruments because they are not validated for counting nucleated cells in fluid samples. The instrument manufacturer should include a method for counting cells in fluids if it is appropriate and validated.
  - Degree of cellularity can be determined by reviewing a direct preparation of fluid (see Figure 19.3a–c).
  - The WBC count estimate method discussed in Chapter 6 is not valid for estimating a nucleated cell count in fluids. Cellularity evaluation is a qualitative assessment.
  - It is recommended to submit fluid samples for a full fluid analysis and pathologists review if the microscopic evaluation of the fluid reveals sufficient cellularity, atypical cells, or possible unusual microorganisms or to document and confirm in-house findings.
- Prepare a cytology slide for staining and evaluation of the cellular elements. Always prepare a direct cytology preparation from the fluid and then, if needed, a preparation from a sedimented sample.
  - For the direct preparations:
    - Prepare a cytology preparation using either the blood film method as described in Chapter 6 for samples that appear bloody or a pull preparation as described for the buffy coat in Chapter 5.
  - If the fluid is clear or slightly hazy,

(a)

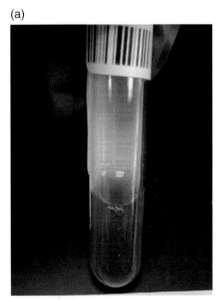

(b)

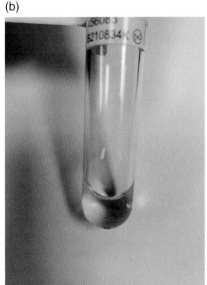

(c)

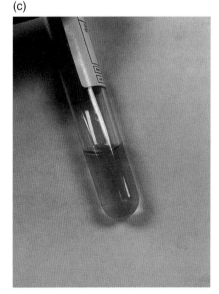

Figure 19.2 (a) Red, cloudy pericardial fluid from a dog; (b) clear, light yellow abdominal fluid from a dog; (c) light yellow slightly cloudy abdominal fluid from a cat. *Source:* Jeremy Bessett (Contributor).

(a)

(b)

(c)

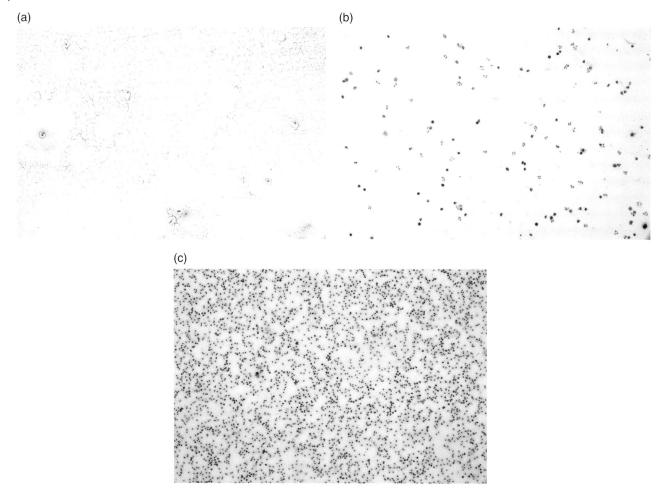

Figure 19.3 (a) High-protein/protein-rich effusion with low cellularity (thoracic fluid from a cat); (b) high-protein/protein-rich effusion with moderate cellularity (abdominal fluid from a dog); (c) high-protein, highly cellular fluid (abdominal fluid from a dog). *Source:* Jeremy Bessett (Contributor).

- prepare a line preparation as described in Chapter 15 for urine sediment.
- a sediment preparation can be made as described in Chapter 15 for urine sediment: a drop of the sediment is then placed on a glass slide and a pull preparation from the resuspended sediment can be made as described for buffy coat preparations.
- Stain the cytology preparation using one of the three staining protocols described in Chapter 5.

19.5 Time Estimate to Perform Test

Twenty minutes.

19.6 Procedural Tips and Troubleshooting

Clear colorless or slightly yellow fluid has low cellularity and evaluation of the fluids can be done easily in-house.

A fluid total protein and review of a sediment preparation is usually all that is needed to confirm the fluid is a transudate. It is rare to see any significant cellular changes to warrant submission to a reference laboratory. However, if any atypical cells are seen, submission of the fluid and any cytological preparations made in-house is recommended.

Body cavity fluid should always be collected in a tube with EDTA anticoagulant, even if it appears to be a transudate. A transudate can contain protein that will precipitate or clot if collected without an anticoagulant and can alter the total protein concentration. In high-protein/protein-rich fluids, this can result in trapping of any cellular elements in the clot. An evaluation of the cellularity of the fluid will not be possible in these preparations. A squash prep of the clot can be made for evaluation but may be too thick for cytological evaluation.

A good cytology reference text at bench-side is extremely valuable for the identification of cells and microorganisms and for the interpretation of findings.

Table 19.1 Categorization of body cavity fluids.

	Total protein (g/dl)	Nucleated cell count (μl)
Transudate	<2.0	<5000
High-protein/ protein-rich effusion	>2.0 but usually < 4.0	<5000
Exudate	>2.0 and usually >3.5	>5000

Source: Modified from Stockham, Scott, and EBSCOhost [1].

19.7 Interpreting Test Results

Most references use the following values to categorize body cavity fluids (see Table 19.1).

19.7.1 Transudates

Transudates are formed by increased hydrostatic pressure within the venules and capillaries of the mesothelial lining of the body cavities "pushing" excessive fluid into the interstitial tissue or increased hydrostatic pressure within the lymphatic system preventing return of the normal amount of fluid that enters the interstitial tissue with normal vascular hydrostatic pressure. It can also be seen with decreased plasma oncotic pressure as a result of hypoalbuminemia. The total protein and cellularity of transudates is low because there is usually no change in vascular permeability to proteins or cells. The cells present in transudates are small numbers of nondegenerate neutrophils, macrophages, and mesothelial cells and, occasionally small lymphocytes (see Figure 19.4). The background staining of transudates is colorless to slightly eosinophilic due to the low total protein.

19.7.2 High-Protein/Protein-Rich Effusions

High-protein/protein-rich effusions are formed by similar processes as seen in transudates with increased vascular permeability to proteins. This occurs most often secondary to significant cardiac disease, especially in association with right heart failure. Right heart failure secondary to heartworm disease commonly results in high-protein effusions. The nucleated cell counts are less than 5000/μl in these effusions. The nucleated cells seen in these effusions are the same as those seen in transudates with increased numbers of nondegenerate neutrophils. The change in number and distribution of the cells may indicate a change in vascular permeability to cells and protein or may be a mild inflammatory response to the presence of the fluid within the body cavity (see Figure 19.5).

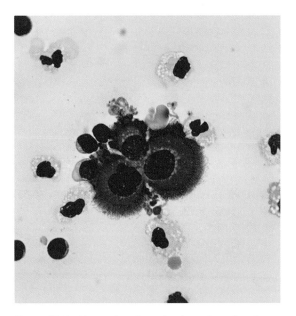

Figure 19.4 Transudate from the thoracic cavity of a cat (sediment preparation). Note the large mesothelial cells with a bright brush border, small lymphocytes, nondegenerate neutrophils, and macrophage with mild vacuolation. *Source:* Jeremy Bessett (Contributor).

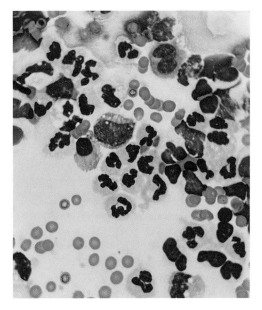

Figure 19.5 Sediment preparation of peritoneal fluid from a dog. The fluid was protein-rich with low to moderate cellularity. Note the mixture of macrophages (some are reactive with increased cytoplasmic basophilia) and increased numbers of nondegenerate neutrophils. *Source:* Jeremy Bessett (Contributor).

19.7.3 Inflammatory Exudates

Exudates are formed when there is significant inflammation present within the mesothelial lining of the body cavity. Inflammatory mediators are responsible for increased vascular permeability in the vessels of the mesothelium with movement of the cells and protein into the body cavity space. Exudates can be septic or sterile. The type of nucleated cells seen in exudates is dependent on the inciting cause. Neutrophils are the predominant cell type in nonseptic conditions and sepsis due to bacterial agents. A mixture of neutrophils and macrophages with a variable component of small lymphocytes and occasional plasma cells can be seen with fungal agents and foreign bodies or endogenous substances (bile and urine). Eosinophils can be a significant component of the response to fungal agents and parasites.

Sepsis due to bacteria that produce cytotoxins are associated with significant neutrophil degenerative change. Degenerative change in neutrophils is characterized by swollen nuclei with lighter basophilic staining compared with normal neutrophils. When degenerative change is seen in the neutrophils, a thorough examination for microorganisms is necessary (see Figures 19.6 and 19.7). The lack of degenerative change *does not* rule out sepsis. Culture of the fluid is always warranted whenever a neutrophilic or pyogranulomatous (mixed) inflammatory exudate is present.

Nonseptic causes of inflammatory effusions include inflammation secondary to gall bladder rupture and urinary bladder rupture. The chemical composition of bile and urine are strong irritants that cause cellular injury to the mesothelium and elicit an inflammatory reaction with movement of variable amounts of proteins and cells into the abdomen. The cells usually seen in both bile peritonitis and uroabdomen are consistent with a chronic mixed inflammation, neutrophils, macrophages, and fewer lymphocytes.

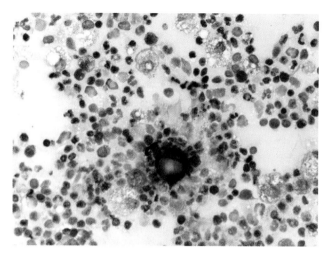

Figure 19.7 Thoracic fluid from a cat, pyogranulomatous exudate. Note the large deeply basophilic spherule of *Coccidioides spp.* surrounded by inflammatory cells. The fluid had marked cellularity and high total protein. *Source:* Jeremy Bessett (Contributor).

Because of the caustic nature of these fluids, neutrophils are often degenerate. Bilirubin crystals may be found in the fluid with bile peritonitis. If uroabdomen is suspected, measurement of fluid creatinine can be done to compare with serum creatinine. If the creatinine concentration of the fluid is greater than 2× that of the serum, uroabdomen is confirmed. Both uroabdomen and bile peritonitis can be septic, in which case, the cellularity and protein will be consistent with an exudate.

The effusions secondary to pancreatitis are primarily suppurative. The release of pancreatic enzymes results in significant necrosis of the tissue of the pancreas and organs surrounding the pancreas. Lipid droplets and lipid-laden macrophages can also be seen due to the saponification of the peripancreatic fat.

19.7.4 Hemorrhagic Effusions

Hemorrhagic effusion can occur in the thorax, pericardium, and abdomen. They are indicative of active hemorrhage into these body cavities (hemoabdomen, hemopericardium, and hemoperitoneum). The simple presence of erythrocytes in an effusion does not indicate active hemorrhage and these effusions are not categorized as hemorrhagic. Erythrocyte diapedesis can occur in any inflamed tissue including the mesothelium and will result in small to moderate numbers of erythrocytes in any inflammatory effusion or exudate. Hemorrhagic effusions are characterized by a PCV at least greater than 25% of the peripheral blood PCV and, in some cases, can exceed the peripheral blood PCV due to reabsorption of the fluid and protein from the abdominal cavity. As a result,

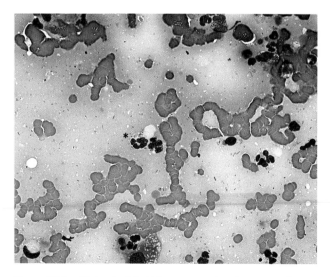

Figure 19.6 Abdominal fluid from a cat, chronic suppurative exudate. Note the degenerate neutrophil with intracellular bacteria and the rod-shaped bacteria throughout the background. The fluid had a high total protein and high cellularity. *Source:* Jeremy Bessett (Contributor).

(a)

(b)

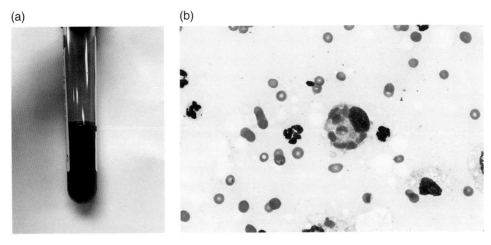

Figure 19.8 (a) Hemorrhagic effusion. Pericardial fluid from a dog. Fluid PCV 15%, peripheral blood PCV 44%; (b) hemorrhagic effusion. Note the large macrophage with numerous intracytoplasmic erythrocytes. *Source:* Jeremy Bessett (Contributor).

hemorrhage into the body cavities may or may not be associated with hypoproteinemia. Erythrocytes can also be removed from the effusion with reclamation of iron. Even with recurrent hemorrhage into the abdominal cavity, iron deficiency is not seen. The nucleated cells associated with hemorrhagic effusion are variable numbers of neutrophils, macrophages, and mesothelial cells. Erythrophagia and intracellular pigments (hemosiderin and hematoidin) are usually seen as well (see Figure 19.8a and b).

19.7.5 Chylous and Lymphocytic Effusions

Chylous effusions are white opaque effusion that accumulate in body cavities (primarily the thorax) secondary to either rupture of a large lymphatic duct or significant lymphatic obstruction (usually from mass lesions impinging on lymphatic vasculature). The white opaque appearance is due to the presence of chyle (see Figure 19.9). The total protein of chylous effusion is often difficult to determine. Lipid in the fluid will artificially increase the total protein by refractometry. The cells present in chylous effusions are small, normal-appearing lymphocytes. Long-standing chylous effusions will have increased numbers of neutrophils and macrophages. The macrophages may show variable numbers of small discrete lipid droplets and small clear droplets may be seen in the basophilic staining background. While chylous effusions are often quite striking, the lack of a milky appearance does not rule out a chylous effusion. Triglyceride concentration of the fluid can be measured; a triglyceride concentration greater than 100 mg/dl is confirmatory of chylous effusion.

Lymphocytic effusions are those effusions that do not contain chyle, will not have a significant triglyceride concentration, but have lymphocytes as the predominant nucleated cell type (see Figure 19.10). These effusions are

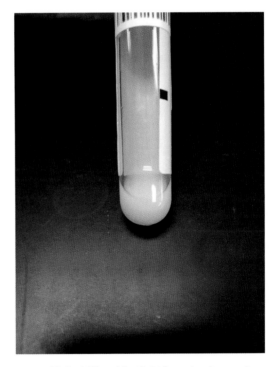

Figure 19.9 Milky white fluid from the thorax of a cat consistent with chylous effusion. Triglyceride concentration was 250 mg/dl. *Source:* Jeremy Bessett (Contributor).

usually secondary to changes in lymphatic hydrostatic pressure secondary to cardiac disease. The lymphocytes present are small, normal-appearing lymphocytes. Small cell lymphoma cannot be ruled out in patients with lymphocytic effusion. If a lymphocytic effusion is found, a search for possible mass lesions in the thorax or abdomen is warranted. The fluid can also be submitted to a reference laboratory to determine if the lymphocyte population is clonal or polyclonal. A monoclonal population is indicative of a neoplastic lymphocyte population.

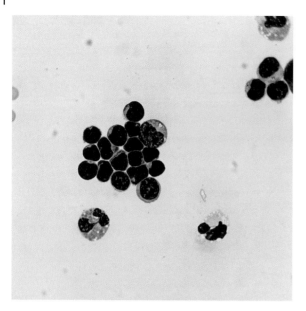

Figure 19.10 Thoracic fluid from a dog. Note the numerous small, normal-appearing lymphocytes. Lymphocytic effusion. *Source:* Jeremy Bessett (Contributor).

Figure 19.11 Direct preparation of thoracic fluid from a dog with multiple pulmonary masses. Histopathology revealed pulmonary adenocarcinoma with multiple intrapulmonary metastatic lesions. Note the large cohesive sheets of pleomorphic epithelial cells. Neoplastic effusion. *Source:* Jeremy Bessett (Contributor).

19.7.6 Neoplastic Effusions

Neoplasia within the thorax, abdomen, and pericardium can result in shedding of neoplastic cells into the thoracic fluid. The neoplastic masses often result in fluid accumulation because the masses obstruct both venous and lymphatic vessels. The character of neoplastic effusion varies considerably from transudates to exudates. Masses that result in hemodynamic changes cause transudates or high-protein/protein-rich effusions. Necrotic neoplastic masses will elicit a significant inflammatory response and can result in an exudate. Hemorrhagic effusions are often seen secondary to rupture of vascular tumors or if the tumor erodes into a major vessel. Neoplasia within the body cavity should always be included in the differential for any effusion. The cellularity and the character of the cellular response is as varied as the type of effusion. Epithelial tumors and round cell tumors, especially lymphoma, are the most common type of tumors to shed cells into effusions (see Figure 19.11). Mesenchymal tumors do not shed cells consistently because they often have significant extracellular matrix.

Care must be taken when making a diagnosis of neoplastic effusion. Atypical cells present in an inflammatory effusion should be interpreted with caution. Mesothelial hyperplasia occurs with the long-standing presence of effusion and can be difficult to differentiate from carcinoma or adenocarcinoma. Inflammatory effusion secondary to the fungal disease can have reactive mesenchymal cells shed into the fluid and be concerning for sarcoma. Whenever there is suspicion for neoplasia on the evaluation of fluid cytology, it is recommended to submit that fluid for a full fluid analysis and pathology review.

19.8 Clinical Case Example(s)

See Part 6, cases #4 and #9.

19.9 Add-On Tests That You May Need to Consider and Their Additive Value

Culture of any exudative body cavity fluid is recommended regardless of whether or not microorganisms are seen. Both aerobic and anaerobic and, if the inflammation is mixed or pyogranulomatous, fungal culture is appropriate.

Triglyceride concentration of any fluid suspected to be chylous in origin is recommended to confirm the presence of chyle (triglyceride concentration > 100 mg/dl) [2].

Glucose concentration of exudative fluids with clinical signs of sepsis and no microorganisms found on cytology can assist in supporting a septic process. A glucose concentration in the fluid greater than 20 mg/dl below serum glucose is suggestive of sepsis [3].

Lactate concentration of the fluid can also support sepsis in exudative body cavity fluids. A fluid lactate concentration greater than 2.5 mmol/l if fluid lactate concentration is greater than blood lactate concentration is supportive of sepsis in the dog. Fluid lactate was not found to be useful in the cat [4].

Flow cytometer of body cavity fluids or polymerase chain reaction for antigen receptor rearrangement (PARR) is recommended if there is suspicion of small or intermediate cells lymphoma when a lymphocytic effusion is identified on fluid analysis. Flow cytometry can also be used to assist in identifying the lineage of myeloproliferative neoplasms.

Body cavity fluid creatinine concentration for comparison with serum creatinine is confirmatory for uroabdomen.

Body cavity fluid bilirubin concentration for comparison with serum bilirubin is confirmatory for bile peritonitis.

19.10　Key Takeaways

- In-house microscopic evaluation of body cavity fluids can provide valuable information to help direct initial treatment, especially in cases where sepsis is a differential.
  - One of the most valuable cytology skills is the ability to review a fluid cytology and determine if the process is most likely inflammatory or noninflammatory and to identify common microorganisms in a fluid sample.
  - If the sample is consistent with an inflammatory process, it can be submitted to a reference laboratory for culture at the same time as the fluid analysis and save valuable time.
  - If sepsis is suspected, serum and fluid glucose and lactate can be performed to provide additional support for sepsis or prognostic value.
- A quick total protein determination and direct preparation can provide sufficient information to prioritize differentials for the underlying cause of the fluid accumulation.
  - Clear, low-protein, low cellular fluid is consistent with fluid accumulation due to alterations in hemodynamic or plasma protein concentration resulting in a pure transudate suggesting possible underlying cardiac, renal, or GI disease.
  - Cloudy, high-protein, high cellular fluid is consistent with inflammation and may warrant concurrent culture of the fluid if the predominant cell types are inflammatory or evaluation by a pathologist if there are significant numbers of atypical cells.
  - High-protein/low-cell or low-protein/high-cell fluid suggests processes such as vasculitis, low-grade sepsis, cardiac disease, liver disease.
  - Hemorrhagic effusions can prompt evaluation for possible bleeding masses within the cavity or coagulation testing for underlying coagulation factor deficiencies (i.e. rodenticide poisoning).

References

1 Stockham, S.L. and Scott, M.A. & EBSCOhost(2008). *Fundamentals of veterinary clinical pathology*, 2e. Ames, Iowa: Blackwell Pub.

2 Tyler, R.D. and Cowell, R.L. (1989). Evaluation of pleural and peritoneal effusions. *Veterinary Clinics of North America: Small Animal Practice* 19 (4): 743–768.

3 Koenig, A. and Verlander, L.L. (2015). Usefulness of whole blood, plasma, peritoneal fluid, and peritoneal fluid supernatant glucose concentrations obtained by a veterinary point-of-care glucometer to identify septic peritonitis in dogs with peritoneal effusion. *Journal of the American Veterinary Medical Association* 247 (9): 1027–1032.

4 Levin, G.M., Bonczynski, J.J., Ludwig, L.L. et al. (2004). Lactate as a diagnostic test for septic peritoneal effusions in dogs and cats. *Journal of the American Animal Hospital Association* 40 (5): 364–371.

Suggested Bench-Side References

Valenciano, A.C. and Cowell, R.L. (2019). *Cowell and Tyler's Diagnostic Cytology and Hematology of the Dog and Cat-E-Book*. Elsevier Health Sciences.

Sharkey, L.C., Radin, M.J., and Seelig, D. (ed.) (2020). *Veterinary Cytology*. Wiley.

Part 6

Clinical Cases

20

Clinical Cases

Jeremy Bessett, with support from Sharon M. Dial

1 Case #1

1.1 Signalment

Fred, 11-year-old castrated male German Shephard dog

1.2 History

Current on vaccinations, receives monthly heartworm preventative/anthelminthic combination, and monthly flea and tick prevention. Receives yearly inhouse CBC/ Biochemistry/UA, and combination ELISA test for Heartworm, *Ehrlichia* spp., *Anaplasma* spp., and *Borrelia Burgdorferi*. His previous laboratory work has always been within the reference intervals and his yearly infectious disease testing has previously been negative.

1.3 Presentation

Fred presents for recent onset of lethargy and anorexia.

1.4 Physical Exam Findings

Temp: 100.1 °F (37.8 °C), HR: 148, RR: 60, MM: Pale, CRT: two seconds, Hydration status: ~5% Dehydration, BCS: 4/9

Cardiopulmonary: Normal bronchovesicular sounds in all fields, a grade 2/6 systolic left-sided heart murmur, and strong synchronous pulses.

Abdomen: Marked splenomegaly and hepatomegaly
Lymph: Mild peripheral lymphadenomegaly
HEENT: No abnormal findings
Urogenital: No abnormal findings
Integument: No abnormal findings
Neurologic: No abnormal findings
Musculoskeletal: No abnormal findings

Initial Data (History/Signalment/Physical Exam) Questions

1 Given the clinical data, what is the differential diagnosis?

2 What diagnostics ideally would you like to perform (given no resource boundaries) and why?

3 What low-cost diagnostics could you perform in this patient that might give you similar information to your ideal list?

4 What information are you expecting to receive from these diagnostics? In other words, what differential do you expect to rule in or rule out with these diagnostics?

5 What results, given the patient's signalment/history/ clinical exam findings, would you expect in this patient?

Initial Data (History/Signalment/Physical Exam) Answers

1 Given the clinical data, what is the differential diagnosis?
   a *Tachycardia, tachypnea, and pale mucous membranes with a normal CRT indicate the presence of anemia. A systolic murmur could be the result of anemia or the result of cardiac valvular insufficiency. Marked splenomegaly and hepatomegaly with the presence of anemia are supportive of infectious diseases (i.e. Mycoplasma spp., Leptospira spp.,*

Babesia spp.), neoplasia, marked extramedullary hematopoiesis or immune-mediated disease (i.e. IMHA). Acute lethargy and anorexia could be the result of numerous conditions and are vague clinical signs.

2 What diagnostics ideally would you like to perform (given no resource boundaries) and why?

a *Ideally performing a CBC, biochemical profile (including ALT, AST, GGT, ALP, total bilirubin, and bile acids if bilirubin is within the reference interval), urinalysis, radiographs, and abdominal ultrasound would be ideal to perform. Depending on the results,*

fine needle aspiration and or histopathology may be indicated.

3 What low-cost diagnostics could you perform in this patient that might give you similar information to your ideal list?

a *PCV/TPP, blood film evaluation, BUN, urinalysis would be a good low-cost starting point. From here, we can better target further diagnostics if needed.*

4 What information are you expecting to receive from these diagnostics? In other words, what differential do you expect to rule in or rule out with these diagnostics?

Hematology				
Test	**Result**	**Units**	**Reference Interval**	**Units**
PCV	15 (0.15)	% (L/L)	35-57 (0.35-0.57)	% (L/L)
Polychromasia	None			
nRBC	0	#/100 WBC	0-2	#/100 WBC
WBC Estimate	106,000	#/uL	5,000-15,500	#/uL
Segmented Neturophils	4	%	NA	%
Band Neutrophils	0	%	NA	%
Metamyelocytes	0	%	NA	%
Lymphocytes	2	%	NA	%
Monocytes	1	%	NA	%
Eosinophils	0	%	NA	%
Basophils	0	%	NA	%
Large Unclassified Cells	93	%	NA	%
Absolute Segmented Neutrophils	4,240	#/uL	2,500-10,750	#/uL
Absolute Band Neutrophils	0	#/uL	0-150	#/uL
Absolute Metamyelocytes	0	#/uL	0	#/uL
Absolute Lymphocytes	2,120	#/uL	850-4,500	#/uL
Absolute Monocytes	1,060	#/uL	150-1,100	#/uL
Absolute Eosinophils	0	#/uL	50-1,500	#/uL
Absolute Basophils	0	#/uL	0-100	#/uL
Large Unclassified Cells	98,580	#/uL	0	#/uL
WBC Morphology Comment	Large unclassified cells present are consistent with neoplastic origin.			
Platelet Estimate	~450,000	#/uL	150,000-450,000	#/uL
Platelet Comment	Large platelets present			

Case Figure 1.1 Hematologic data. Absolute leukocyte values are based on WBC estimate and differential count.

a *PCV, TPP, and blood film are going to be helpful in assessing red blood cell mass (confirming anemia), leukocyte concentration, and differential (supporting inflammatory disease or neoplasia), evaluate for hemoparasites (i.e. Mycoplasma spp., or Babesia spp.), plasma protein status (possibly supporting inflammatory disease or neoplasia). BUN and urinalysis will help assess renal function (supporting or refuting Leptospira spp., or other diseases).*

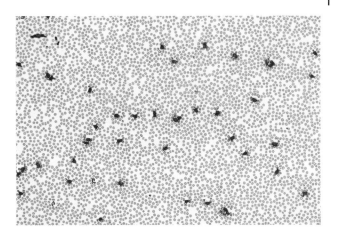

Case Figure 1.4 Blood film (Diff–Quick, 200×).

5 What results, given the patient's signalment/history/clinical exam findings, would you expect in this patient?
  a *In this patient, a decreased PCV would be expected with or without signs of regeneration on the blood film. We may also see leukocytosis depending on the underlying cause of the anemia. A stress leukogram caused by increased circulating endogenous glucocorticoids can be expected in sick patients. Otherwise, there are no other results that can be predicted at this point.*

Diagnostic Data Interpretation Questions

1 Given the diagnostic results, what abnormalities do you identify? What is your interpretation of these findings?

2 Are any of these diagnostic results surprising/unexpected?

3 What are the broad mechanisms by which these abnormalities occur?

4 In this case, what is/are the top differential diagnoses based on the current diagnostic data?

5 What diagnostic results are most supportive for each of the differential diagnoses?

6 What additional diagnostics would you need to confirm/refute the top differentials for this case?

7 In patients with the condition depicted in this case, why is bicytopenia or pancytopenia a frequent finding?

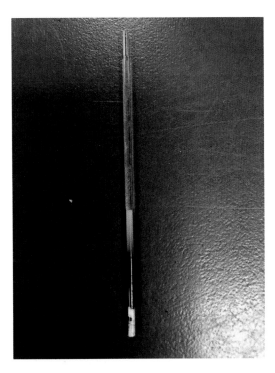

Case Figure 1.2 Hematocrit tube gross image. *Source:* Image courtesy of Laurie Holm, BS, CVT.

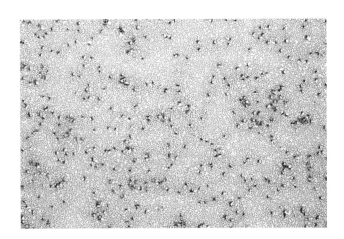

Case Figure 1.3 Blood film (Diff–Quick, 100×).

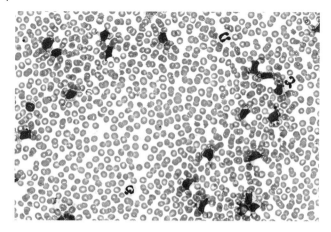

Case Figure 1.5 Blood film (Diff–Quick, 500×).

Diagnostic Data Interpretation Answers

1 Given the diagnostic results, what abnormalities do you identify? What is your interpretation of these findings?

   a *Moderate to marked anemia (PCV 15%), marked leukocytosis with 93% of nucleated cells being large unclassified cells, and thrombocytosis. There is no evidence of erythroid regeneration (no polychromasia or nucleated erythrocytes). BUN is normal with an adequately concentrated USG is consistent with adequate renal function. Mild proteinuria is commonly seen in concentrated urine in the dog. Trace bilirubinuria is normal in dogs.*

2 Are any of these diagnostic results surprising/ unexpected?

   a *There are very few cases where a marked leukocytosis is expected. In this case the estimated WBC count was 98,000/ul. In general, inflammatory leukograms are commonly associated with pyrexia, especially with leukocyte concentrations of this magnitude, which wasn't seen in this case.*

3 What are the broad mechanisms by which these abnormalities occur?

   a *Marked leukocytosis, in this case, is the result of neoplastic hematopoietic cells circulating within the peripheral blood. Neoplastic cells proliferate in the bone marrow, begin circulating in peripheral blood, and can accumulate in other organs (i.e. spleen, liver, lymph nodes, etc.)*

   b *Anemia occurs for three primary reasons: erythrocytes are destroyed (hemolysis), they are used/consumed, or they are not adequately produced. In this case, there is no evidence of hemolysis (spherocytes, ghost cells, etc.) upon reviewing the blood film. There is also no evidence of loss or consumption since we do not see an indication of hemorrhage (i.e. clinical findings, decreased total plasma protein) in this patient. There is evidence of inadequate bone marrow response to anemia (lack of polychromasia or nucleated erythrocytes) supporting replacement of hematopoietic tissue by the neoplastic leukocytes.*

   c *Thrombocytosis occurs as a result of megakaryocyte stimulation to produce platelets. Thrombocytosis can be due to tumor associated inflammation with release of inflammatory cytokines that promote thrombopoiesis, the most common cause, or as a paraneoplastic syndrome due to tumor specific prothrombopoietic mechanisms.*

4 In this case, what is/are the top differential diagnoses based on the current diagnostic data?

   a *Acute leukemia with bone marrow suppression likely due to myelophthisis and infiltration of neoplastic cells into the spleen and liver.*

5 What diagnostic results are most supportive for each of the differential diagnoses?

   a *The most compelling finding is the extreme leukocytosis caused by large numbers of atypical nucleated cells. Although the large cells appear morphologically similar to lymphoid cells, their lineage cannot be definitively determined on a routinely stained blood film. A reactive lymphocytosis is very unlikely considering the absolute number and morphologic characteristics of these large unclassified cells.*

6 What additional diagnostics would you need to confirm/refute the top differentials for this case?

   a *In this case, there are several diagnostics that should be pursued to confirm the diagnosis of acute leukemia. Flow cytometry should be performed to identify the origin of the neoplastic cells (myeloid vs. lymphoid). Aspiration of the spleen and liver should be performed to confirm infiltration of neoplastic cells in these tissues. Bone marrow core biopsy should be performed to confirm that neoplastic cells have infiltrated the bone marrow resulting in myelopthisis. Bone marrow aspiration cytology is not as helpful as core biopsy due to the degree of leukocytosis in this patient and the amount of blood contamination in these samples. The same would hold true for the* liver and spleen aspirates.

Chemistry

Test	Result	Units	Reference Interval	Units
Total Plasma Protein:	8.5 (85)	g/dL (g/L)	6.0-7.5 (60-75)	g/dL (g/L)
Plasma Color:	Clear			
BUN (Azostix®):	15-26 (5.36-9.28)	mg/dL (mmol/L)	<30 (10.71)	mg/dL (mmol/L)
USG:	1.042			
Urine Protein:	Trace			
Urine Glucose:	Negative			
Urine Ketone:	Negative			
Urine pH:	6.5			
Urine Bilirubin	Trace			
Urine Sediment:	0-1 Hyaline casts	#/lpf		#/lpf

Case Figure 1.6   Biochemistry and urinalysis data. Urinalysis sample by cystocentesis.

7   In patients with the condition depicted in this case, why is bicytopenia or pancytopenia a frequent finding?

a   *Patients with acute leukemias typically develop marked cytopenias due to myelophthisis. The replacement of normal hematopoietic tissue by neoplastic cells greatly reduces the ability to maintain normal blood cell concentrations in the peripheral blood.*

2   Case #2

2.1   Signalment

Bella, 6-year-old spayed female Golden Retriever dog.

2.2   History

Current on vaccinations, does not currently receive heartworm preventatives, anthelminthics, or flea/tick preventatives. Currently receiving sulfamethoxazole-trimethoprim antimicrobial therapy for a urinary tract infection. Today was the last treatment in a 14-day course of the antimicrobials.

2.3   Presentation

Bella presents for acute collapse, lethargy, and panting.

2.4   Physical Exam Findings

Temp: 103.1 °F (39.5 °C), HR: 132, RR: 80, MM: Pale yellow, CRT: <2 seconds, Hydration status: <5% Dehydrated, BCS: 6/9

Cardiopulmonary: No murmurs on auscultation, strong synchronous pulses, lungs auscultate normally. Abdomen: Moderate splenomegaly on palpation.

Lymph: No abnormal findings.

HEENT: Icteric sclera, pinnae, and oral mucosa.

Urogenital: Icteric vulvar mucosa.

Integument: No abnormal findings.

Neurologic: No abnormal findings.

Musculoskeletal: No abnormal findings.

Initial Data (History/Signalment/Physical Exam) Questions

1   Given the clinical data, what is the differential diagnosis?

2   What diagnostics ideally would you like to perform (given no resource boundaries) and why?

3   What low-cost diagnostics could you perform in this patient that might give you similar information to your ideal list?

4   What information are you expecting to receive from these diagnostics? In other words, what differential do you expect to rule in or rule out with these diagnostics?

5   What results, given the patient's signalment/history/ clinical exam findings, would you expect in this patient?

Initial Data (History/Signalment/Physical Exam) Answers

1 Given the clinical data, what is the initial differential diagnosis?

  a *The primary differentials in this case are:*

  i) *Prehepatic icterus due to hemolytic anemia supported by pale yellow mucous membranes, tachycardia, and tachypnea, with strong peripheral pulses, normal CRT, and splenomegaly.*

  ii) *Hepatic or posthepatic icterus with secondary anemia supported by pale icteric mucous membranes.*
  Differentiation of the primary cause of icterus cannot be determined by clinical findings alone and requires additional diagnostic tests. With the history of sulfonamide administration, idiosyncratic hepatocellular injury or secondary immune-mediated hemolytic anemia should be considered.

2 What diagnostics ideally would you like to perform (given no resource boundaries) and why?

  a *Ideally a CBC (including blood film review), biochemical profile, and urinalysis would be a good initial diagnostic plan. It is also beneficial to perform abdominal ultrasonography to examine the liver, biliary tract, and spleen. If there is evidence of erythrocyte aggregation on examination of the blood collection tube, a saline dispersion test should be performed to differentiate nonspecific aggregation from immune agglutination.*

  b *CBC would confirm anemia, determine the bone marrow response, and identify changes in other blood cell lineages.*

  c *Blood film review is critical in these cases! Erythrocyte morphology is the most direct way to identify the cause of anemia. The presence of spherocytes, ghost cells, Heinz bodies, and eccentrocytes can all be associated with hemolytic anemia. It is important to interpret all physical and laboratory findings together when evaluating blood cell morphology.*

  d *Biochemical profile is important in making the distinction between prehepatic, hepatic, or posthepatic icterus, as well as identifying potential causes.*

  e *Urinalysis is critical for adequate interpretation of the biochemistry profile and other clinical pathology data.*

  f *Abdominal ultrasonography is the best noninvasive way to differentiate hepatic from posthepatic icterus. In addition, ultrasonographic evaluation and fine needle aspiration is useful in identifying the cause in cases of hepatosplenomegaly.*

An important note, the Coombs test or Direct Antiglobulin may not be helpful in cases of hemolytic anemia due to low sensitivity and specificity of this test.

3 What low-cost diagnostics could you perform in this patient that might give you similar information to your ideal list?

  a *The low-cost diagnostics that could be performed in this case would be PCV, TPP, blood film, BUN, and urinalysis.*

4 What information are you expecting to receive from these diagnostics? In other words, what differential do you expect to rule in or rule out with these diagnostics?

  a *PCV would determine if the patient is anemic to help rule in or out prehepatic icterus. In addition, evaluation of buffy coat size might help identify the presence of leukocytosis or thrombocytosis.*

  b *TPP would help support hydration status findings. High total plasma protein may suggest nonspecific aggregation of erythrocytes versus immune agglutination.*

  c *Blood film review would identify spherocyte formation, or other RBC abnormalities consistent with hemolytic anemia and allow evaluation of leukocytes and platelets.*

  d *BUN is an evaluator of both renal glomerular filtration rate and hepatic function. In the icteric patient, a decreased BUN would suggest decreased hepatic function. Since a potential differential in the icteric dog is leptospirosis, renal injury is also a concern warranting BUN monitoring.*

  e *Urinalysis is critical in monitoring the renal function in any ill patient and adequate interpretation of the biochemical profile.*

5 What results, given the patient's signalment/history/clinical exam findings, would you expect in this patient?

  a *In this case, bilirubinuria and icteric plasma is expected since the patient is grossly icteric. Given the tachycardia, tachypnea, slightly pale mucous membranes, normal CRT, and normal pulse quality, anemia is likely. Since the patient's history of sulfonamide antimicrobial administration significantly increases the probability of an immune mechanism for the anemia, spherocyte formation would be an expected finding on the blood film. Because immune-mediated hemolytic anemia is usually regenerative, polychromasia is an expected finding. Leukocytosis of varying magnitude can be expected due to either inflammation, increased circulating glucocorticoids, or both.*

Hematology				
Test	**Result**	**Units**	**Reference Interval**	**Units**
PCV	22 (0.22)	% (L/L)	35-57 (0.35-0.57)	% (L/L)
RBC Morphology:	Polychromasia 2+, Anisocytosis 3+, Spherocytes 2+			
nRBC	15	#/100 WBC	0-2	#/100 WBC
WBC Estimate	17,600	#/uL	5,000-15,500	#/uL
Segmented Neturophils	78	%	NA	%
Band Neutrophils	5	%	NA	%
Metamyelocytes	1	%	NA	%
Lymphocytes	4	%	NA	%
Monocytes	11	%	NA	%
Eosinophils	1	%	NA	%
Basophils	0	%	NA	%
Absolute Segmented Neutrophils	13,728	#/uL	2,500-10,750	#/uL
Absolute Band Neutrophils	880	#/uL	0-150	#/uL
Absolute Metamyelocytes	176	#/uL	0	#/uL
Absolute Lymphocytes	704	#/uL	850-4,500	#/uL
Absolute Monocytes	1,936	#/uL	150-1,100	#/uL
Absolute Eosinophils	176	#/uL	50-1,500	#/uL
Absolute Basophils	0	#/uL	0-100	#/uL
Toxic Change	2+ (Moderate)			
Platelet Estimate	~605,000	#/uL	150,000-450,000	#/uL
Platelet Comment	Large platelets present			
Total Protein:	7.2	g/dL	6.0-8.0	g/dL
Plasma Color:	Yellow/ Icteric			

Case Figure 2.1 Hematologic data. *Absolute leukocyte values are based on WBC estimate and differential count.

Diagnostic Result Interpretation

1 Given the diagnostic results, what abnormalities do you identify? What is your interpretation of these findings?

2 Would the icterus in this patient be considered prehepatic, hepatic, or posthepatic in origin?

3 What are the broad mechanisms by which these abnormalities occur?

4 In this case, what is/are the top differential diagnoses based on the current diagnostic data?

5 What diagnostic results are most supportive for each of the differential diagnoses?

6 What additional diagnostics would you need to confirm/refute the top differentials for this case?

7 Why do we typically see signs of regeneration in cases of extravascular hemolytic anemia but not in intravascular hemolytic anemias? Does the presence of regeneration completely rule in or out either?

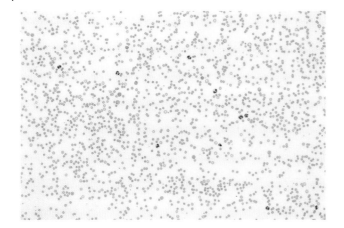

Case Figure 2.2 Blood film (Wrights–Giemsa, 200×).

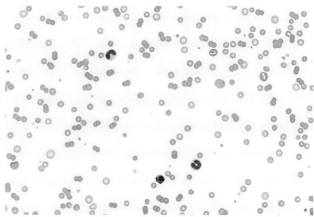

Case Figure 2.5 Blood film (Wrights–Giemsa, 500×).

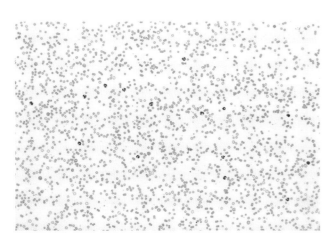

Case Figure 2.3 Blood film (Wrights–Giemsa, 200×).

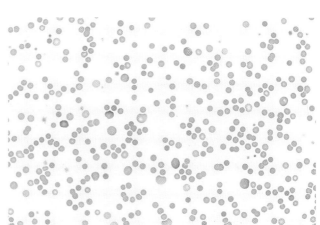

Case Figure 2.6 Blood film (Wrights–Giemsa, 500×).

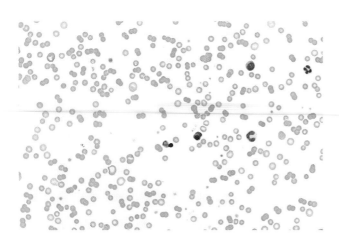

Case Figure 2.4 Blood film (Wrights–Giemsa, 500×).

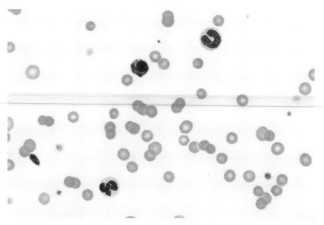

Case Figure 2.7 Blood film (Wrights–Giemsa, 1000×).

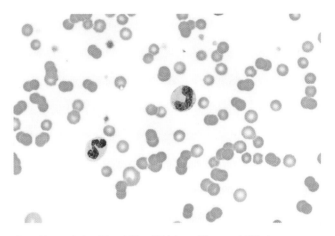

Case Figure 2.8 Blood film (Wrights–Giemsa, 1000×).

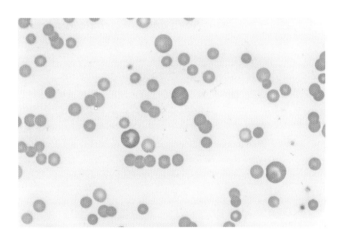

Case Figure 2.9 Blood film (Wrights–Giemsa, 1000×).

Diagnostic Result Interpretation

1 Given the diagnostic results, what abnormalities do you identify? What is your interpretation of these findings?

   a *There is moderate anemia present, with evidence of regeneration (2+ polychromasia, 15 nRBC/100WBC). There is moderate spherocytosis which is supportive of IMHA in this case. Mild leukocytosis with significant shift to immaturity (to metamyelocytes) is present supporting an inflammatory process, i.e. IMHA. Mild thrombocytosis is present, which is consistent with regenerative response to anemia or stimulation of thrombopoiesis by inflammatory cytokines.*

   b *The lack of hemoglobinemia and hemoglobinuria in the presence of icterus and spherocytes is consistent with extravascular hemolytic anemia.*

   c *BUN is within the reference interval and USG is within the range of adequate concentration, which supporting normal renal function.*

   d *Bilirubinuria and icteric plasma are consistent with the grossly evident icterus.*

2 Would the icterus in this patient be considered prehepatic, hepatic, or posthepatic in origin?

   a *In this case given the patient's history, physical exam findings, and evidence of hemolytic anemia, icterus is most likely of prehepatic origin.*

Chemistry				
Test	**Result**	**Units**	**Reference Interval**	**Units**
Total Plasma Protein:	7.2 (72)	g/dL (g/L)	6.0-7.5 (60-75)	g/dL (g/L)
Plasma Color:	Clear			
BUN (Azostix®):	15-26 (5.36-9.28)	mg/dL (mmol/L)	<30 (10.71)	mg/dL (mmol/L)
USG:	1.035			
Urine Protein:	Negative			
Urine Glucose:	Negative			
Urine Ketone	Negative			
Urine pH:	6.5			
Urine Bilirubin	2+			
Urine Sediment:	No casts/ crystals seen	#/lpf		#/lpf

Case Figure 2.10 Biochemistry and urinalysis data. Urinalysis sample by cystocentesis.

3 What are the broad mechanisms by which these abnormalities occur?

a *In cases of extravascular immune hemolysis (i.e. IMHA) erythrocytes are removed from circulation by macrophages predominantly in the spleen and liver. As these macrophages phagocytose erythrocytes, hemoglobin is ultimately converted into unconjugated bilirubin and released for processing by the liver. The liver quickly becomes overwhelmed, which leads to significant hyperbilirubinemia, icterus, and bilirubinuria. The resulting anemia leads to decreased oxygen availability for the tissues and release of erythropoietin. Stimulation of the bone marrow erythroid lineage by erythropoietin results in a regenerative response to anemia. Erythropoietin has thrombopoietic effects and secondarily increases platelet numbers. Inflammatory cytokines stimulated by erythrocyte immune lysis leads to increased leukocyte production and subsequent leukocytosis and can stimulate thrombopoiesis.*

4 In this case, what is/are the top differential diagnoses based on the current diagnostic data?

a *In this case, the primary differential diagnoses are:*

i) *Primary immune-mediated hemolytic anemia (autoimmune)*

ii) *Secondary immune-mediated hemolytic anemia*

1) *Idiosyncratic sulfonamide reaction*

2) *Infectious origin*

a) Babesia *spp.,* Leishmania *spp.,* Dirofilaria immitis, Bartonella *spp., and* Anaplasma phagocytophilum *have been associated with secondary IMHA in the dog.*

5 What diagnostic results are most supportive of each of the differential diagnoses?

a *Currently, there is not enough evidence to allow the distinction between primary and secondary immune-mediated hemolytic anemia. Since there is insufficient evidence, both mechanisms should be considered.*

6 What additional diagnostics would you need to confirm/refute the top differentials for this case?

a *Additional diagnostics are required to determine the origin of IMHA in this patient. Serologic or molecular diagnostics would be beneficial in ruling out infectious causes since primary IMHA and secondary IMHA due to idiosyncratic drug reaction are both diagnoses of exclusion.*

b *Given the history of the patient, administration of a potential IMHA inciting drug treatment should be ceased with continued monitoring. Resolution of*

disease with drug discontinuation is highly supportive of a drug reaction over primary IMHA.

7 Why do we typically see signs of regeneration in cases of extravascular hemolytic anemia but not in intravascular hemolytic anemias? Does the presence of regeneration completely rule in or out either?

a *It is important to remember it takes ~5 days to see evidence of regeneration from the bone marrow. Most commonly, the regenerative response is moderate to marked with extravascular hemolysis and nonregenerative or mildly regenerative with intravascular hemolysis. The main difference between the two types of hemolysis is the time point at which the disease is recognized by the owner. Patients with intravascular hemolysis usually have acute hemolytic crises with rapid onset of significant clinical disease. Because their clinical signs are acute, the bone marrow has not had time to respond prior to presentation. With extravascular hemolysis, the duration of the disease process is more chronic than intravascular hemolysis. There is a more gradual decrease in erythrocyte mass with extravascular hemolysis rather than the precipitous drop with intravascular hemolysis.*

3 Case #3

3.1 Signalment

Benji, a 2-year-old castrated male Staffordshire terrier mix dog

3.2 History

Current on all vaccinations, receives a monthly heartworm preventative/anthelminthic combination, but is not on flea/tick preventatives. Last week, Benji had his yearly physical exam, Heartworm/*Ehrlichia*/*Anaplasma*/*Borellia* ELISA testing, and updated his vaccinations.

3.3 Presentation

Benji presents today on emergency after his owners found him collapsed in their backyard and panting. Currently, the temperature outside is 106°F (41.1°C).

3.4 Physical Exam Findings

Temp: 108.6°F (42.5°C), HR: 160, RR: 100 (Panting), MM: Brick red/Injected, CRT: <2 seconds, Hydration Status: ~8% Dehydrated, BCS 4/9

Cardiopulmonary: Adventitious lung sounds in the bronchovesicular regions bilaterally, fine crackles audible bilaterally. The heart auscults normally, peripheral pulses are rapid but weak.

Integument: Skin feels hot to the touch with diffuse erythema present.

Lymph: No abnormal findings.

Abdomen: No abnormal findings.

Neuro: Obtunded mentation, laterally recumbent, mydriasis present OU.

Musculoskeletal: Muscle tremors present.

HEENT: All mucosal surfaces are brick red/hyperemic, hypersalivation present, episcleral injection OU.

NIBP: 65 mmHg (systolic)

Questions for Part 1 of Case

1 Is echinocytosis commonly associated with dehydration? If so, why was echinocytosis not seen in this patient's blood film?

Answers for Part 1 of Case

1 Is echinocytosis commonly associated with dehydration? If so, why was echinocytosis not seen in this patient's blood film?
   a Echinocytosis can be associated with numerous causes such as EDTA artifact, envenomation, etc. However, dehydration is not commonly associated with echinocytosis.

Hematology				
Test	**Result**	**Units**	**Reference Interval**	**Units**
PCV	72 (0.72)	% (L/L)	35-57 (0.35-0.57)	% (L/L)
Polychromasia	None			
nRBC	0	#/100 WBC	0-2	#/100 WBC
WBC Estimate	33,000	#/uL	5,000-15,500	#/uL
Segmented Neturophils	79	%	NA	%
Band Neutrophils	0	%	NA	%
Metamyelocytes	0	%	NA	%
Lymphocytes	8	%	NA	%
Monocytes	13	%	NA	%
Eosinophils	0	%	NA	%
Basophils	0	%	NA	%
Absolute Segmented Neutrophils	26,070	#/uL	2,500-10,750	#/uL
Absolute Band Neutrophils	0	#/uL	0-150	#/uL
Absolute Metamyelocytes	0	#/uL	0	#/uL
Absolute Lymphocytes	2,640	#/uL	850-4,500	#/uL
Absolute Monocytes	4,290	#/uL	150-1,100	#/uL
Absolute Eosinophils	0	#/uL	50-1,500	#/uL
Absolute Basophils	0	#/uL	0-100	#/uL
Toxic Change	None			
Platelet Estimate	160,000	#/uL	150,000-450,000	#/uL
Platelet Comment	Few large platelets present			

Case Figure 3.1 Hematologic data. *Absolute leukocyte values are based on WBC estimate and differential count.

Case Figure 3.2 Blood film (Wrights–Giemsa, 100×).

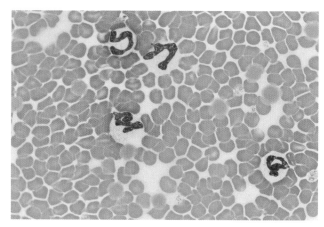

Case Figure 3.5 Blood film (Wrights–Giemsa, 1000×).

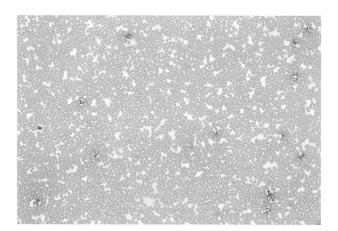

Case Figure 3.3 Blood film (Wrights–Giemsa, 200×).

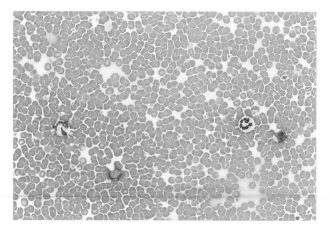

Case Figure 3.4 Blood film (Wrights–Giemsa, 500×).

Follow-up: After treatment for heat stroke, Benji's temperature returned to a normal range, his mental status improved, and neurologic signs resolved. Benji's respiratory effort has improved, and he is no longer dyspneic.

Four hours later you perform a recheck examination on Benji. Overnight and this morning, the patient has had hemorrhagic diarrhea.

3.5 Follow-Up Physical Exam Findings

Temp: 102.7 °F (39.3 °C), HR: 112, RR: 48, MM: Pink, CRT: <2 seconds, Hydration status: 5% Dehydrated

Cardiopulmonary: On auscultation, the heart ausculs normally, and there are strong synchronous peripheral pulses. Adventitious lung sounds in the bronchovesicular region, improved

Integument: Petechiae and purpura noted on the ventrum

Lymph: No abnormal findings

Abdomen: Abdomen tense and painful.

Neuro: Patient is aware, but depressed. Ambulates normally and has normal conscious proprioceptive responses and nociceptive responses. A brief cranial nerve exam is within normal limits.

Musculoskeletal: No abnormal findings

HEENT: Petechiae noted on oral mucosa and pinna. Mild hyphema identified OS on ophthalmic exam.

Initial Data (History/Signalment/Physical Exam) Questions

1 Given the clinical data what is the differential diagnosis?

2 What diagnostics ideally would you like to perform (given no resource boundaries) and why?

3 What low-cost diagnostics could you perform in this patient that might give you similar information to your ideal list?

Chemistry

Test	Result	Units	Reference Interval	Units
Total Plasma Protein:	8.8 (88)	g/dL (g/L)	6.0-7.5 (60-75)	g/dL (g/L)
Plasma Color:	Clear			
BUN (Azostix®):	50-80 (17.85-28.57)	mg/dL (mmol/L)	<30 (10.71)	mg/dL (mmol/L)
Blood Glucose:	32 (1.8)	mg/dL (mmol/L)	65-200 (3.6-11.1)	mg/dL (mmol/L)
Lactate:	9.7	mmol/L	<2.5	mmol/L
ACT:	75	sec	<80	sec
USG:	1.060			
Urine Protein:	1+			
Urine Glucose:	Negative			
Urine Ketone	Negative			
Urine pH:	6.0			
Urine Bilirubin	Negative			
Urine Sediment:	No casts/ crystals seen	#/lpf	0-1 Hyaline Casts	#/lpf

Case Figure 3.6   Biochemistry and urinalysis data. Urinalysis sample by cystocentesis.

4   What results, given the patient's signalment/history/clinical exam findings, would you expect in this patient?

Initial Data (History/Signalment/Physical Exam) Answers

1   Given the clinical data what is the differential diagnosis?
   a   *Given the clinical presentation and physical exam, the primary differential is heat stroke. Heat stroke patients present with a constellation of signs, severe hyperthermia, severe dehydration/hypovolemia, evidence of coagulopathy (typically petechiae), and gastrointestinal signs (typically diarrhea).*

2   What diagnostics ideally would you like to perform (given no resource boundaries) and why?
   a   *In this patient performing a CBC, biochemical profile, arterial or venous blood gas analysis, lactate, urinalysis, coagulation profile (PT, aPTT, TCT, fibrinogen, antithrombin, FDPs, and D-dimers), and blood pressure measurement would be ideal in this case.*

   b   *CBC is especially important for evaluating erythrocyte morphology, leukocyte concentration, platelet concentration. Patients with heat stroke commonly have severe thrombocytopenia. It is important to monitor these parameters since DIC and Systemic Inflammatory Response Syndrome (SIRS) are common sequelae of heat stroke.*
   c   *Serum biochemical profile is important because heat stroke can lead to severe metabolic derangements and multiorgan failure.*
   d   *Blood gas analysis is important for initial stabilization and monitoring of these patients. Patients with heat stroke can present with metabolic acidosis, respiratory alkalosis, and mixed acid–base abnormalities*
   e   *Lactate is usually elevated in patients with heat stroke and is often moderate to markedly increased.*
   f   *Urinalysis is important because acute kidney injury is a common sequela to heat stroke due to acute tubular injury. Urinalysis is also critical to the adequate interpretation of a biochemical profile.*
   g   *Coagulation profiles are valuable in managing heat stroke cases. Coagulopathy secondary to DIC is common sequelae of heat stroke.*

h *Blood pressure measurement is important in the acute management of heat stroke cases. Marked dehydration and vascular injury in patients lead to severe hypovolemia and inadequate organ perfusion due to low blood pressure.*

3 What low-cost diagnostics could you perform in this patient that might give you similar information to your ideal list?

a *In this case, PCV/TPP, blood film evaluation, ACT, BUN, blood glucose, lactate, and urinalysis should be performed.*

4 What results, given the patient's signalment/history/ clinical exam findings, would you expect in this patient?

a *In this patient we would expect to see hyperlactatemia, erythrocytosis/hemoconcentration, hyperproteinemia, azotemia, and hypoglycemia. We could also see thrombocytopenia or a prolonged activated clotting time.*

NIBP: 115 mmHg (Systolic)

Hematology

Test	Result	Units	Reference Interval	Units
PCV	51 (0.51)	% (L/L)	35-57 (0.35-0.57)	%
Polychromasia	1+			
nRBC	60	#/100 WBC	0-2	#/100 WBC
WBC Estimate	22,000	#/uL	5,000-15,500	#/uL
Segmented Neturophils	75	%	NA	%
Band Neutrophils	12	%	NA	%
Metamyelocytes	0	%	NA	%
Lymphocytes	3	%	NA	%
Monocytes	9	%	NA	%
Eosinophils	1	%	NA	%
Basophils	0	%	NA	%
Absolute Segmented Neutrophils	16,500	#/uL	2,500-10,750	#/uL
Absolute Band Neutrophils	2,640	#/uL	0-150	#/uL
Absolute Metamyelocytes	0	#/uL	0	#/uL
Absolute Lymphocytes	660	#/uL	850-4,500	#/uL
Absolute Monocytes	1,980	#/uL	150-1,100	#/uL
Absolute Eosinophils	220	#/uL	50-1,500	#/uL
Absolute Basophils	0	#/uL	0-100	#/uL
Toxic Change	2+ (Dohle bodies & Toxic Granulation)			
Platelet Estimate	~30,000	#/uL	150,000-450,000	#/uL
Platelet Comment	Few large platelets present			
Plasma Color:	Clear			

Case Figure 3.7 Hematologic data four hours post presentation. *Absolute leukocyte values are based on WBC estimate and differential count.

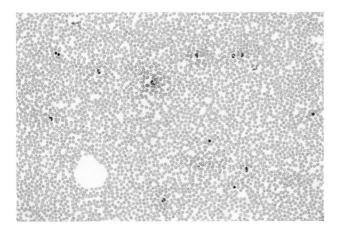

Case Figure 3.8 Blood film (Wrights–Giemsa, 200×).

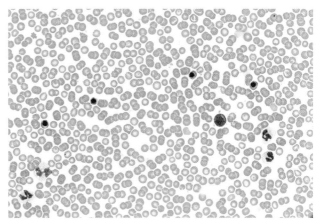

Case Figure 3.11 Blood film (Wrights–Giemsa, 500×).

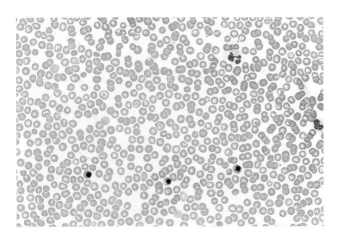

Case Figure 3.9 Blood film (Wrights–Giemsa, 500×).

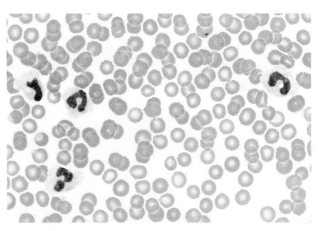

Case Figure 3.12 Blood film (Wrights–Giemsa, 1000×).

Diagnostic Result Interpretation Questions

1 Given the diagnostic results, what is your interpretation of the abnormalities identified?

2 Are any of these diagnostic results surprising/unexpected?

3 What are the broad mechanisms by which the abnormalities in question 1 occur?

4 In this case, what is/are the top differential diagnoses based on the current diagnostic data?

5 What additional diagnostics would you need to confirm or refute the top differentials for this case?

6 What is the significance of metarubricytosis in the absence of anemia?

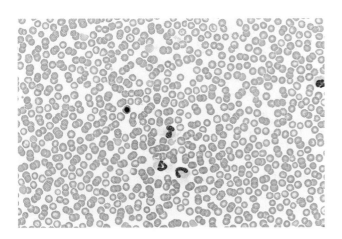

Case Figure 3.10 Blood film (Wrights–Giemsa, 500×).

Chemistry

Test	Result	Units	Reference Interval	Units
Total Plasma Protein:	7.5 (75)	g/dL (g/L)	6.0-7.5 (60-75)	g/dL (g/L)
Plasma Color:	Clear			
BUN (Azostix®):	50-80 (17.85-28.57)	mg/dL (mmol/L)	<30 (10.71)	mg/dL (mmol/L)
Blood Glucose:	130 (7.2)	mg/dL (mmol/L)	65-200 (3.6-11.1)	mg/dL (mmol/L)
Lactate:	6.9	mmol/L	<2.5	mmol/L
ACT:	125	sec	<80	sec
USG:	1.010			
Urine Protein:	2+			
Urine Glucose:	2+			
Urine Ketone	Negative			
Urine pH:	7.0			
Urine Bilirubin	Negative			
Urine Sediment:	0-2 granular casts	#/lpf	0-1 Hyaline Casts	#/lpf

Case Figure 3.13   Biochemistry and urinalysis data. Urinalysis sample by cystocentesis.

7   Why was it important to perform follow-up diagnostics within a relatively short time frame?

Diagnostic Result Interpretation Answers

1   Given the diagnostic results, what is your interpretation of the abnormalities identified?

 a   *The patient on initial presentation had marked erythrocytosis/hemoconcentration, hyperproteinemia, azotemia, hypersthenuria, all of which are consistent with severe dehydration. Marked hyperlactatemia and hypoglycemia are consistent with the clinical presentation of heat stroke.*

 b   *The changes from the initial diagnostics are persistent azotemia and hyperlactatemia despite appropriate fluid therapy, metarubricytosis, leukocyte shift to immaturity, evidence of a stress leukogram, precipitous decline in platelet count, glucosuria, cylindruria, and proteinuria.*

 c   *Mild leukocytosis characterized by neutrophilia with a significant shift to immaturity, and monocytosis are consistent with inflammation. Lymphopenia and monocytosis is likely secondary to increased circulating glucocorticoids from stress. Marked thrombocytopenia is also present in this patient as well as prolonged ACT, consistent with*

coagulopathy. Persistent azotemia despite appropriate fluid therapy to correct for dehydration/hypovolemia, proteinuria, glucosuria, and cylindruria indicate acute kidney injury. Persistent hyperlactatemia in the presence of normal blood pressure suggests inadequate peripheral perfusion and persistent anaerobic metabolism.

2   Are any of these diagnostic results surprising/ unexpected?

 a   *The leukocytosis is not surprising and is likely the result of stress considering the presence of lymphopenia and monocytosis. None of the other diagnostics on initial presentation are surprising or unexpected since they are common findings in patients with heat stroke.*

 b   *The persistent azotemia despite correction of dehydration/hypovolemia is unexpected. We would expect that since our patient was significantly dehydrated and initially had adequate urine-concentrating ability indicating prerenal azotemia that correction of the fluid deficiency should correct the azotemia. The same is true for the hyperlactatemia. Some of the patient's leukogram changes are not entirely surprising (i.e. lymphopenia and monocytosis associated with stress) but the significant shift to immaturity is unexpected unless there is development of sepsis. The inappropriate metarubricytosis is not surprising due to hyperthermic injury to the splenic and bone marrow vasculature resulting in increased release of metarubricytes from the bone marrow and decreased clearing of metarubricytes from the blood by the spleen.*

3 What are the broad mechanisms by which the abnormalities in question 1 occur?

a *Hypoglycemia resulting from heat stroke is likely multifactorial, resulting from increased consumption and decreased mobilization.*

b *Increased PCV/TPP is the result of dehydration from increased water loss from the vascular space.*

c *Azotemia is often both prerenal and renal in origin. For the prerenal aspect, severe dehydration decreases glomerular perfusion resulting in decreased GFR and increased serum concentration of nitrogenous waste products. For the renal aspect, injury to renal tubules from hyperthermia is likely multifactorial. Thermal injury, decreased tissue oxygen tension from decreased perfusion, and compounds released from injury to other tissues (i.e. myoglobin from rhabdomyolysis) are all potential contributors to renal injury.*

d *Hyperlactatemia occurs as a result of increased anaerobic metabolism that is due to hypoxemia (primarily) and hypoglycemia. Inadequate oxygen prevents aerobic cellular respiration resulting in decreased ATP production through glycolysis producing lactic acid is a byproduct.*

e *Thrombocytopenia is the result of severe platelet consumption, which has multiple causes. With severe hyperthermia, there is widespread vascular endothelial injury, which is a potent stimulus for platelet activation and clotting. In addition, tissue damage releases procoagulants from the tissue (i.e. Factor III), which further contributes to platelet and coagulation factor activation and consumption.*

f *Prolongation of activated clotting time is caused by severe depletion of secondary hemostatic factors. This is a result of widespread activation of the coagulation cascade. Note: Platelet numbers needed to prolong activated clotting time are extremely low ($<10,000/\mu l$).*

g *Cylindruria is the result of renal tubular necrosis with sloughing of tubular epithelial cells and formation of cellular casts that are shed into the urine.*

h *Glucosuria in the absence of hyperglycemia above the renal threshold is the result of renal tubular necrosis. Tubular injury prevents the reabsorption of glucose from renal filtrate and allows excretion in the urine.*

i *Proteinuria occurs as a result of the proximal renal tubule's inability to reabsorb the small amount of protein normally found in the glomerular filtrate.*

j *Inappropriate metarubricytosis in this case is the result of bone marrow and splenic sinusoidal injury from hyperthermia. Injured bone marrow and splenic sinusoids inappropriately releases immature cells (i.e. nRBCs) into circulation.*

k *Leukocytosis characterized by neutrophilia, significant shift to immaturity, and toxic change indicate an inflammatory process. This could be the result of bacterial translocation from the GI tract secondary to hyperthermic injury, the result of inflammation secondary to tissue necrosis or direct bone marrow injury secondary to heat stroke. Injured bone marrow inappropriately releases immature cells (i.e. band neutrophils) into circulation.*

4 In this case, what is/are the top differential diagnoses based on the current diagnostic data?

a *Disseminated intravascular coagulopathy, acute renal injury, and bone marrow injury secondary to heat stroke.*

5 What additional diagnostics would you need to confirm or refute the top differentials for this case?

a *Based on the clinical presentation, there is enough information to confirm the clinical diagnosis of heat stroke.*

i) *No additional information would be needed to confirm acute kidney injury and bone marrow injury secondary the heat stroke. However, to provide the best supportive care and monitoring for additional changes in organ function, a full CBC, biochemical profile, urinalysis, and coagulation profile with d-dimers should be performed.*

6 What is the significance of metarubricytosis in the absence of anemia?

a *Inappropriate metarubricytosis is a clinicopathologic finding with relatively few differential diagnoses. Most commonly, this finding relates to bone marrow injury (i.e. heat stroke, lead poisoning, etc.), splenic dysfunction, or traumatic release into the vascular space (i.e. long bone fracture).*

7 Why was it important to perform follow-up diagnostics within a relatively short time frame?

a *Severe hyperthermia due to heat stroke directly injures multiple organs. The injury may not be evident in laboratory data early in the process. Although treatment returns the patient to a normothermic state, injury may be ongoing and does not stop once the patient is cooled or adequately rehydrated.*

4 Case #4

4.1 Signalment

Mittens, a 10-month-old castrated male Siamese cat

4.2 History

Mittens is current on vaccinations and receives a monthly flea/tick preventative. Mittens was neutered at ~4 months of age by the shelter where he was adopted. Mittens came home from the shelter with severe diarrhea that resolved after three days.

4.3 Presentation

Patient presents for lethargy and hyporexia. The owners also report Mittens "feels hot".

4.4 Physical Exam Findings

Temp: 104.9°F (40.5°C), HR: 212, RR: 32, MM: Pale Pink/ Tacky, CRT: two seconds, Hydration status: ~5% Dehydrated, BCS: 3/9

Cardiopulmonary: No murmurs on auscultation, strong synchronous pulses, lungs auscultate normally.

Abdomen: Mild abdominal distension with fluid wave present and mild splenomegaly on palpation.

Lymph: No abnormalities identified.

HEENT: No abnormalities identified.

Urogenital: No abnormalities identified.

Integument: No abnormalities identified.

Neurologic: Patient is QAR, ambulates normally and has normal conscious proprioceptive responses and nociceptive responses. A brief cranial nerve exam is within normal limits.

Musculoskeletal: No abnormalities identified.

Initial Data (History/Signalment/Physical Exam) Questions

1 Given the clinical data what is the differential diagnosis?

2 What diagnostics ideally would you like to perform (given no resource boundaries) and why?

3 What low-cost diagnostics could you perform in this patient that might give you similar information to your ideal list?

4 What information are you expecting to receive from these diagnostics? In other words, what differential do you expect to rule in or rule out with these diagnostics?

5 What results, given the patient's signalment/history/ clinical exam findings, would you expect in this patient?

Initial Data (History/Signalment/Physical Exam) Answers

1 Given the clinical data, what is the differential diagnosis?

   a *From the clinical data the primary differential would be feline infectious peritonitis (FIP) due to the high fever, abdominal distension, and palpable fluid wave. Given the temperature and splenomegaly, hemotropic mycoplasma infection should be included as a differential. Fever indicates there is an inflammatory process occurring. Therefore, any compatible inflammatory diseases would be an appropriate differential. Otherwise, the clinical signs are nonspecific.*

2 What diagnostics ideally would you like to perform (given no resource boundaries) and why?

   a *It would be ideal to perform a CBC, biochemistry profile, urinalysis, FELV/FIV testing, and abdominocentesis w/fluid analysis. If fluid analysis is supportive of inflammation, bacterial culture and sensitivity, as well as, PCR for feline coronavirus would be ideal to perform. Depending on findings of the initial CBC, it may be beneficial to perform PCR for* Mycoplasma *spp., or other infectious organisms.*

   b *The CBC is part of any minimum database. The patient has pale pink mucous membranes, and slight tachycardia. It is important to evaluate if the patient is simply dehydrated or truly anemic. Leukogram evaluation may support an inflammatory process.*

   c *Biochemistry profile will help rule out or indicate potential causes of the abdominal effusion. Common differentials for abdominal effusion are inflammatory exudation (i.e. peritonitis), decreased vascular* oncotic pressure (i.e. hypoproteinemia), and increased vascular hydrostatic pressure (i.e. heart failure). Biochemistry profile will evaluate plasma proteins, liver function, and renal function, important differentials for abdominal effusion. Serum bilirubin measurement is important and increases may raise suspicion for infection with hemotropic mycoplasmas or liver dysfunction.

d Urinalysis is critical for adequate interpretation of a serum biochemistry profile and should always be performed.

e FELV/FIV testing would help rule in or out retroviral infection in this patient. Retroviral status is important to establish in all feline patients with significant inflammatory disease.

f Abdominal fluid analysis +/− infectious disease testing would be beneficial in this patient to investigate potential causes of effusion. The characterization of the fluid would help support the possibility of FIP.

Abdominal radiographs would be less helpful in this case because fluid within the peritoneal cavity obscures radiographic detail. Abdominal ultrasound and thoracic radiographs may be beneficial to perform.

3 What low-cost diagnostics could you perform in this patient that might give you similar information provided by your ideal list of diagnostics?

a *PCV/TPP, blood film review, BUN, urinalysis, and abdominal fluid analysis would be appropriate low-cost diagnostics.*

4 What information are you expecting to receive from these diagnostics? In other words, what differential do you expect to rule in or rule out with these diagnostics?

a *PCV/TPP will confirm if the patient is anemic. If anemic, the total plasma protein can help determine the cause of the anemia. Total plasma protein may provide insight into disease process such as dehydration, hypoproteinemia, or inflammation.*

Hematology

Test	Result	Units	Reference Interval	Units
PCV	32 (0.32)	% (L/L)	30-45 (0.30-0.45)	% (L/L)
Ecchinocytes	2+			
RBC Comment:	Marked Rouleaux, Protein crescents frequent			
WBC Estimate	4,500	#/uL	5,000-15,500	#/uL
Segmented Neturophils	89	%	NA	%
Band Neutrophils	0	%	NA	%
Metamyelocytes	0	%	NA	%
Lymphocytes	7	%	NA	%
Monocytes	1	%	NA	%
Eosinophils	3	%	NA	%
Basophils	0	%	NA	%
Absolute Segmented Neutrophils	4,005	#/uL	2,500-10,750	#/uL
Absolute Band Neutrophils	0	#/uL	0-150	#/uL
Absolute Metamyelocytes	0	#/uL	0	#/uL
Absolute Lymphocytes	315	#/uL	850-4,500	#/uL
Absolute Monocytes	45	#/uL	150-1,100	#/uL
Absolute Eosinophils	135	#/uL	50-1,500	#/uL
Absolute Basophils	0	#/uL	0-100	#/uL
Toxic Change	WBC morphology appears normal			
Platelet Estimate	400,000	#/uL	150,000-450,000	#/uL
Platelet Comment	Platelet morphology appears normal			

Case Figure 4.1 Hematologic data. *Absolute leukocyte values are based on WBC estimate and differential count.

Case Figure 4.2 Blood film (Wrights–Giemsa, 100×).

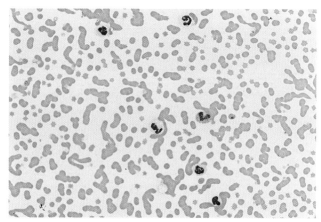

Case Figure 4.5 Blood film (Wrights–Giemsa, 500×).

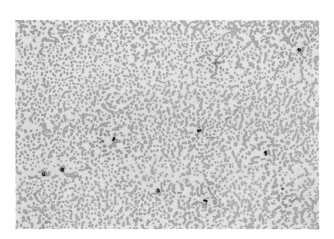

Case Figure 4.3 Blood film (Wrights–Giemsa, 200×).

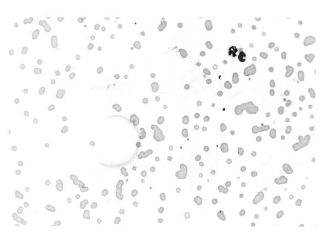

Case Figure 4.6 Blood film (Wrights–Giemsa, 500×).

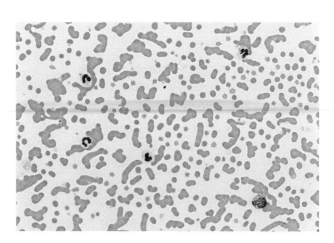

Case Figure 4.4 Blood film (Wrights–Giemsa, 500×).

b *Blood film evaluation can support evidence of an inflammatory process. Potentially, hemotropic mycoplasmas or other erythroparasites may be found to assist in determining the cause of anemia if present.*

c *BUN will help support possible dehydration and may provide insight into the origin of the abdominal effusion if there is other evidence of renal insufficiency.*

d *Urinalysis is necessary for adequate interpretation any biochemistry profile and BUN in this case. Urinalysis may also provide insight into potential causes of abdominal effusion if there is significant proteinuria.*

e *Abdominal fluid analysis will classify the effusion and provide insight into potential causes of the effusion.*

Fluid Analysis

Test	Result	Units
Sample:	Abdominal Effusion	NA
Sample Container:	EDTA (Purple Top) Tube	NA
Sample Color	Slightly orange	NA
Sample Clarity:	Mildly Turbid	NA
Sample Consistency:	Low viscosity	NA
PCV:	<2	%
PCV:	<0.02	L/L
TP:	7.6	g/dL
Cellularity Estimate From Direct Preparation:	Mild Cellularity	
%Neutrophils	13	%
%Lymphocytes	7	%
%Monocytes	79	%
%Eosinophils	1	%
%Basophils	0	%
%Other	0	%
Comment:	Macrophages are predominately large and activated with vacuolated cytoplasm. Neutrophils are mildly degenerate. No infectious organisms identified	

Case Figure 4.7 Fluid analysis data.

Chemistry

Test	Result	Units	Reference Interval	Units
Total Plasma Protein:	>12 (120)	g/dL (g/L)	6.0-7.5 (60-75)	g/dL (g/L)
Plasma Color:	Slight Icterus			
BUN (Azostix®):	15-26 (5.36-9.28)	mg/dL (mmol/L)	<30 (10.71)	mg/dL (mmol/L)
Urine Color:	Bright Yellow			
USG:	1.045			
Urine Protein:	Negative			
Urine Glucose:	Negative			
Urine Ketone:	Negative			
Urine pH:	7.0			
Urine Bilirubin	1+			
Urine Sediment:	No casts/ crystals seen	#/lpf	0-1 Hyaline Casts	#/lpf

Case Figure 4.8 Biochemistry and urinalysis data. Urinalysis sample by cystocentesis.

5 What results, given the patient's signalment/history/clinical exam findings, would you expect in this patient?

   a *In this patient, a normal BUN with a USG in the hypersthenuric range (patient is ~5% dehydrated) is expected. An inflammatory leukogram, stress (glucocorticoid) leukogram, or both would be expected considering the presence of fever in this patient. Abdominal effusion may reveal an exudate or protein-rich effusion considering the presence of fever. However, a transudate or protein-poor cellular infiltrate could be possible. Given the patient's pale mucous membranes and slight tachycardia, the PCV may be decreased. Given the abdominal effusion and fever, the total plasma protein may be high due to increased inflammatory proteins, possible dehydration. Since there is no clinical evidence of blood loss, hypoproteinemia is less likely.* However, hypoproteinemia due to protein loss through the gastrointestinal tract or kidney is possible.*

Diagnostic Result Interpretation Questions

1 Given the diagnostic results, what abnormalities do you identify? What is your interpretation of these findings?

2 Are any of these diagnostic results surprising/unexpected?

3 What are the broad mechanisms by which these abnormalities occur?

4 Is rouleaux normally seen in cats? If so, is it ever of diagnostic value when present?

5 How can we distinguish rouleaux from erythrocyte agglutination? Why is it important to make the distinction between the two?

6 What is the reason we see bilirubinuria and mildly icteric plasma in this patient? Is bilirubinuria ever normal in cats?

7 In this case, what is/are the top differential diagnoses based on the current diagnostic data?

8 What diagnostic results are most supportive for each of the differential diagnoses?

9 What additional diagnostics would you need to confirm/refute the top differentials for this case?

Diagnostic Result Interpretation Answers

1 Given the diagnostic results, what abnormalities do you identify? What is your interpretation of these abnormalities?

   a *The PCV is within the reference interval, indicating the patient's pale mucous membranes are more likely due to poor perfusion and not anemia.*

   b *The total plasma protein is markedly increased. Considering the inflammatory process evident in the fluid analysis, the markedly increased total plasma protein is most likely due to inflammation. A less likely possibility would be an immunoglobulin producing plasma cell neoplasm. The degree of dehydration is unlikely to cause this degree of hyperproteinemia.*

   c *The WBC estimate is mildly decreased, the neutrophil count is within the reference interval. The mild leukopenia is likely the result of lymphopenia, and monocytopenia. Lymphopenia is likely secondary to increased circulating glucocorticoid (cortisol) concentration. Monocytopenia is not a clinically significant finding.*

   d *The BUN is normal and urine specific gravity shows adequate urine-concentrating ability. Therefore, the patient likely has normal renal function.*

   e *There is mild bilirubinuria, which supports the mildly icteric plasma appearance. Bilirubinuria in combination with icteric plasma confirms that this patient is hyperbilirubinemic. In this case, the increase in plasma bilirubin concentration is not of a magnitude that is resulting in grossly evident jaundice. There is not enough information to definitively determine the cause of icterus in this patient.*

   f *The abdominal fluid analysis shows a very high-protein effusion. There are predominantly large, activated macrophages with low numbers of neutrophils and lymphocytes and no infectious agents identified. This finding is very consistent with chronic inflammation and is commonly seen in patients with feline infectious peritonitis (FIP).*

2 Are any of these diagnostic results surprising/unexpected?

   a *The icteric plasma and bilirubinuria was unexpected, but not surprising. It was unexpected because the patient did not have gross evidence of icterus. Generally, serum bilirubin concentrations have to be >2.5 mg/dL to be visibly evident as* *icteric mucous membranes. However, increased plasma bilirubin concentration is a common finding in cats with FIP.*

b *The markedly increased total plasma protein was also unexpected but not surprising. In cats, marked immunologic responses, can be common with certain inflammatory conditions. This degree of hyperglobulinemia is common with FIP. Feline infectious peritonitis is a major differential to consider in cases of marked hyperproteinemia caused by markedly increased globulin concentration.*

c *In this case, the relatively normal leukogram is surprising because of the presence of significant fever and inflammatory abdominal effusion. However, it is important to remember that even in cases of significant tissue inflammation you may not see leukocytosis or neutrophilia.*

3 What are the broad mechanisms by which these abnormalities occur?

a *In this case, prehepatic icterus is unlikely since the PCV is within reference interval. The icterus is most likely hepatic in origin, although a posthepatic component cannot definitively be ruled out without abdominal ultrasound. Icterus of hepatic origin is likely the result of vasculitis and subsequent hepatocellular injury, a common sequela of FIP.*

b *Lymphopenia is the result of increased plasma glucocorticoid (cortisol) concentration. Glucocorticoids have many effects on lymphocytes: induction of lympholysis, reduced egress from lymph nodes, and decreased lymphocyte proliferation. All of these can contribute to lymphopenia due to glucocorticoid (cortisol) response.*

c *Increases in total plasma protein can have several mechanisms including increased production of proteins or loss of plasma water effectively concentrating proteins. It is unlikely that this patient's hyperproteinemia is the result of the dehydration present. Hyperproteinemia in this case is most likely the result of increased production of immunoglobulins and acute phase proteins such as fibrinogen, C-reactive protein, Serum Amyloid A, and other alpha and beta globulins.*

d *High-protein, low cell effusion is the result of cavitary protein and water exudation, but little loss of cells into the fluid. Widespread vasculitis is a common cause of protein and fluid loss from the vascular space into the cavitary space. Fluid cellularity can be mild to moderate, mainly due to the adhesion of inflammatory cells to endothelium and inflammation secondary to necrosis. The inflammatory cell*

population is predominantly activated macrophages, which in the case in FIP occurs as a result of virus-mediated macrophage proliferation.

4 Is rouleaux normally seen in cats? If so, is it ever of diagnostic value when present?

a *Rouleaux can be a normal finding in cats when examining the blood film; however, rouleaux to the degree seen in this case is abnormal. This degree is supportive of a markedly increased plasma protein concentration. Increased plasma proteins lead to increased erythrocyte attraction by altering surface charge. If there is marked rouleaux and markedly increased plasma protein, there are relatively few conditions that should be considered depending on clinical signs (i.e. Plasma cell neoplasia, severe inflammatory response, etc.).*

5 How can we distinguish rouleaux from erythrocyte agglutination? Why is it important to make the distinction between the two?

a *Erythrocyte agglutination and rouleaux can be challenging to distinguish by morphology alone.*
Performing a saline agglutination test allows for distinction between the two entities. When performed, the dilution of the plasma protein will usually allow the erythrocyte surface charge to become more normal. This allows the stacked erythrocytes to "disperse" from each other. In the case of true erythrocyte agglutination, the saline will not disperse the cells, and they will remain aggregated.

It is critical to distinguish these two entities from each other. Erythrocyte agglutination has more significant implications than rouleaux. Erythrocyte agglutination indicates immune-mediated hemolytic anemia, where rouleaux can be normal or simply indicate increased plasma protein concentration.

6 What is the reason we see bilirubinuria and mildly icteric plasma in this patient? Is bilirubinuria ever normal in cats?

a In cats, bilirubinuria is never "normal" and by itself is indicative of hyperbilirubinemia. The bilirubinuria and mildly icteric plasma are both consistent with hyperbilirubinemia. In cats with no signs of jaundice on physical exam, a positive urine bilirubin should be confirmed, to ensure the result is not erroneous. In this case, the presence of icteric plasma confirms the urinalysis result is correct.

*Note: Bilirubinuria is normal in dogs because they have a lower renal threshold for bilirubin and can conjugate and secrete bilirubin in the kidney.

7 In this case, what is/are the top differential diagnoses based on the current diagnostic data?

    a *FIP is the primary differential. Other differentials to consider are FELV, FIV, Hemotropic Mycoplasma, or other infectious diseases. Concurrent diseases cannot be ruled out.*

8 What diagnostic results are most supportive for each of the differential diagnoses?

    a *The most likely differential is FIP, supported by the marked hyperproteinemia, high-protein and mild cellularity effusion, and evidence of hepatic disease. Other causes of vasculitis should be considered as well. FELV/FIV should always be considered in ill patients with evidence of inflammatory or infectious disease. Hemotropic mycoplasma infection also cannot be entirely ruled out at this time because of the observed splenomegaly and icteric plasma. The anemia associated with hemotropic mycoplasmas can be periodic. Currently, we don't have enough information to rule in other disease, that may be more apparent with a full minimum database.*

9 What additional diagnostics would you need to confirm/refute your top differentials for this case?

    a *In this case, complete fluid analysis with quantification of the nucleated cell count and Feline Coronavirus PCR on the abdominal effusion would assist in confirming or refuting the diagnosis of FIP. It is important in a case like this to rule out other potential causes i.e. FELV, Mycoplasma, etc. therefore, PCR testing for a variety of infectious agents may be helpful in efficiently identifying a cause for the patient's signs. It would also be helpful to perform serum protein electrophoresis to differentiate a monoclonal gammopathy (secondary to neoplasia) from a polyclonal gammopathy (secondary to marked inflammation). Infectious diseases typically result in a polyclonal gammopathy; however, in rare cases, infectious disease may result in monoclonal gammopathies (i.e. Ehrlichiosis in dogs and FIP in cats).*

5 Case #5

5.1 Signalment

Star, a 9-week-old intact female Australian Shepherd dog

5.2 History

Star was adopted by her family yesterday from an online ad. She came with no documentation of vaccinations, previous veterinary visits, or fecal examination.

5.3 Presentation

Star presents for a wellness exam and vaccinations. This morning the owners noticed that Star was not acting like she was yesterday. She is depressed, will not eat, has bloody diarrhea and is vomiting.

5.4 Physical Exam Findings

Temp: 102.9°F (39.4°C), HR: 124, RR: 28, MM: Pink/Tacky, CRT: three seconds, Hydration status: 5% Dehydrated, BCS: 4/9

Cardiopulmonary: No murmurs on auscultation, strong synchronous pulses, lungs auscultate normally. Abdomen: Abdomen appears painful on palpation, patient moans when attempted.

Lymph: No abnormalities identified.

HEENT: No abnormalities identified.

Urogenital: No abnormalities identified.

Integument: No abnormalities identified.

Neurologic: Patient is QAR, ambulates normally and has normal conscious proprioceptive responses and nociceptive responses. A brief cranial nerve exam is within normal limits.

Musculoskeletal: No abnormalities identified.

Initial Data (History/Signalment/Physical Exam) Questions

1 Given the clinical data what is the differential diagnosis?

2 What diagnostics ideally would you like to perform (given no resource boundaries) and why?

3 What low-cost diagnostics could you perform in this patient that might give you similar information to your ideal list?

4 What information are you expecting to receive from these diagnostics? In other words, what differential do you expect to rule in or rule out with these diagnostics?

5 What results, given the patient's signalment/history/ clinical exam findings, would you expect in this patient?

Initial Data (History/Signalment/Physical Exam) Answers

1 Given the clinical data what is the differential diagnosis?
  a Canine parvoviral enteritis, canine distemper virus, giardiasis, or intestinal parasitism are the top differentials.

2 What diagnostics ideally would you like to perform (given no resource boundaries) and why?
  a *Ideally in this patient, a CBC, biochemistry profile, urinalysis, fecal direct smear, fecal flotation, and rapid antigen testing for Canine parvovirus (CPV) and Giardia would be ideal.*
  b *The CBC is important to assess for evidence of inflammation. If this patient has a CPV infection, leukocyte concentration is an important prognostic indicator.*
  c *A biochemical profile would be valuable in assessing electrolyte/acid–base status. It will also be important for treatment monitoring and adjustment based on changes in parameters related to renal function and hydration status (i.e. BUN and creatinine).*
  d *Urinalysis is critical for adequate interpretation of the serum biochemical profile and they should always be performed together.*
  e *Fecal direct smear will allow us to evaluate for motile parasites (i.e. Giardia) and the population of microorganisms present.*
  f *Fecal flotation would allow evaluation for the presence of GI parasites, which are common in puppies. It is needed to rule out the possibility of hookworms, roundworms, and whipworms as a cause of the diarrhea.*
  g *Rapid antigen testing would rule in or out the possibility of CPV or Giardia. Although a fecal direct smear would allow for diagnosis of Giardia if organisms were identified, this is not a sensitive test. In any young patient with an unknown vaccination status and diarrhea, parvoviral enteritis must be the primary differential until its presence or absence is confirmed.*

3 What low-cost diagnostics could you perform in this patient that might give you similar information to your ideal list?
  a *In this case PCV/TPP, blood film evaluation, blood glucose, BUN, urinalysis, fecal direct smear, and fecal flotation should be performed.*

4 What information are you expecting to receive from these diagnostics? In other words, what differential do you expect to rule in or rule out with these diagnostics?
  a *The PCV/TPP will help assess the patient's hydration status both before and after treatment, and assess for anemia.*
  b *Blood film evaluation is helpful in estimating patient leukocyte concentration. This is important because leukopenia is a negative prognostic indicator for patients with parvoviral enteritis.*
  c *Blood glucose is a critical parameter to monitor in any patient with diarrhea and the potential for sepsis (i.e. CPV). Hypoglycemia puts patients at higher risk for mortality.*
  d *BUN will help assess the patient's hydration status and renal function during treatment.*
  e *Urinalysis will help interpret the BUN, assess hydration, and may help guide adjustment of fluid therapy according to patient response.*
  f *See the answers to Question 2 for rationale behind performing a fecal direct smear and fecal flotation.*

5 What results, given the patient's signalment/history/ clinical exam findings, would you expect in this patient?
  a Based on the current clinical findings, the leukocyte count may be low, normal, or high, depending on the cause of the clinical signs. In the case of canine parvovirus, a low or normal leukocyte count can be expected. Regardless of the leukocyte count, there may be a shift to immaturity present. The PCV may be decreased, normal, or increased depending on the underlying disease. Considering the presence of hematochezia, the PCV and total plasma protein may be decreased or within the reference interval. Considering the age of the patient, acute hemorrhagic diarrhea syndrome (formerly known as hemorrhagic gastroenteritis) is unlikely. Blood glucose may be low, especially since the patient is lethargic, anorexic, and has the potential for sepsis. BUN may be increased since there is evidence of dehydration and GI blood loss.

Hematology

Test	Result	Units	Reference Interval	Units
PCV	45 (0.45)	% (L/L)	35-57 (0.35-0.57)	% (L/L)
RBC Comment	Smudging present from lipemia			
nRBC	0	#/100 WBC	0-2	#/100 WBC
WBC Estimate	4600	#/uL	5,000-15,500	#/uL
Segmented Neturophils	53	%	NA	%
Band Neutrophils	30	%	NA	%
Metamyelocytes	1	%	NA	%
Lymphocytes	7	%	NA	%
Monocytes	9	%	NA	%
Eosinophils	0	%	NA	%
Basophils	0	%	NA	%
Absolute Segmented Neutrophils	2438	#/uL	2,500-10,750	#/uL
Absolute Band Neutrophils	1380	#/uL	0-150	#/uL
Absolute Metamyelocytes	46	#/uL	0	#/uL
Absolute Lymphocytes	322	#/uL	850-4,500	#/uL
Absolute Monocytes	414	#/uL	150-1,100	#/uL
Absolute Eosinophils	0	#/uL	50-1,500	#/uL
Absolute Basophils	0	#/uL	0-100	#/uL
Toxic Change	**1+ (Dohle bodies present)**			
WBC Comment	Circulating mast cells commonly observed (~0-1/50X Field)			
Platelet Estimate	~400,000	#/uL	150,000-450,000	#/uL
Platelet Comment	Few Large platelets present			

Case Figure 5.1 Hematologic data. *Absolute leukocyte values are based on WBC estimate and differential count.

Case Figure 5.2 Blood film (Wrights–Giemsa, 200×).

Case Figure 5.3 Blood film (Wrights–Giemsa, 200×).

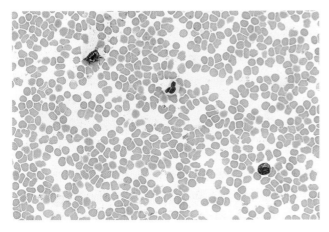

Case Figure 5.4 Blood film (Wrights–Giemsa, 500×).

Diagnostic Result Interpretation Questions

1 Given the diagnostic results, what abnormalities do you identify? What is your interpretation of these findings?

2 Are any of these diagnostic results surprising/ unexpected?

3 What are the broad mechanisms by which these abnormalities occur?

4 Why does this patient have mastocytemia?

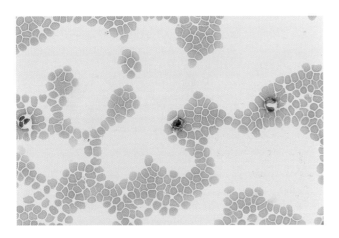

Case Figure 5.5 Blood film (Wrights–Giemsa, 500×).

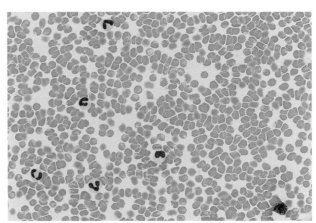

Case Figure 5.6 Blood film (Wrights–Giemsa, 500×).

Chemistry				
Test	**Result**	**Units**	**Reference Interval**	**Units**
Total Plasma Protein:	5.3 (53)	g/dL (g/L)	6.0-7.5 (60-75)	g/dL (g/L)
Plasma Color:	1+ Lipemia			
BUN (Azostix®):	30-40 (10.71-14.28)	mg/dL (mmol/L)	<30 (10.71)	mg/dL (mmol/L)
Blood Glucose:	50 (2.8)	mg/dL (mmol/L)	65-200 (3.6-11.1)	mg/dL (mmol/L)
USG:	1.040			
Urine Protein:	Negative			
Urine Glucose:	Negative			
Urine Ketone	Trace			
Urine pH:	6.5			
Urine Bilirubin	Negative			
Urine Sediment:	No casts/ cyrstals seen	#/lpf	0-1 Hyaline Casts	#/lpf

Case Figure 5.7 Biochemistry and urinalysis data. Urinalysis sample by cystocentesis.

Fecal Analysis		
Test	**Result**	**Units**
Sample Consistency:	Liquid, mucous present	NA
Sample Color	Beige, hemorrhagic	NA
Fecal Direct Smear:	No motile parasites seen	
Fecal Floatation (Sugar Centrifugation)	No ova or parasites seen	

Case Figure 5.8 Fecal analysis data.

5   In this patient, monitoring for resolution of leukopenia and transition from a degenerative to a regenerative shift to immaturity is prognostically important. How long before we would expect to start to see evidence of a bone marrow response in this patient?

6   In this case, what is/are the top differential diagnoses based on the current diagnostic data?

7   What diagnostic results are most supportive of the top differential diagnosis?

8   What additional diagnostics would you need to confirm/refute the top differentials for this case?

Diagnostic Result Interpretation Answers

1   Given the diagnostic results, what abnormalities do you identify? What is your interpretation of these abnormalities?
   a   *There is mild leukopenia present, the segmented neutrophil count is just barely below the reference interval, and there is a significant shift to immaturity. These findings are consistent with an uncompensated shift to immaturity. Lymphopenia is present, which may be consistent with stress or lympholysis due to viral disease. There are circulating mast cells present, which can occur with severe acute gastrointestinal disease in the dog.*
   b   *The total plasma protein is decreased, this is likely secondary to loss of protein into the gastrointestinal tract secondary to mucosal injury and hemorrhage.*
   c   *The lipemia present is nonspecific but may indicate mobilization of lipid from adipose secondary to anorexia. If the mild ketonuria is pathologic in origin, in conjunction with lipemia, it supports a negative energy balance in this patient.*

   d   *The blood glucose is low, which is not uncommon in sick puppies when anorexic and can be seen with underlying sepsis.*
   e   *The BUN is increased in conjunction with adequate urine-concentrating ability, supporting prerenal origin of the azotemia. In addition, the presence of hematochezia may be contributing to the increased BUN.*
   f   *Fecal smear and flotation reveal no evidence of parasitic disease. Although this does not completely rule out endoparasites, it does increase the suspicion for CPV.*

2   Are any of these diagnostic results surprising/ unexpected?
   a   *In this case, the mastocytemia was unexpected, but not surprising. The most common cause of mastocytemia in the dog is gastrointestinal inflammation. The lipemia and ketonuria in this patient was also unexpected. The most likely explanation is that the patient's anorexia created a negative energy balance. With inadequate glucose, the body starts to generate ketones from lipid as an energy source. It is mildly surprising that there were no parasites identified on fecal flotation or direct smear considering the patient's history.*

3   What are the broad mechanisms by which these abnormalities occur?
   a   *Leukopenia is common in cases of canine parvovirus, which is suspected in this case and can occur from two mechanisms. The first is hematopoietic injury directly from canine parvovirus infection of hematopoietic precursors in the bone marrow. Canine parvovirus infects and causes necrosis of both hematopoietic and lymphoid cells. This injury dramatically alters the body's hematopoietic ability, which has a rapid impact on circulating leukocyte numbers. In addition*

to the hematopoietic injury, there is also significant tissue demand and consumption of leukocytes secondary to gastrointestinal tract injury. The leukocytes in circulation and bone marrow storage pool are rapidly consumed leading to leukopenia and a shift to immaturity.

b *Decreased total plasma protein is the result of gastrointestinal injury and inflammation; this causes loss of proteins into the gastrointestinal lumen.*

c *Decreased blood glucose can occur for two reasons. The first reason is that young animals do not have large glycogen stores and limited capacity for gluconeogenesis. During periods of anorexia, there is little glycogen to mobilize to create glucose, and their liver has limited ability to synthesize glucose from amino acids leading to hypoglycemia. Another cause of hypoglycemia in this case could be sepsis. With severe injury to the gastrointestinal tract, bacteria can easily translocate from the lumen into the vascular space leading to sepsis. Sepsis often results in liver dysfunction and decreased insulin degradation which can contribute to the hypoglycemia.*

d *Prerenal azotemia occurs as a result of dehydration associated hypovolemia. There is decreased perfusion to the glomerulus, which decreases GFR and collectively leads to increased concentrations of nitrogenous waste within the blood. Hemorrhage into the gastrointestinal tract leads to increased protein digestion and subsequent increases in BUN, as would be seen with any protein meal.*

e *Ketonuria and lipemia occur secondary to metabolism shift from carbohydrates to lipids.*

4 Why does this patient have mastocytemia?

a *Mastocytemia in the dog is most commonly seen with severe acute gastrointestinal inflammation, of which CPV is the most common. This finding should not be surprising in a puppy with bloody diarrhea.*

5 In this patient, monitoring for resolution of leukopenia and transition from a degenerative to a regenerative shift to immaturity is prognostically important. When would you expect to see the leukocyte count within the reference interval in a leukopenic patient that is responding favorably to treatment?

a *In the case of viral enteritis due to CPV, if a puppy's leukocyte count returns to within the reference interval within 24–48 hours, they have a higher probability for survival* [1].

6 In this case, what is/are the top differential diagnoses based on the current diagnostic data?

a *The top differential is canine parvovirus associated enteritis. Canine distemper virus, intestinal parasitic disease, or other infectious causes of gastrointestinal disease cannot be entirely ruled out at this time.*
Canine distemper virus (CDV) can result in similar signs, (enteritis, leukopenia, etc.), which means that it must remain a differential until there is more information. Canine distemper virus, unlike CPV, is classically associated with respiratory disease followed by neurologic signs without significant hemorrhagic diarrhea.

7 What diagnostic results are most supportive of the top differential diagnosis?

a *The constellation of clinical findings (lack of vaccine history, acute onset lethargy, vomiting, and bloody diarrhea) with the diagnostic findings (leukopenia, mastocytemia, negative fecal flotation, and direct smear) is strongly supportive of canine parvovirus as the most likely diagnosis.*

8 What additional diagnostics would you need to confirm/refute the top differentials for this case?

a *It would be ideal to perform antigen testing for canine parvovirus. If negative PCR may be necessary, in which case checking for multiple antigens (i.e. CPV, CDV, etc.) would be the most efficient way to rule out other potential causes of this patient's clinical signs. If the diagnostic tests for underlying viral disease are negative, it would also be beneficial to repeat fecal flotation, direct smear, and Giardia antigen testing as well to help eliminate those as potential entities contributing to the patient's signs.*

6 Case #6

6.1 Signalment

Earl, a 5-year-old castrated male Labrador Retriever dog.

6.2 History

Earl is current on vaccinations and gets a monthly flea/tick preventative. Owners have previously declined heartworm preventatives or anthelminthics.

6.3 Presentation

Earl presents for routine physical exam. The owners report that Earl has had an intermittent cough and exercise intolerance over the past year.

6.4 Physical Exam Findings

Temp: 100.1°F (37.8°C), HR: 124, RR: 36, MM: Pink, CRT: <2 seconds, Hydration status: <5% Dehydrated, BCS: 5/9

Cardiopulmonary: Grade 2/6 murmur loudest over the Tricuspid valve on auscultation, strong synchronous pulses. Mild adventitious lung sounds in the bronchovesicular regions.

Abdomen: Mild hepatomegaly on palpation.
Lymph: No abnormalities identified.
HEENT: No abnormalities identified.
Urogenital: No abnormalities identified.
Integument: No abnormalities identified.
Neurologic: No abnormal findings.
Musculoskeletal: No abnormalities identified.

Initial Data (History/Signalment/Physical Exam) Questions

1 Given the clinical data, what is the differential diagnosis?

2 What diagnostics ideally would you like to perform (given no resource boundaries) and why?

3 What low-cost diagnostics could you perform in this patient that might give you similar information to your ideal list?

4 What information are you expecting to receive from these diagnostics? In other words, what differential do you expect to rule in or rule out with these diagnostics?

5 What results, given the patient's signalment/history/ clinical exam findings, would you expect in this patient?

6 Do patients with right-sided heart failure typically experience signs of pulmonary disease?

Initial Data (History/Signalment/Physical Exam) Answers

1 Given the clinical data, what is the differential diagnosis?

a *The primary differential to rule out in this case would be heartworm infestation. Other differentials to consider would be Dipetalonema infestation, fungal infections (i.e. coccidioidomycosis, blastomycosis, etc.), neoplasia, or cardiac disease. It is uncommon for any of the pathogens in the canine infectious respiratory disease complex to cause clinical signs for this length of time.*

2 What diagnostics ideally would you like to perform (given no resource boundaries) and why?

a *Ideally, three view thoracic radiographs should be performed in conjunction with a CBC, biochemistry profile, urinalysis, and heartworm antigen test. If there are findings compatible with fungal disease on radiographs, serologic testing should be performed. If there is evidence of neoplasia on radiographs, ultrasound-guided aspirate of any accessible lesions should be performed.*

b *Three view thoracic radiographs would allow evaluation of intrathoracic structures and help identify radiographic features of heartworm infestation, other cardiac diseases, fungal infection, or neoplasia.*

c *CBC/biochemistry/UA are all part of the minimum database. It is ideal to perform them in all patients with systemic illness. Information collected from the minimum database may help guide future diagnostics and treatment depending on their results.*

d *Review of a blood film may show circulating microfilariae if this patient has a patent heartworm infestation.*

e *Heartworm antigen test is the most sensitive test that we can perform to rule in or out heartworm infestation.*

3 What low-cost diagnostics could you perform on this patient that might give you similar information to your ideal list?

a *In this case performing a PCV/TPP, blood film evaluation, BUN, and urinalysis would be a good starting point. If there are no microfilaria identified on the blood film, performing an evaluation of the buffy coat or examination of the plasma just above the buffy coat in a hematocrit tube would be recommended.*

4 What information are you expecting to receive from these diagnostics? In other words, what differential do you expect to rule in or rule out with these diagnostics?

a *Anemia secondary to erythrocyte fragmentation can be seen depending on parasite burden, which may be evident on PCV/TPP examination.*

b *Blood film evaluation would allow us to screen for the presence of microfilaria.*

c *BUN should also be performed in all patients if a biochemistry profile cannot be performed. Monitoring renal function, especially in patients with suspected cardiac disease, is an important factor to consider in the development of a treatment plan.*

d *Urinalysis is critical for adequate interpretation of BUN.*

5 What results, given the patient's signalment/history/clinical exam findings, would you expect in this patient?

a *Given the clinical signs in this patient (cough, exercise intolerance, and right-sided heart murmur) and the lack of heartworm prevention, one expected finding is the presence of microfilaria on examination of the blood film. In addition, possible hemolytic anemia secondary to erythrocyte fragmentation, or nonregenerative anemia secondary to chronic inflammatory disease may be seen. If the patient has heartworm disease, significant proteinuria may be seen secondary to glomerular injury from antigen–antibody complexes that can form with many infectious diseases.*

6 Do patients with right-sided heart failure typically experience signs of pulmonary disease?

a *No, typically pulmonary disease is associated with left-sided heart failure not right. Right-sided heart failure is typically associated with signs of systemic venous congestion and hepatomegaly. Although right-sided heart failure is not typically associated with pulmonary signs, it is possible to see disease on both sides of the heart concurrently.*

Diagnostic Result Interpretation Questions

1 Given the diagnostic results, what abnormalities do you identify? What is your interpretation of these findings?

2 Are any of these diagnostic results surprising/unexpected?

3 What are the broad mechanisms by which these abnormalities occur?

4 Eosinophilia/basophilia are commonly associated with parasitic infections. Do we have to see eosinophilia/basophilia to know that these inflammatory responses are occurring in tissues?

Rapid Diagnostic Screening

Test	Result	Units	Reference Interval	Units
PCV	43 (0.43)	% (L/L)	35-57 (0.35-0.57)	% (L/L)
Total Plasma Protein:	6.3 (63)	g/dL (g/L)	6.0-7.5 (60-75)	g/dL (g/L)
Plasma Color:	Clear			
BUN (Azostix®):	15-26 (5.36-9.28)	mg/dL (mmol/L)	<30 (10.71)	mg/dL (mmol/L)
Urine Color:	Yellow			
USG:	1.035			
Urine Protein:	Negative			
Urine Glucose:	Negative			
Urine Ketone	Negative			
Urine pH:	7.0			
Urine Bilirubin	Negative			
Urine Sediment:	No casts/ crystals seen	#/lpf	0-1 Hyaline Casts	#/lpf

Case Figure 6.1 Rapid basic diagnostic results.

Case Figure 6.2   Blood film (Wrights–Giemsa, 100×).

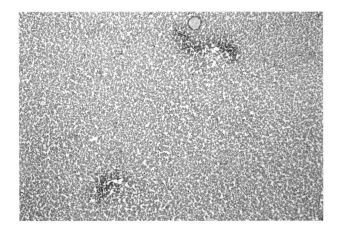

Case Figure 6.3   Blood film (Wrights–Giemsa, 100×).

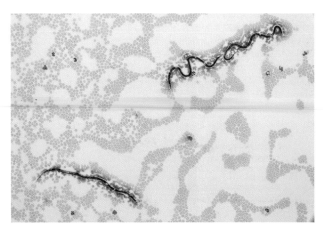

Case Figure 6.4   Blood film (Wrights–Giemsa, 200×).

5   Microfilariae are not always found in blood films of heartworm-infected patients. What are some possible techniques to increase the likelihood of identifying microfilaria?

6   In this case, what is/are the top differential diagnoses based on the current diagnostic data?

7   What diagnostic results are most supportive of each of the differential diagnoses?

8   What additional diagnostics would you need to confirm/refute the top differentials for this case?

Diagnostic Result Interpretation Answers

1   Given the diagnostic results, what abnormalities do you identify? What is your interpretation of these abnormalities?
    a   *PCV, TPP, and BUN are all within the reference interval. Blood film examination reveals numerous microfilariae. While differentiating Dirofilaria immitis from Dipetalonema microfilaria is not possible on a blood film, Dipetalonema is not associated with clinical disease. A heartworm antigen test is necessary to confirm heartworm disease.*

2   Are any of these diagnostic results surprising/ unexpected?
    a   *None of the findings in this case were surprising. In dogs not receiving heartworm preventatives, signs of right-sided heart failure (i.e. right-sided murmur, hepatomegaly, etc.) in conjunction with pulmonary signs (i.e. cough) is highly suggestive of heartworm infestation.*

3   What are the broad mechanisms by which these abnormalities occur?
    a   *In cases of canine heartworm infestation, microfilariae are readily produced once juvenile worms reach sexual maturity (~6–7 months post infection). This leads to a significant microfilaria burden, making identification on the blood film common in patent infections.*

4   Eosinophilia/basophilia are commonly associated with parasitic infections. Does the absence of eosinophilia/ basophilia rule out parasitic infections?
    a   *No, while it is common to see eosinophilia +/− basophilia in cases of heartworm infestations, this does not mean that these changes must be seen. There can*

be significant inflammatory responses within tissues that are not reflected by similar changes in the blood. The presence of a classic inflammatory response is merely supportive and the lack of one cannot rule out the diagnosis of infection.

5 Microfilaria are not always found in blood films of heartworm-infected patients. What are some possible techniques to increase the likelihood of identifying microfilaria?

   a *If antigen tests for heartworm are not available, blood film evaluation can be used to screen for heartworm infestation but is less sensitive. In some patients with a patent heartworm infestation, no microfilariae are found on a blood film. Evaluation of a buffy coat preparation or of the plasma just above the buffy coat allows for concentration of the microfilaria and may increase the likelihood of detection.*

6 In this case, what is/are the top differential diagnoses based on the current diagnostic data?

   a *In this case, there is enough information to come to a definitive diagnosis of heartworm infestation. However, depending on radiographic findings, it may be beneficial to rule out other concurrent infections with dimorphic fungal organisms (i.e. Coccidioides spp., Histoplasma capsulatum, Blastomyces dermatitidis).*

7 What additional diagnostics would you need to confirm/refute the top differentials for this case?

   a *In this case, it would be ideal to perform three view thoracic radiographs, and heartworm antigen testing to confirm patent heartworm infestation resulting in right-sided heart disease. Serologic testing for other infectious agents may be appropriate depending on radiographic findings.*

7 Case #7

7.1 Signalment

Sammy, a 7-year-old spayed female Giant Schnauzer dog.

7.2 History

Sammy is current on vaccinations, receives monthly heartworm/anthelminthic combination as well as a monthly flea and tick preventative. Her owners have noticed that she has been polydipsic, polyuric, and polyphagic for about two months.

7.3 Presentation

Sammy presents today for examination due to orange discoloration of urine, as well as polyuria, polydipsia, polyphagia, and stranguria.

7.4 Physical Exam Findings

Temp: 102.4°F (39.1°C), HR: 112, RR: 44, MM: Pink, CRT: <2 seconds, Hydration status: <5% Dehydrated, BCS: 4/9

   Cardiopulmonary: No murmurs on auscultation, strong synchronous pulses, lungs auscultate normally.

   Abdomen: Mild splenomegaly and hepatomegaly appreciated.

   Lymph: No abnormalities identified.

   HEENT: No abnormalities identified.

   Urogenital: No abnormalities identified.

   Integument: No abnormalities identified.

   Neurologic: No abnormal findings.

   Musculoskeletal: No abnormalities identified.

Initial Data (History/Signalment/Physical Exam) Questions

1 Given the clinical data, what is the differential diagnosis?

2 What diagnostics ideally would you like to perform (given no resource boundaries) and why?

3 What low-cost diagnostics could you perform in this patient that might give you similar information to your ideal list?

4 What information are you expecting to receive from these diagnostics? In other words, what differential do you expect to rule in or rule out with these diagnostics?

5 What results, given the patient's signalment/history/clinical exam findings, would you expect in this patient?

Initial Data (History/Signalment/Physical Exam) Answers

1 Given the clinical data, what is the differential diagnosis?

   a *In this case, the primary differentials would be diabetes mellitus, hyperadrenocorticism, bacterial* *cystitis, impaired renal function (primary or secondary renal disease), or urolithiasis.*

2 What diagnostics ideally would you like to perform (given no resource boundaries) and why?
   a *CBC, biochemistry profile, urinalysis, and abdominal radiographs would be indicated.*
   b *The CBC is part of a normal minimum database. Alterations in erythrogram and leukogram may indicate an inflammatory process.*
   c *Biochemistry profile is necessary to rule in or out the metabolic diseases listed as differential diagnoses. Evaluation of serum glucose concentrations would help rule in or out diabetes mellitus. Evaluation of hepatic enzymes may assist in evaluating for primary or secondary hepatic disease, including the effects of endocrinopathy on the liver. Evaluation of BUN, creatinine, and SDMA may provide insight into the role renal function may play in this patient's polyuria and polydipsia.*

d *Urinalysis is critical for adequate interpretation of a biochemistry profile. Primary or secondary renal disease and endocrine disorders like diabetes mellitus, hyperadrenocorticism, or hypoadrenocorticism, which may result in changes in the urinalysis, and support the biochemistry findings.*
e *Abdominal radiographs are beneficial to evaluate the liver, spleen, and kidneys as well as for the presence of urolithiasis as a possible cause for stranguria in this patient.*
f *Depending on the results of the previously mentioned diagnostics, additional testing may be warranted including tests to evaluate endocrine function.*

3 What low-cost diagnostics could you perform in this patient that might give you similar information to your ideal list?
   a *PCV/TPP, blood film evaluation, BUN, blood glucose, and urinalysis would be an appropriate initial low-cost diagnostic plan.*

Hematology				
Test	**Result**	**Units**	**Reference Interval**	**Units**
PCV	47 (0.47)	% (L/L)	35–57 (0.35–0.57)	% (L/L)
RBC Morphology:	RBC morphology appears normal			
WBC Estimate	13400	#/uL	5,000–15,500	#/uL
Segmented Neturophils	87	%	NA	%
Band Neutrophils	0	%	NA	%
Metamyelocytes	0	%	NA	%
Lymphocytes	3	%	NA	%
Monocytes	10	%	NA	%
Eosinophils	0	%	NA	%
Basophils	0	%	NA	%
Absolute Segmented Neutrophils	11658	#/uL	2,500–10,750	#/uL
Absolute Band Neutrophils	0	#/uL	0–150	#/uL
Absolute Metamyelocytes	0	#/uL	0	#/uL
Absolute Lymphocytes	402	#/uL	850–4,500	#/uL
Absolute Monocytes	1340	#/uL	150–1,100	#/uL
Absolute Eosinophils	0	#/uL	50–1,500	#/uL
Absolute Basophils	0	#/uL	0–100	#/uL
Toxic Change	WBC morphology appears normal			
Platelet Estimate	430,000	#/uL	150,000–450,000	#/uL
Platelet Comment	Platelet morphology appears normal			

Case Figure 7.1 Hematologic data. *Absolute leukocyte values are based on WBC estimate and differential count.

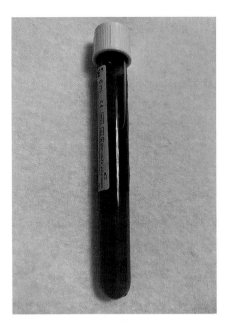

Case Figure 7.2 Gross urine appearance, precentrifugation.

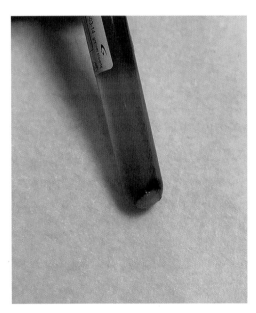

Case Figure 7.3 Gross urine appearance, postcentrifugation.

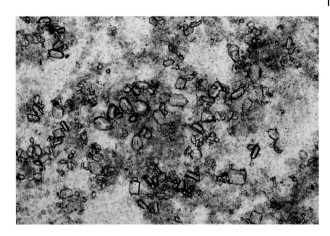

Case Figure 7.4 Urine sediment, wet mount (unstained, 100×).

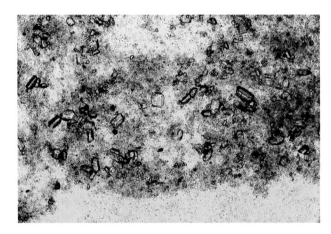

Case Figure 7.5 Urine sediment, wet mount (unstained, 100×).

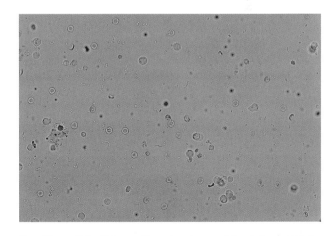

Case Figure 7.6 Urine sediment, wet mount (unstained, 400×).

4 What information are you expecting to receive from these diagnostics? In other words, what differential do you expect to rule in or rule out with these diagnostics?

   a *PCV/TPP will allow evaluation for possible anemia (i.e. anemia of chronic disease) and hydration status.*

   b *Blood film evaluation will identify underlying changes in leukocyte concentration and distribution as well as platelet mass.*

   c *BUN will assist in evaluation of kidney function in a polyuric patient.*

   d *Blood glucose will support or elimination diabetes mellitus as a differential diagnosis for the polydipsia, polyuria, and polyphagia.*

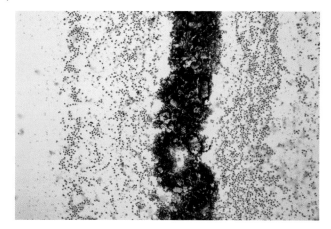

Case Figure 7.7 Urine sediment, dry mount (Wrights–Giemsa, 100×).

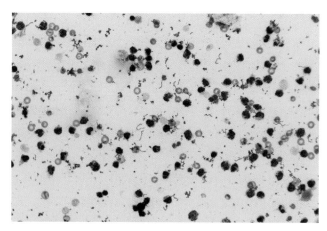

Case Figure 7.10 Urine sediment, dry mount (Wrights–Giemsa, 500×).

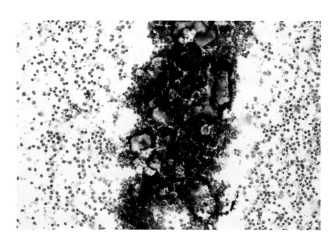

Case Figure 7.8 Urine sediment, dry mount (Wrights–Giemsa, 200×).

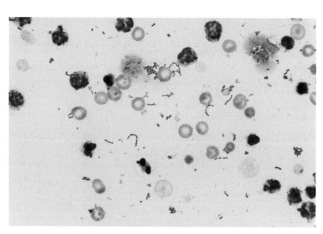

Case Figure 7.11 Urine sediment, dry mount (Wrights–Giemsa, 1000×).

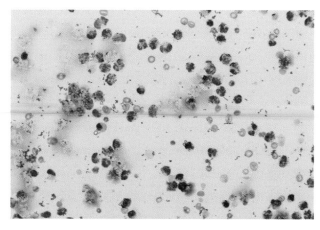

Case Figure 7.9 Urine sediment, dry mount (Wrights–Giemsa, 500×).

e *Urinalysis is necessary for the interpretation of BUN and blood glucose results. In addition, any possible inflammatory process may be identified along with bacteriuria if present.*

5 What results, given the patient's signalment/history/clinical exam findings, would you expect in this patient?

a *With polyuria, polydipsia, and polyphagia, increased blood glucose consistent with diabetes mellitus with or without hyperadrenocorticism would be expected. In the presence of stranguria, a positive heme reaction and RBCs in the urine sediment would be expected. Urinalysis may show evidence of urinary tract infection since diabetes mellitus is a major risk factor for this disease process. Urine specific gravity may show isosthenuria or be within the range of minimal concentration if there is underlying endocrine disease.*

		Chemistry			
Test	**Result**	**Units**	**Reference Interval**	**Units**	
Total Plasma Protein:	7.3 (73)	g/dL (g/L)	6.0-7.5 (60-75)	g/dL (g/L)	
Plasma Color:	Clear				
BUN (Azostix®):	15-26 (5.36-9.28)	mg/dL (mmol/L)	<30 (10.71)	mg/dL (mmol/L)	
Blood Glucose:	651 (36.2)	mg/dL (mmol/L)	65-200 (3.6-11.1)	mg/dL (mmol/L)	
Urine Color:	Amber				
USG:	1.020				
Urine Protein:	3+				
Urine Heme:	2+				
Urine Glucose:	3+				
Urine Ketone:	1+				
Urine pH:	8.5				
Urine Bilirubin	Negative				
Casts/ Crystals:	>10 Struvite	#/lpf	0-1 Hyaline Casts	#/lpf	
RBC:	30-50	#/hpf	0-5	#/hpf	
WBC:	10-30	#/hpf	0-3	#/hpf	
Bacteria:	>50	#/hpf	0	#/hpf	
Bacteria Morphology:	Cocci (Strep morphology)				

Case Figure 7.12 Biochemistry and urinalysis data. Urinalysis sample by cystocentesis.

Diagnostic Result Interpretation Questions

1 Given the diagnostic results, what abnormalities do you identify? What is your interpretation of these abnormalities?

2 Are any of these diagnostic results surprising/ unexpected?

3 What are broad mechanisms by which these abnormalities occur?

4 Does the presence of crystalluria definitively tell us a patient has urolithiasis?

5 How can various urine collection methods impact the degree of bacterial contamination in a urine sample?

6 In this case, what is the primary differential diagnoses based on the current diagnostic data?

7 What additional diagnostics would you need to confirm/refute the top differentials for this case?

Diagnostic Result Interpretation Answers

1 Given the diagnostic results, what abnormalities do you identify? What is your interpretation of these abnormalities?

  a *PCV and TPP are both within the reference interval.*

  b *Blood film evaluation shows a mature neutrophilia, monocytosis, lymphopenia, and eosinopenia. This constellation of leukocyte abnormalities is consistent with increased circulating glucocorticoids (cortisol). Platelet estimate is within the reference interval.*

  c *BUN is within the reference interval.*

  d *There is marked hyperglycemia consistent with diabetes mellitus. Marked glycosuria, ketonuria, and urine specific gravity in the hypersthenuric range are supportive of diabetes mellitus as well.*

  e *Urinalysis reveals alkaluria, pyuria, hematuria, bacteriuria, and struvite crystalluria. These findings are consistent with bacterial cystitis and secondary struvite crystalluria.*

2 Are any of these diagnostic results surprising/ unexpected?

   a *These findings are all consistent with the differential diagnosis in this case and are not surprising.*

3 What are broad mechanisms by which these abnormalities occur?

   a *A stress leukogram results from increased circulating glucocorticoids (cortisol). Cortisol increases neutrophil production and reduces marginating ability, which results in a mature neutrophilia. Monocytosis is common with increased circulating glucocorticoids, but the mechanism for this change is unknown. Lymphopenia results from several glucocorticoids effects including induction of lympholysis, reduced egress from lymph nodes, and decreased lymphocyte proliferation. The mechanism for eosinopenia in the stress leukogram is not well understood.*

   b *In dogs, diabetes mellitus is the most likely cause of this degree of hyperglycemia. Diabetes mellitus in dogs occurs due to hypoinsulinemia. Insufficient insulin prevents circulating blood glucose from being utilized at the cellular level leading to significantly increased plasma glucose concentrations. Marked hyperglycemia exceeds the renal glucose threshold and allows glucose to be excreted into urine in large quantities. Ketone production occurs due to the utilization of fat for energy production instead of carbohydrates, resulting in ketosis. This increase in ketones leads to excretion of ketones in the urine (ketonuria). Unless there is concurrent diabetes mellitus, dogs with hyperadrenocorticism should not be glycosuric, ketonuric, or ketonemic.*

   c *Marked glycosuria promotes the development of bacterial cystitis. Glucose in the urine provides an excellent source of energy for bacteria, allowing increased proliferation of bacteria. Bacteria that produce urease increase urine pH which greatly increases the risk of struvite crystal formation.*

4 Does the presence of crystalluria definitively tell us a patient has urolithiasis?

   a *The presence of crystalluria does not always correlate to the presence of a urolith. For this reason, radiographs are critical in assessing for the presence of uroliths. The presence of crystalluria and compatible clinical signs may increase the suspicion for urolithiasis.*

5 How can various urine collection methods impact the degree of bacterial contamination in a urine sample?

   a *Collection methods vary in their potential for bacterial contamination. Cystocentesis has the lowest chance of bacterial contamination; samples collected by this method are considered sterile. Urine collection via catheterization can be sterile but may contain small amounts of bacteria that are introduced during retrograde catheter movement into the bladder. Urine collection via free catch often contains large amounts of normal bacteria that are shed in the urine as it moves through the urogenital tract.*

   b *If bacteria are seen on a free-catch urine sample, either catheterization or, preferably, cystocentesis should be performed to confirm the presence of bacteria and provide a sterile sample for bacterial culture and sensitivity.*

6 In this case, what is the primary differential diagnosis based on the current diagnostic data?

   a *The primary differential diagnosis is diabetes mellitus with secondary bacterial cystitis and struvite crystalluria. At this time, concurrent hyperadrenocorticism cannot be entirely ruled out. If the diabetes mellitus is refractory to medical management, additional endocrine testing is indicated.*

7 What additional diagnostics would you need to confirm/refute the top differentials for this case?

   a *Performing abdominal radiographs to assess for urolithiasis would be important to perform. Abdominal ultrasound would also be beneficial in this case to assess the hepatosplenomegaly. Urine culture and sensitivity testing should be done to speciate the bacteria present and select appropriate antimicrobial drugs.*

8 Case #8

8.1 Signalment

Coffee, 5-year-old spayed female domestic shorthaired (DSH) cat

8.2 History

Coffee is current on vaccinations and does not receive any medications. Coffee presents for anorexia and vomiting of six days duration. The owners have noted that Coffee has become polydipsic, polyuric, and polyphagic.

8.3 Presentation

Yesterday, they noticed a yellow hue to his skin, and made an appointment to have him examined.

8.4 Physical Exam Findings

Temp: 97.6°F (36.4°C), HR: 228, RR: 44, MM: Icteric and Pale/moist, CRT: <2 seconds, Hydration status: <5% Dehydrated, BCS: 9/9

Cardiopulmonary: No murmurs on auscultation, strong synchronous pulses, lungs auscultate normally.

Abdomen: There is moderate hepatomegaly on palpation.

Lymph: No abnormalities identified.

HEENT: OU icteric sclera.

Urogenital: No abnormalities identified.

Integument: Diffusely icteric skin, grossly evident along the ventrum and peri-aural regions.

Neurologic: Patient is QAR, reluctant to ambulate but will if stimulated, has normal conscious proprioceptive responses and nociceptive responses. A brief cranial nerve exam is within normal limits.

Musculoskeletal: No abnormalities identified.

Initial Data (History/Signalment/Physical Exam) Questions

1 Given the clinical data, what is the differential diagnosis?

2 What diagnostics ideally would you like to perform (given no resource boundaries) and why?

3 What low-cost diagnostics could you perform in this patient that might give you similar information to your ideal list?

4 What information are you expecting to receive from these diagnostics? In other words, what differential do you expect to rule in or rule out with these diagnostics?

5 What results, given the patient's signalment/history/clinical exam findings, would you expect in this patient?

Initial Data (History/Signalment/Physical Exam) Answers

1 Given the clinical data what is the differential diagnosis?

a *The primary differentials in this case would be primary or secondary hepatic disease, diabetes mellitus, pancreatitis, gastrointestinal foreign body, or gastrointestinal neoplasia. Although less likely, causes of pre-hepatic icterus should be considered.*

2 What diagnostics ideally would you like to perform (given no resource boundaries) and why?

a *A CBC, biochemistry profile, urinalysis, and abdominal radiographs would be appropriate initial diagnostics. Abdominal ultrasound may be indicated depending on the results of the initial diagnostics.*

b *CBC is an important component of any minimum database. Results may be supportive of inflammation or stress.*

c *Biochemistry profile will be critical for evaluating organ function and refining the differential diagnosis. Evaluation of liver function and hepatic enzymes will help support or refute primary or secondary hepatic disease as a differential. Evaluation of blood glucose will help support or refute diabetes mellitus as a differential. Increases in amylase or lipase are not specific or sensitive, but elevations with compatible clinical signs and other diagnostics would be supportive of pancreatitis.*

d *Urinalysis is critical for adequate interpretation of any biochemistry profile. Evaluation may also help support or refute diabetes as a differential diagnosis.*

e *Abdominal radiographs are an important diagnostic to perform. A six-day history of vomiting warrants radiographs to evaluate for a possible GI foreign body.*

3 What low-cost diagnostics could you perform in this patient that might give you similar information to your ideal list?

a *PCV/TPP, blood film examination, BUN, blood glucose, and urinalysis would be appropriate low-cost initial diagnostics.*

4 What information are you expecting to receive from these diagnostics? In other words, what differential do you expect to rule in or rule out with these diagnostics?

a *PCV/TPP will identify anemia as a possible cause of the pale mucous membranes, tachycardia, and tachypnea.*

b *Blood film examination will help assess erythrocyte morphology that may relate to the cause of the patient's anemia if present. Leukocyte morphology and differential will allow evaluation for* *inflammatory changes. Platelet concentration can be assessed as well.*

c *BUN will allow assessment of renal function and potentially hepatic function, as causes of underlying polyuria, polydipsia, or icterus.*

d *Blood glucose measurement will help rule in or out diabetes mellitus as a differential for the polyuria and polydipsia.*

e *Urinalysis will allow adequate interpretation of the BUN result and will also help support or refute diabetes mellitus as a differential diagnosis.*

5 What results, given the patient's signalment/history/ clinical exam findings, would you expect in this patient?

a *Icteric plasma and bilirubinuria should be expected since the patient is grossly icteric. This patient likely has hyperglycemia, which may be from stress or diabetes mellitus given the patient's history. Based on the*

pale mucous membranes, tachycardia, and tachypnea, anemia is an expected finding.

Diagnostic Result Interpretation Questions

1 Given the diagnostic results, what abnormalities do you identify? What is your interpretation?

2 What are the broad mechanisms by which these abnormalities occur?

3 In this patient, the blood glucose reading was >750 mg/ dL or 41.7 mmol/L. Can we dilute the patient's sample to try to get an exact glucose reading?

4 Is this patient's hyperglycemia the result of stress from systemic illness or due to diabetes mellitus? How do you know?

Hematology

Test	Result	Units	Reference Interval	Units
PCV	14 (0.14)	% (L/L)	30-45 (0.30-0.45)	% (L/L)
Polychromasia:	None seen			
RBC Morphology:	RBC morphology appears normal			
WBC Estimate	8900	#/uL	5,000-15,500	#/uL
Segmented Neturophils	80	%	NA	%
Band Neutrophils	0	%	NA	%
Metamyelocytes	0	%	NA	%
Lymphocytes	12	%	NA	%
Monocytes	7	%	NA	%
Eosinophils	1	%	NA	%
Basophils	0	%	NA	%
Absolute Segmented Neutrophils	7120	#/uL	2,500-10,750	#/uL
Absolute Band Neutrophils	0	#/uL	0-150	#/uL
Absolute Metamyelocytes	0	#/uL	0	#/uL
Absolute Lymphocytes	1068	#/uL	850-4,500	#/uL
Absolute Monocytes	623	#/uL	150-1,100	#/uL
Absolute Eosinophils	89	#/uL	50-1,500	#/uL
Absolute Basophils	0	#/uL	0-100	#/uL
Toxic Change	WBC morphology appears normal			
Platelet Estimate	350,000	#/uL	150,000-450,000	#/uL
Platelet Comment	Platelet morphology appears normal			

Case Figure 8.1   Hematologic data. *Absolute leukocyte values are based on WBC estimate and differential count.

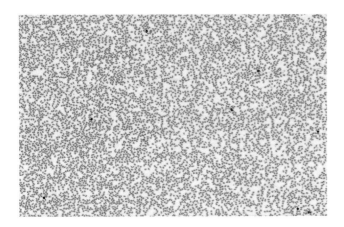

Case Figure 8.2   Blood film (Wrights–Giemsa, 200×).

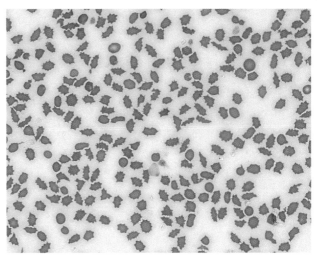

Case Figure 8.5   Blood film (Wrights–Giemsa, 800×).

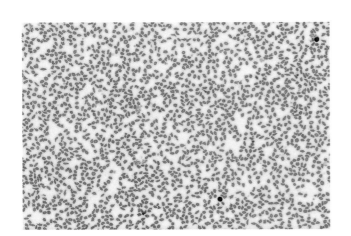

Case Figure 8.3   Blood film (Wrights–Giemsa, 400×).

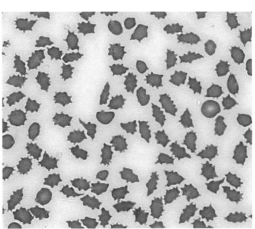

Case Figure 8.6   Blood film (Wrights–Giemsa, 1000×).

5   In this case, what is/are the top differential diagnoses based on the current diagnostic data?

6   What diagnostic results are most supportive for each of the differential diagnoses?

7   What additional diagnostics would you need to confirm/refute the top differentials for this case?

Diagnostic Result Interpretation Answers

1   Given the diagnostic results, what abnormalities do you identify? What is your interpretation?

   a   *The PCV reveals an anemia with no evidence of regeneration and no evidence of an inflammatory response is seen on examination of the blood film.*

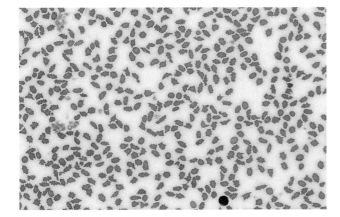

Case Figure 8.4   Blood film (Wrights–Giemsa, 800×).

Chemistry				
Test	**Result**	**Units**	**Reference Interval**	**Units**
Total Plasma Protein:	5.6 (56)	g/dL (g/L)	6.0–7.5 (60–75)	g/dL (g/L)
Plasma Color:	Dark Yellow (3+ Icterus)			
BUN (Azostix®):	5–15 (1.79–5.36)	mg/dL (mmol/L)	<30 (10.71)	mg/dL (mmol/L)
Blood Glucose:	>750 (41.7)	mg/dL (mmol/L)	65–200 (3.6–11.1)	mg/dL (mmol/L)
Urine Color:	Orange			
USG:	1.016			
Urine Protein:	Negative			
Urine Heme:	Negtaive			
Urine Glucose:	3+			
Urine Ketone:	2+			
Urine pH:	7.0			
Urine Bilirubin	3+			
Casts/ Crystals:	0–2 Bilirubin crystals	#/lpf	0–1 Hyaline Casts	#/lpf
RBC:	0–3	#/hpf	0–5	#/hpf
WBC:	0–2	#/hpf	0–3	#/hpf
Bacteria:	0	#/hpf	0	#/hpf

Case Figure 8.7 Biochemistry and urinalysis data. Urinalysis sample by cystocentesis.

b *Blood film shows marked ovaloacanthocytosis, and Heinz bodies are frequently observed. Ovaloacanthocytes are commonly observed in cases of hepatic lipidosis or renal disease. Heinz body formation is commonly seen with oxidative injury to erythrocytes in diseases such as hepatic lipidosis and diabetes mellitus.*

c *Icteric plasma in addition to marked bilirubinuria is highly supportive of hyperbilirubinemia.*

d *BUN is decreased, which is suggestive of decreased hepatic function.*

e *Marked hyperglycemia, glycosuria, and ketonuria are supportive of diabetes mellitus.*

2   What are broad mechanisms by which these abnormalities occur?

a *Diabetes mellitus in cats occurs due to insulin resistance resulting in marked hyperglycemia. Obesity changes adipose-associated hormone expression, leading to decreased insulin receptor responsiveness or density. These changes lead to insulin resistance and increases in plasma glucose concentration. Marked hyperglycemia exceeds the renal glucose threshold and allows glucose to be excreted into urine*

in large quantities. In cats, insufficient insulin responsiveness prevents circulating blood glucose from being utilized at the cellular level leading to significantly increased plasma glucose concentrations. Ketone production occurs due to the utilization of fat for energy production instead of carbohydrates, resulting in ketosis. This increase in ketones leads to excretion of ketones in the urine (ketonuria). Hepatic disease, specifically, hepatic lipidosis can also contribute to ketonemia and ketonuria.

b *Moderate anemia with the presence of Heinz bodies and icterus, without evidence of intravascular hemolysis, indicates an extravascular hemolytic anemia. The lack of regeneration is likely the result of concurrent illness that may be suppressing the bone marrow's ability to respond. Heinz bodies are indicative of oxidative injury, which can occur secondary to diabetes mellitus and has been associated with hepatic lipidosis in cats.*

c *Erythrocyte shape changes (i.e. ovaloacanthocyte formation) occur secondary to changes in erythrocyte membrane lipid.*

d *Icterus in this case is likely a combination of prehepatic and hepatic icterus. Severe hepatocyte swelling* *due to lipid accumulation results in intrahepatic canalicular cholestasis and interferes with bilirubin excretion. In addition, the prehepatic mechanisms increase unconjugated bilirubin production overwhelming the liver's ability to take-up, conjugate, and secrete bilirubin into the canaliculi, further contributing to hyperbilirubinemia and icterus.*

  e *BUN is decreased secondary to decreased hepatic function or anorexia.*

  f *Hypoproteinemia is likely secondary to decreased hepatic function, which results in decreased protein synthesis.*

3 In this patient, the blood glucose reading was >750 mg/dl or 41.7 mmol/l. Can we dilute the patient's sample to try to get an exact glucose reading?

  a You cannot dilute the sample for a handheld glucometer. It is critical to follow the manufacturer's procedure exactly for accurate blood glucose measurement. In addition, dilution to obtain an exact glucose concentration is likely of little value for treatment or prognosis of any patient.

4 Is this patient's hyperglycemia the result of stress from systemic illness or due to diabetes mellitus? How do you know?

  a This patient's hyperglycemia is secondary to diabetes mellitus. Systemic illness leads to an increase in plasma glucocorticoids (cortisol) known as a stress response. Stress responses do not cause hyperglycemia of the magnitude seen in this case. In the cat, stress hyperglycemia may sufficiently increase plasma glucose to exceed the renal glucose threshold and cause glycosuria; however, stress is not associated with ketonemia or ketonuria.

5 In this case, what is/are the top differential diagnoses based on the current diagnostic data?

  a In this case, the primary differential diagnoses would be diabetes mellitus with secondary hepatic lipidosis. An additional differential would be pancreatitis, which is a common comorbidity in patients with diabetes mellitus and with hepatic disease, most commonly hepatic lipidosis in the cat.

6 What diagnostic results are most supportive of each of the differential diagnoses?

  a Marked hyperglycemia, glycosuria, and ketonuria are consistent with diabetes mellitus in this case.

  b Decreased BUN, ovaloacanthocytosis, icterus, and bilirubinuria, with a compatible clinical history, are highly supportive of hepatic disease including hepatic lipidosis.

7 What additional diagnostics would you need to confirm/refute the top differentials for this case?

  a In this case, it would be ideal to perform a CBC, biochemistry profile, and urinalysis. In addition, measurement of feline pancreas specific lipase, and abdominal ultrasound would be ideal to evaluate for hepatic lipidosis and to rule out pancreatitis as a concurrent disease process. Fine needle aspiration of the liver is recommended to confirm hepatic lipidosis.

9 Case #9

9.1 Signalment

Dexter, a 10-year-old intact male Golden Retriever dog

9.2 History

Dexter is current on vaccinations, receives a monthly flea and tick preventative, but no other medications. Dexter first collapsed yesterday but about five minutes later got up and acted normal. Today the owners noticed that Dexter had collapsed again, and his abdomen was distended.

9.3 Presentation

Dexter presents as an emergency for acute collapse and abdominal enlargement.

9.4 Physical Exam Findings

Temp: 99.5°F (37.5°C), HR: 160, RR: 80, MM: Pale/Moist, CRT: four seconds, Hydration status: 5–7% Dehydrated, BCS: 4/9

Cardiopulmonary: No murmurs on auscultation of the chest, faint synchronous pulses palpated, lungs auscultate normally.

Abdomen: There is moderate abdominal distension and fluid wave present.

Lymph: No abnormalities identified.

HEENT: No abnormalities identified.

Urogenital: No abnormalities identified.

Integument: No abnormalities identified.

Neurologic: Patient is laterally recumbent and aware, will move to sternal position for a brief time if stimulated. A brief cranial nerve exam is within normal limits.

Musculoskeletal: No abnormalities identified.

Initial Data (History/Signalment/Physical Exam) Questions

1 Given the clinical data, what is the differential diagnosis?

2 What diagnostics ideally would you like to perform (given no resource boundaries) and why?

3 What low-cost diagnostics could you perform in this patient that might give you similar information to your ideal list?

4 What information are you expecting to receive from these diagnostics? In other words, what differential do you expect to rule in or rule out with these diagnostics?

5 What results, given the patient's signalment/history/clinical exam findings, would you expect in this patient?

Initial Data (History/Signalment/Physical Exam) Answers

1 Given the clinical data, what is the differential diagnosis?
   a *The primary differential in this case would be hemoabdomen due to the history of acute recurrent collapse, acute abdominal distension, and clinical signs of pale mucous membranes, tachycardia, and tachypnea. The most common causes of hemoabdomen would be:*
      i) *Ruptured splenic mass (hemangioma, hematoma, hemangiosarcoma, regenerative nodule, etc.)*
      ii) *Coagulopathy (i.e. rodenticide toxicity)*
      iii) *Trauma*
   b *Other causes of abdominal effusion should still be considered; however, these are less likely given the clinical signs of pale mucous membranes, tachycardia, tachypnea, and hypovolemia (prolonged CRT and faint pulses), as well as the rapid onset of clinical signs.*

2 What diagnostics ideally would you like to perform (given no resource boundaries) and why?
   a *It would be ideal to perform a full CBC, biochemistry profile, urinalysis, lactate, PT and aPTT, abdominal ultrasonography, three view thoracic radiographs, and abdominal fluid analysis.*

   b *CBC is important to assess for potential causes of hemorrhage, i.e. thrombocytopenia. In addition, CBC would allow assessment of RBC mass and degree of regeneration since anemia cannot be confirmed by the current physical exam findings (pale mucous membranes with poor pulse quality and prolonged CRT) alone. Leukocyte evaluation may aid in refining the differential diagnosis if changes are noted in the leukogram.*
   c *Biochemistry profile is part of the "minimum database". Hemoabdomen patients may require surgical intervention; therefore, it is critical to know organ function, metabolic state, acid–base status, and electrolyte status when planning for anesthesia and surgical management.*
   d *Lactate indicates the presence of inadequate tissue perfusion. In cases of shock, lactate will increase. Therefore, lactate measurement is a good analyte for endpoint assessment for treatment and monitoring of shock patients.*
   e *PT and aPTT measurements are critical in the evaluation of a patient with hemoabdomen, especially if there is concern for rodenticide toxicity. Patients with rodenticide toxicity should have prolonged PT and aPTT. Some patients with ruptured splenic masses may have prolongation of clotting times associated with disseminated intravascular coagulopathy.*
   f *Abdominal ultrasonography will aid in locating the source of abdominal hemorrhage (i.e. ruptured neoplasm).*
   g *Thoracic radiographs are important to perform in patients with hemoabdomen. Radiographs aid in screening for potential heart-base masses (i.e. atrial hemangiosarcoma) as well as metastatic neoplasia or evidence of hemorrhage into the thoracic cavity, which supports coagulopathy over neoplasia.*
   h *Abdominal fluid analysis is critical to perform in cases where effusion is present. Characterization of the effusion is necessary to confirm the presence of hemoabdomen versus another type of effusion (i.e. exudate), which is necessary to refine the differential diagnosis.*
   * Abdominal radiographs could be performed but are not ideal. Large amounts of fluid within the peritoneum obscure radiographic detail, making interpretation challenging or impossible.

3 What low-cost diagnostics could you perform in this patient that might give you similar information to your ideal list?

Hematology

Test	Result	Units	Reference Interval	Units
Sample:	EDTA Whole Blood			
PCV	27 (0.27)	% (L/L)	35-57 (0.35-0.57)	% (L/L)
RBC Morphology:	Ecchinocytes 2+, Rare Codocytes (Target Cells)			
nRBC	0	#/100 WBC	0-2	#/100 WBC
WBC Estimate	11,600	#/uL	5,000-15,500	#/uL
Segmented Neturophils	63	%	NA	%
Band Neutrophils	0	%	NA	%
Metamyelocytes	0	%	NA	%
Lymphocytes	15	%	NA	%
Monocytes	21	%	NA	%
Eosinophils	1	%	NA	%
Basophils	0	%	NA	%
Absolute Segmented Neutrophils	7,308	#/uL	2,500-10,750	#/uL
Absolute Band Neutrophils	0	#/uL	0-150	#/uL
Absolute Metamyelocytes	0	#/uL	0	#/uL
Absolute Lymphocytes	1,740	#/uL	850-4,500	#/uL
Absolute Monocytes	2,436	#/uL	150-1,100	#/uL
Absolute Eosinophils	116	#/uL	50-1,500	#/uL
Absolute Basophils	0	#/uL	0-100	#/uL
Toxic Change	None			
WBC Comment	WBC morphology appears normal			
Platelet Estimate	~150,000 minimum	#/uL	150,000-450,000	#/uL
Platelet Comment	Platelet Clumping Present			

Case Figure 9.1   Hematologic data. *Absolute leukocyte values are based on WBC estimate and differential count.

a   *PCV/TPP, blood film examination, BUN, lactate, activated clotting time (ACT), and urinalysis would be appropriate initial low-cost diagnostics in this case.*

4   What information are you expecting to receive from these diagnostics? In other words, what differential do you expect to rule in or rule out with these diagnostics?

   a   *PCV/TPP would confirm anemia and assist in determining its origin.*

   b   *Blood film examination would allow evaluation of leukocyte concentration and distribution. In addition, it would allow for platelet estimation, which may indicate if thrombocytopenia is contributing to this patient's clinical signs of possible intra-abdominal hemorrhage.*

   c   *BUN is important to help establish the patient's renal function, which should be considered in both medical management and anesthetic approach.*

   d   *Lactate will assess the patient's perfusion status since the patient is showing clinical signs of shock and hypovolemia. It will also be beneficial in monitoring effectiveness of shock treatments and to aid in anesthetic management.*

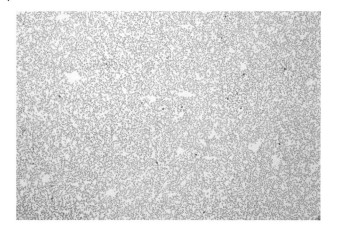

Case Figure 9.2   Blood film (Wrights–Giemsa, 100×).

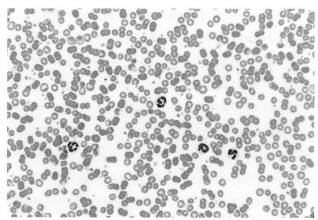

Case Figure 9.5   Blood film (Wrights–Giemsa, 500×).

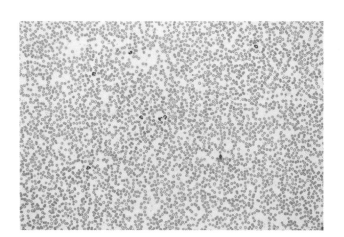

Case Figure 9.3   Blood film (Wrights–Giemsa, 200×).

Fluid Analysis

Test	Result	Units
Sample:	Abdominal Effusion	
Sample Container:	Zero additive tube (White top tube)	
Sample Color:	Hemorrhagic	
Sample Clarity:	Opaque	
Sample Consistency:	Low viscosity	
PCV:	29 (0.29)	% (L/L)
TP:	5.5 (55)	g/dL (g/L)
%Neutrophils	63	%
%Lymphocytes	15	%
%Monocytes	21	%
%Eosinophils	1	%
%Basophils	0	%
%Other	0	%
Platelet Estimate:	0	#/uL
Comment:	Sample does not clot in zero additive tube	

Case Figure 9.6   Fluid analysis data.

e *Activated clotting time (ACT) is critical to perform to assess for the presence of coagulopathy. If ACT is prolonged, coagulopathy should be thoroughly investigated.*

f *Urinalysis is required for adequate interpretation of BUN results.*

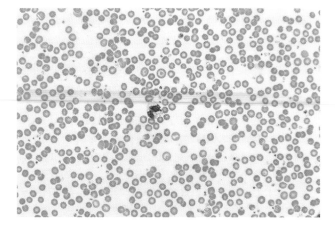

Case Figure 9.4   Blood film (Wrights–Giemsa, 500×).

Chemistry				
Test	**Result**	**Units**	**Reference Interval**	**Units**
Total Plasma Protein:	5.8 (58)	g/dL (g/L)	6.0-7.5 (60-75)	g/dL (g/L)
Plasma Color:	Clear			
BUN (Azostix®):	30-40 (10.71-14.28)	mg/dL (mmol/L)	<30 (10.71)	mg/dL (mmol/L)
Lactate:	5.1	mmol/L	<2.5	mmol/L
ACT:	70	sec	≤80	sec
USG:	1.035			
Urine Protein:	Negative			
Urine Glucose:	Negative			
Urine Ketone:	Negative			
Urine pH:	6.0			
Urine Bilirubin:	Negative			
Urine Sediment:	No casts/ crystals seen	#/lpf	0-1 Hyaline Casts	#/lpf

Case Figure 9.7 Biochemistry and urinalysis data. Urinalysis sample by cystocentesis.

5 What results, given the patient's signalment/history/ clinical exam findings, would you expect in this patient?
a *Decreased PCV with variable TPP (decreased or within the reference interval) would be expected in this patient considering clinical signs of consistent with hemorrhage and secondary hemoabdomen. Azotemia may be seen because the patient is dehydrated. Hyperlactatemia will likely be present since the patient is exhibiting clinical signs of shock.*

Diagnostic Result Interpretation Questions

1 Given the diagnostic results, what abnormalities do you identify?

2 What are the broad mechanisms by which these abnormalities occur?

3 What is the significance in comparing the platelet estimate of the whole blood and the abdominal hemorrhage?

4 Is it possible through evaluation of the abdominal hemorrhage to determine this condition is the result of malignant neoplasia?

5 Is it important that the PCV of the whole blood and abdominal fluid are of similar values? If the PCV of the abdominal fluid was lower than the blood, would we be able to say that this is strictly hemoabdomen?

6 In this case, what is/are the top differential diagnoses based on the current diagnostic data?

7 What breeds are most commonly associated with this condition?

8 What diagnostic results are most supportive for each of the differential diagnoses?

9 What additional diagnostics would you need to confirm/refute the top differentials for this case?

Diagnostic Result Interpretation Answers

1 Given the diagnostic results, what abnormalities do you identify?
a *Moderate decreased PCV with mild hypoproteinemia is consistent with anemia secondary to internal hemorrhage. The platelet estimate shows adequate platelet concentration in the peripheral blood. Note that due to platelet clumping observed on the blood film, the platelet estimate reflects the minimum platelet*

concentration in peripheral blood. Mild to moderate echinocytosis is present, which is likely an artifact.

b Azotemia is present in conjunction with adequate urine concentration, indicating that renal function is likely normal. The azotemia seen in this case is consistent with prerenal origin associated with dehydration.

c Activated clotting time is within the reference interval making coagulopathy a less likely differential at this time.

d Lactate is mildly increased consistent with hypoperfusion of tissue secondary to shock.

2 What are broad mechanisms by which these abnormalities occur?

a Anemia can occur due to three mechanisms: lack of production, loss, and hemolysis. The primary mechanism for anemia in this case is erythrocyte loss into the abdominal cavity and fluid shift from the interstitium into the vascular space to compensate for decreased vascular volume. As a result, the remaining erythrocytes and plasma proteins are diluted within the vascular space decreasing PCV and total plasma protein. Total plasma protein may not decrease with internal hemorrhage because the peritoneum is capable of reclaiming proteins. This is in contrast to external hemorrhage, where total plasma protein is decreased due to loss from the body.

b Azotemia and hyperlactatemia occur secondary to decreased tissue perfusion and dehydration. Hypovolemia (from both dehydration and hemorrhage) leads to decreased glomerular perfusion and subsequent decrease in GFR and increase in nitrogenous waste products in the blood. Tissue hypoperfusion secondary to hypovolemia causes decreases in tissue oxygen tension and initiation of anaerobic metabolism, which produces lactate.

c Abdominal fluid analysis is consistent with a hemorrhagic effusion due to hemorrhage into the abdominal cavity.

3 What is the significance in comparing the platelet estimate of the whole blood and the abdominal hemorrhage?

a Comparison of blood platelet estimate and abdominal fluid platelet estimate is of no significant value. Platelets and clotting factors are rapidly consumed after hemorrhage into the abdominal cavity. Contact with the peritoneal surface initiates the coagulation cascade leading to rapid consumption of platelets and clotting factors. This leaves the remaining

hemorrhagic fluid devoid of platelets and clotting factors. Therefore, there is no perceivable significance or benefit to this comparison.

4 Is it possible through evaluation of the abdominal hemorrhage to determine if hemoabdomen is the result of malignant neoplasia?

a When examining samples of cavitary hemorrhage from ruptured neoplasms, severe blood admixture makes finding neoplastic cells very difficult. In addition, finding one or two atypical cells is not sufficient for making a diagnosis of malignancy. This method for evaluation has poor sensitivity and specificity for diagnosing neoplasia and is an inefficient diagnostic choice to screen for neoplasia.

5 Is it important that the PCV of the whole blood and abdominal fluid are similar? If the PCV of the abdominal fluid was lower than the blood, would this decrease the probability of hemoabdomen?

a Comparing the PCV of the whole blood to the abdominal fluid is important in determining if the effusion is primarily hemorrhage by rhexis (rupture of a vessel or vascular mass) versus an effusion with hemorrhage by diapedesis (loss of erythrocytes through intact vascular walls). If the abdominal fluid PCV was significantly less than the PCV of peripheral blood, it would be prudent to evaluate for potential causes of effusion other than hemorrhage. However, it is important to remember that hemorrhage into the peritoneum will incite mesothelial reaction and inflammation, which can dilute the abdominal fluid and mildly decrease the PCV of the abdominal fluid. If the PCV of the abdominal fluid is at least 25% of the peripheral blood PCV, hemorrhage is the primary differential.

6 In this case, what is/are the top differential diagnoses based on the current diagnostic data?

a The differential diagnosis for hemoabdomen would be traumatic or nontraumatic hemoabdomen. Differentials for nontraumatic hemoabdomen include a coagulopathy or ruptured splenic mass. Given that there is no history or external indication of trauma, the most likely cause would be nontraumatic hemoabdomen. Because the ACT was within the reference interval, coagulopathy associated nontraumatic hemoabdomen is considered less likely. However, because ACT is highly insensitive and requires consumption of >95% of coagulation factors to show prolongation outside the reference interval, coagulopathy cannot be entirely ruled out at this time.

7 What breeds are most commonly associated with this condition?

  a *Most commonly, nontraumatic hemoabdomen is associated with Golden Retrievers, Labrador Retrievers, and German Shepherds* [2].

8 What diagnostic results are most supportive of each of the differential diagnoses?

  a *There is no clinical history suggesting that hemoabdomen may be of traumatic origin. The patient's signalment, history, and absent clinical indications of coagulopathy (i.e. petechiae, ecchymoses, hemorrhage into other body cavities), support a bleeding mass as the most likely differential in this case. However, coagulopathy cannot be entirely excluded without additional diagnostics with higher sensitivity.*

9 What additional diagnostics would you need to confirm/refute the top differentials for this case?

  a *In this case, it would be ideal to perform a full CBC, biochemistry profile, PT and aPTT, abdominal ultrasonography, and three view thoracic radiographs to evaluate for evidence of neoplasia or hemorrhage into a second body cavity.*

10 Case #10

10.1 Signalment

Tabitha, 13-year-old spayed female Siamese cat

10.2 History

Tabitha is current on vaccinations and does not receive any medications. Tabitha has periodically vomited ever since they adopted her at four years old. Tabitha's vomiting has become progressive, and she has started losing weight over the past two months. Today she is vomiting at a frequency of twice per day. She is polyuric and polydipsic, and has diarrhea.

10.3 Presentation

Tabitha presents for examination due to chronic and progressive vomiting.

10.4 Physical Exam Findings

Temp: 100.5°F (38.0°C), HR: 224, RR: 36, MM: Pale pink/moist, CRT: two seconds, Hydration status: 10% Dehydrated, BCS: 7/9

Cardiopulmonary: No murmurs ausculted, strong synchronous pulses, lungs auscult normally.

Abdomen: No abnormalities identified.

Lymph: No abnormalities identified.

HEENT: No abnormalities identified.

Urogenital: No abnormalities identified.

Integument: No abnormalities identified.

Neurologic: No abnormalities identified.

Musculoskeletal: No abnormalities identified.

Initial Data (History/Signalment/Physical Exam) Questions

1 Given the clinical data what is the differential diagnosis?

2 What diagnostics ideally would you like to perform (given no resource boundaries) and why?

3 What low-cost diagnostics could you perform in this patient that might give you similar information to your ideal list?

4 What information are you expecting to receive from these diagnostics? In other words, what differential do you expect to rule in or rule out with these diagnostics?

5 What results, given the patient's signalment/history/clinical exam findings, would you expect in this patient?

Initial Data (History/Signalment/Physical Exam) Answers

1 Given the clinical data, what is the differential diagnosis?

  a *The primary differentials in this case are alimentary neoplasia, inflammatory bowel disease, and other infectious or noninfectious enteropathies/enteritis.*

2 What diagnostics ideally would you like to perform (given no resource boundaries) and why?

  a *Ideally a CBC, biochemistry profile, urinalysis, fecal direct smear, fecal flotation, and abdominal ultrasound would be indicated as initial diagnostics. The findings of the previously mentioned diagnostics may* warrant performing of fine needle aspiration of any masses or biopsy of the gastrointestinal tract.

b *CBC is part of a minimum database and may identify underlying anemia of chronic disease or leukogram changes suggestive of inflammation and or stress.*

c *Biochemistry profile will allow for evaluation of plasma proteins, which are often affected in patients with gastrointestinal disease. It is important to rule out underlying diseases that may potentially contribute to the patient's clinical condition. A biochemistry profile is warranted given the patient's polyuria and polydipsia, this would rule in or out common differentials for these signs (i.e. chronic kidney disease [CKD] or endocrinopathy).*

d *Urinalysis is critical to adequately interpret the biochemistry profile, especially in a patient that is polyuric. If the patient is hypoproteinemic, it is important to rule out renal protein loss as a differential.*

e *Fecal direct smear would allow identification of motile parasites such as Tritrichomonas foetus.*

f *Fecal flotation would be beneficial in ruling out gastrointestinal parasite infestation as a cause of this patient's clinical signs.*

3 What low-cost diagnostics could you perform in this patient that might give you similar information to your ideal list?

a *PCV/TPP, blood film examination, BUN, blood glucose, urinalysis, fecal flotation, and fecal direct smear would be appropriate initial low-cost diagnostics.*

4 What information are you expecting to receive from these diagnostics? In other words, what differential do you expect to rule in or rule out with these diagnostics?

	Hematology				
Test	**Result**	**Units**		**Reference Interval**	**Units**
PCV	26 (0.26)	% (L/L)		30-45 (0.30-0.45)	% (L/L)
Polychromasia:	None seen				
RBC Morphology:	RBC morphology appears normal				
WBC Estimate	7500	#/uL		5,000-15,500	#/uL
Segmented Neturophils	80	%		NA	%
Band Neutrophils	0	%		NA	%
Metamyelocytes	0	%		NA	%
Lymphocytes	12	%		NA	%
Monocytes	7	%		NA	%
Eosinophils	1	%		NA	%
Basophils	0	%		NA	%
Absolute Segmented Neutrophils	6000	#/uL		2,500-10,750	#/uL
Absolute Band Neutrophils	0	#/uL		0-150	#/uL
Absolute Metamyelocytes	0	#/uL		0	#/uL
Absolute Lymphocytes	900	#/uL		850-4,500	#/uL
Absolute Monocytes	525	#/uL		150-1,100	#/uL
Absolute Eosinophils	75	#/uL		50-1,500	#/uL
Absolute Basophils	0	#/uL		0-100	#/uL
Toxic Change	WBC morphology appears normal				
Platelet Estimate	350,000	#/uL		150,000-450,000	#/uL
Platelet Comment	Platelet morphology appears normal				

Case Figure 10.1 Hematologic data. *Absolute leukocyte values are based on WBC estimate and differential count.

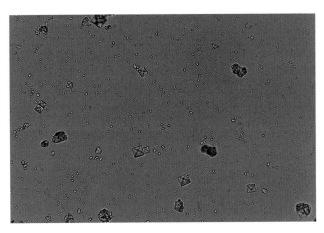

Case Figure 10.2   Urine sediment, wet mount (unstained, 400×).

a *PCV/TPP will help identify anemia and clarify the patient's plasma protein status, which may be affected by conditions like protein-losing enteropathy or nephropathy in a patient with diarrhea.*

b *Blood film examination will evaluate for causes of anemia (if present) as well as degree of regeneration. Examination of a blood film will also evaluate leukocyte concentration and distribution, as well as platelet concentration.*

c *BUN will help establish the patient's renal function, it is critical to rule in or out CKD as a cause of polyuria and polydipsia in this patient.*

d *Blood glucose will help to rule in or out diabetes mellitus as a cause of polyuria and polydipsia in this patient.*

Chemistry

Test	Result	Units	Reference Interval	Units
Total Plasma Protein:	5.1 (51)	g/dL (g/L)	6.0-7.5 (60-75)	g/dL (g/L)
Plasma Color:	Clear			
BUN (Azostix®):	15-26 (5.36-9.28)	mg/dL (mmol/L)	<30 (10.71)	mg/dL (mmol/L)
Blood Glucose:	164 (9.1)	mg/dL (mmol/L)	65-200 (3.6-11.1)	mg/dL (mmol/L)
Urine Color:	Light Yellow			
USG:	1.005			
Urine Protein:	Negative			
Urine Heme:	Negtaive			
Urine Glucose:	Negative			
Urine Ketone:	Negative			
Urine pH:	7.0			
Urine Bilirubin	Negative			
Casts/ Crystals:	1-6 CaOx Dihydrate, Amorphous crystals present	#/lpf	0-1 Hyaline Casts	#/lpf
RBC:	0-3	#/hpf	0-5	#/hpf
WBC:	0-2	#/hpf	0-3	#/hpf
Bacteria:	0	#/hpf	0	#/hpf

Case Figure 10.3   Biochemistry and urinalysis data. Urinalysis sample by cystocentesis.

Case Figure 10.4   Fecal analysis.

Fecal Analysis

Test	Result	Units
Sample Consistency:	Firm	NA
Sample Color	Medium Brown	NA
Fecal Floatation (Sugar Centrifugation)	No ova or parasites seen	
Fecal Direct Smear:	No motile parasites seen	

e *Urinalysis will allow for interpretation of BUN and may help support other diagnostic findings in refining the differential diagnosis.*

f *Fecal direct smear and fecal flotation will help rule out parasitic causes of the patient's clinical signs.*

5 What results, given the patient's signalment/history/clinical exam findings, would you expect in this patient?

a *Given the slightly pale mucous membranes, it would be expected that this patient has a decreased PCV. The presence of polyuria and polydipsia in senior patients make CKD an important condition to rule out. Increased BUN and supporting urinalysis findings such as isosthenuria may be present if the patient has CKD.*

Diagnostic Result Interpretation

1 Given the diagnostic results, what abnormalities do you identify? What is your interpretation of these findings?

2 Are any of these diagnostic results surprising/unexpected?

3 What are the broad mechanisms by which these abnormalities occur?

4 Urine pH is a critical factor in crystal formation; at what pH range do calcium oxalate crystals typically form?

5 In this case, what is/are the top differential diagnoses based on the current diagnostic data?

6 What diagnostic results are most supportive for each of the differential diagnoses?

7 What additional diagnostics would you need to confirm/refute the top differentials for this case?

Diagnostic Result Interpretation Answers

1 Given the diagnostic results, what abnormalities do you identify? What is your interpretation of these findings?

a *The PCV is decreased and there is no polychromasia seen on the blood film, consistent with a* nonregenerative anemia. WBC estimate, differential, and platelet estimate are all within the reference interval.

b *The BUN is within the reference interval and the USG is in the hyposthenuric range supporting normal renal function. Normal BUN with a normal glucose indicates that liver mass is likely adequate and not the cause of the polyuria.*

c *Urinalysis shows hyposthenuria and calcium oxalate dihydrate crystalluria. This finding is suggestive of hypercalciuresis, which may be the result of hypercalcemia or excessive calcium excretion by the kidney. This finding is most consistent with hypercalcemia since the urine pH is not within a range (acidic) that would promote increases in calciuresis in the normocalcemic patient. There is no evidence of renal protein loss ruling out renal disease as the cause of the decreased plasma protein.*

d *The total plasma protein is decreased and there is no evidence of proteinuria, liver dysfunction, or clinical signs of hemorrhage. This finding is most likely consistent with hypoproteinemia secondary to gastrointestinal loss of protein.*

2 Are any of these diagnostic results surprising/unexpected?

a *The finding of calcium oxalate crystalluria was unexpected but not surprising in this case. Calcium oxalate crystalluria in cats is most commonly associated with hypercalcemia. Hypercalcemia is a common paraneoplastic disorder, often referred to as hypercalcemia of malignancy, and is associated with neoplasms like lymphoma, multiple myeloma, and apocrine gland anal sac adenocarcinoma (AGASACA). This finding is supportive of alimentary neoplasia. Given the age of the cat and the clinical signs, alimentary lymphoma is the primary differential.*

3 What are the broad mechanisms by which these abnormalities occur?

a *Mild nonregenerative anemia seen in this case is most likely the result of chronic inflammation associated with gastrointestinal disease. Proinflammatory cytokines downregulate erythropoiesis, which usually results in a mild nonregenerative anemia.*

b *Hyposthenuria occurs secondary to hypercalcemia and increased calciuresis. Increased calcium concentration within the blood inhibits the activity of ADH interfering with the urine-concentrating ability by preventing water reabsorption.*

c *Calcium oxalate crystalluria occurs secondary to hypercalciuresis. Increased calcium concentration in urine increases the likelihood for crystal formation.*

d *Decreased total plasma protein is likely due to increased loss of protein and decreased absorption of protein in the gastrointestinal tract.*

4 Urine pH is a critical factor in crystal formation, at what pH range do calcium oxalate crystals typically form?

a *Acidic urine predisposes patients to the formation of calcium oxalate crystals by increasing calciuresis.*

5 In this case, what is/are the top differential diagnoses based on the current diagnostic data?

a *The primary differential in this case would be alimentary neoplasia (most likely alimentary lymphoma) with secondary hypercalcemia. Other differentials to consider are IBD or other enteropathies with unrelated hypercalciuria.*

6 What diagnostic results are most supportive of each of the differential diagnoses?

a *Calcium oxalate crystalluria is most commonly associated with hypercalcemia and hypercalciuria in the cat. Nonneoplastic enteropathies are not typically associated with hypercalcemia and hypercalciuria; therefore, this finding favors alimentary neoplasia with alimentary lymphoma, which is statistically the most common. It is important to note, hypercalcemia of malignancy can be associated with any neoplasm, but certain types of neoplasia (i.e. lymphoma, multiple myeloma, and AGASACA) are most commonly associated with this paraneoplastic syndrome. In the cat, multiple myeloma and AGASACA are rare.*

7 What additional diagnostics would you need to confirm/refute the top differentials for this case?

a *Additional more sensitive diagnostics are needed in order to make a definitive diagnosis in this case. A full CBC and biochemistry profile should be performed, and if the suspicion of hypercalcemia is confirmed, a hypercalcemia of malignancy profile (ionized calcium, parathyroid hormone, and parathyroid-hormone relate peptide) is necessary to determine the cause of the hypercalcemia. Abdominal ultrasonography and biopsies would be the most appropriate diagnostics to confirm the diagnosis of alimentary lymphoma. Depending on the results of ultrasonography and*

biopsy, ancillary testing may be required to confirm the diagnosis (i.e. PARR to confirm lymphoma). If the patient is normocalcemic, it may be beneficial to perform serum cobalamin, folate, and specific pancreatic lipase testing to evaluate for nonneoplastic enteropathy as the cause of the patient's clinical signs. A deworming trial is beneficial to perform in any patient with diarrhea; this is an inexpensive diagnostic and GI parasites are not always identified via fecal flotation. PCR testing for common enteric pathogens would be beneficial to efficiently rule out their contribution to this patient's clinical signs.

11 Case #11

11.1 Signalment

Ace, a three-month-old castrated male Labrador Retriever puppy

11.2 History

Ace was adopted from a shelter three days ago by his new owners. He has received three vaccinations and is due for his next vaccine in two weeks. When at the shelter, he received a deworming treatment with Pyrantel Pamoate and was treated for coccidiosis with Sulfadimethoxine.

11.3 Presentation

Ace presents for examination due to diarrhea. Yesterday, Ace started having diarrhea and the owners are concerned about the possibility of "Parvo."

11.4 Physical Exam Findings

Temp: 102.1°F (38.9°C), HR: 112, RR: 32, MM: Pink, CRT: <2 seconds, Hydration status: <5% Dehydrated, BCS: 4/9

Cardiopulmonary: No murmurs auscultated, strong synchronous pulses, lungs auscultate normally

Abdomen: On abdominal palpation mild gas distension is appreciated.

Lymph: No abnormalities identified.

HEENT: No abnormalities identified.

Urogenital: No abnormalities identified.

Integument: No abnormalities identified.

Neurologic: No abnormalities identified.

Musculoskeletal: No abnormalities identified.

Initial Data (History/Signalment/Physical Exam) Questions

1 Given the clinical data, what is the differential diagnosis?

2 What diagnostics ideally would you like to perform (given no resource boundaries) and why?

3 What low-cost diagnostics could you perform in this patient that might give you similar information to your ideal list?

4 What results, given the patient's signalment/history/ clinical exam findings, would you expect in this patient?

Initial Data (History/Signalment/Physical Exam) Answers

1 Given the clinical data, what is the differential diagnosis?

    a *The primary differentials in this case are giardiasis or GI parasitic infestation. Other differentials to consider would be dietary indiscretion and canine parvovirus (CPV). Although CPV cannot be ruled out, the vaccination history and lack of lethargy or vomiting, makes it less likely.*

2 What diagnostics ideally would you like to perform (given no resource boundaries) and why?

    a *Ideally fecal flotation, fecal direct smear, fecal antigen testing for CPV and Giardia, as well as a CBC.*

    b *Fecal flotation will help confirm or refute the presence of GI parasites (i.e. hookworm, roundworm, or whipworm infestations).*

    c *Fecal direct smear will allow evaluation for motile parasites (i.e. Giardia).*

    d *Fecal antigen testing would provide the most sensitive testing for CPV and Giardia to help confirm or refute these as differentials.*

    e *CBC would evaluate the patient for anemia and degree of regeneration, as well as identify leukocyte changes consistent with inflammation or stress, and evaluate platelet concentration.*

Hematology				
Test	**Result**	**Units**	**Reference Interval**	**Units**
PCV	54 (0.54)	% (L/L)	35-57 (0.35-0.57)	% (L/L)
Total Plasma Protein:	6.1 (61)	g/dL (g/L)	6.0-7.5 (60-75)	g/dL (g/L)
Plasma Color:	Clear			

Case Figure 11.1　Hematologic data.

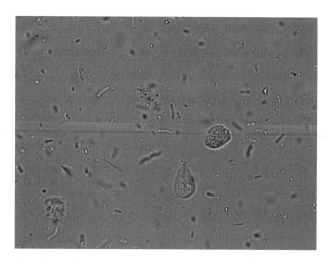

Case Figure 11.2　Fecal direct smear (unstained, 1000×).

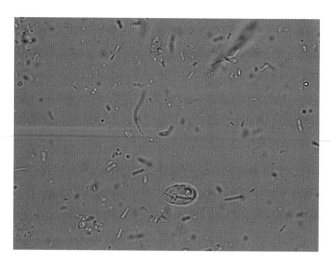

Case Figure 11.3　Fecal direct smear (unstained, 1000×).

Fecal Analysis

Test	Result	Units
Sample Consistency:	Soft, semi liquid	NA
Sample Color	Tan, greasy	NA
Fecal Direct Smear:	Motile flagellate protozoans. Movement appears as a "falling leaf", consistent with Giardia spp., few oocysts identified.	
Fecal Floatation (Sugar Centrifugation)	No ova or parasites seen	
Fecal Floatation (Sodium Nitrate Centrifugation)	Numerous Giardia spp. Trophozoites and cysts identified	

Case Figure 11.4   Fecal analysis data.

3   What low-cost diagnostics could you perform in this patient that might give you similar information to your ideal list?

   a   *The appropriate initial low-cost diagnostics in this case, are almost identical to the ideal diagnostic list. Fecal flotation, fecal direct smear, as well as a PCV/ TPP would be appropriate initial low-cost diagnostics to perform.*

4   What results, given the patient's signalment/history/ clinical exam findings, would you expect in this patient?

   a   *In this patient, identification of either parasite ova on fecal flotation or motile parasites on direct smear would be expected. Because this patient has diarrhea, hypoproteinemia may be seen secondary to loss of protein into the gastrointestinal lumen. If the patient has a heavy intestinal parasite burden, anemia may be seen secondary to iron deficiency.*

Diagnostic Result Interpretation Questions

1   Given the diagnostic results, what abnormalities do you identify? What is your interpretation of these findings?

2   Why were there no *Giardia* cysts or trophozoites identified on the fecal flotation with Sugar solution but numerous with the sodium nitrate solution?

3   If giardiasis or any gastrointestinal parasite infection is suspected in a patient that had negative fecal

diagnostics, can we fully eliminate them as a differential? What could we do that would further evaluate for these two differentials?

4   In this case, what is/are the working diagnosis based on the current diagnostic data?

Diagnostic Result Interpretation Answers

1   Given the diagnostic results, what abnormalities do you identify? What is your interpretation of these findings?

   a   *The diagnostic results are consistent with giardiasis. The identification of flagellate organisms with the "falling leaf" motility pattern is highly supportive of giardiasis. In conjunction with compatible motility, identification of morphologically compatible trophozoites and cysts is diagnostic for Giardiasis.*

2   Why were no *Giardia* spp. cysts or trophozoites identified on the fecal flotation with sugar solution but numerous with the sodium nitrate solution?

   a   *Sheather's sugar solution is extremely hypertonic; this often results in significant distortion of giardia organisms. Therefore, it is likely that the organism cysts and trophozoites were present but not recognizable. The ideal fecal float solution for diagnosis of giardiasis is zinc sulfate; however, a diagnosis can be obtained using sodium nitrate based fecal float solutions. Zinc sulfate and sodium nitrate based fecal solutions will not distort the organisms like Sheather's sugar solution.*

3   If giardiasis or any gastrointestinal parasite infection is suspected in a patient that had negative fecal diagnostics, can we completely eliminate them as a differential? What could we do that would further evaluate for these two differentials?

   a   *Antigen testing is the most sensitive methodology for detecting giardia infections. Commercial patient-side ELSIA tests are available and would help rule out giardiasis if negative. Alternatively, PCR testing for giardia and multiple other enteric pathogens would be a highly sensitive, specific, and efficient diagnostic methodology to determine the cause of this patient's clinical signs. Contact your local veterinary diagnostic laboratory to determine what fecal PCR tests are available.*

4 In this case, what is/are the working diagnosis based on the current diagnostic data?

   a *The primary differential in this case is giardiasis, although concurrent infection with other gastrointestinal pathogens cannot be entirely ruled out (i.e. hookworm or whipworm infestation)*

12 Case #12

12.1 Signalment

Timothy, a 6-month-old intact male Boston Terrier dog

12.2 History

Timothy was found by his owners wandering the Arizona desert at about 12 weeks of age. He is current on vaccinations and receives a monthly flea/tick preventative. He does not currently receive heartworm prevention or anthelminthics.

12.3 Presentation

Timothy presents for examination due to mild lethargy. The owners noticed that yesterday he started acting a little depressed and tired easily.

12.4 Physical Exam Findings

Temp: 100.1°F (37.8°C), HR: 132, RR: 40, MM: Pale Pink, CRT: <2 seconds, Hydration status: <5% Dehydrated, BCS: 4/9

  Cardiopulmonary: No murmurs auscultated, strong synchronous pulses, lungs auscultate normally

  Abdomen: No abnormalities identified.

  Lymph: No abnormalities identified.

  HEENT: No abnormalities identified.

  Urogenital: No abnormalities identified.

  Integument: No abnormalities identified.

  Neurologic: No abnormalities identified.

  Musculoskeletal: No abnormalities identified.

Initial Data (History/Signalment/Physical Exam) Questions

1 Given the clinical data, what is the differential diagnosis?

2 What diagnostics ideally would you like to perform (given no resource boundaries) and why?

3 What low-cost diagnostics could you perform in this patient that might give you similar information to your ideal list?

4 What information are you expecting to receive from these diagnostics? In other words, what differential do you expect to rule in or rule out with these diagnostics?

5 What results, given the patient's signalment/history/clinical exam findings, would you expect in this patient?

Initial Data (History/Signalment/Physical Exam) Answers

1 Given the clinical data, what is the differential diagnosis?

  a *There are many possible differentials in this case given the vague presenting complaint and physical exam findings. However, given the patient's history and possible evidence of anemia, the primary differentials to consider would be GI parasitic infestation, anemia of infectious origin, and coccidioidomycosis (which always must be considered in endemic areas).*

2 What diagnostics ideally would you like to perform (given no resource boundaries) and why?

  a *It would be ideal in this case to perform a CBC, biochemistry profile, urinalysis, fecal flotation, and serology for coccidioidomycosis.*

  b *CBC is part of any minimum database and will be beneficial in narrowing the differential diagnosis. It would allow for the evaluation of RBC mass, confirming anemia, which is suspected based on the physical exam findings (pale pink mucous membranes, tachycardia, and tachypnea). It would also allow the evaluation of leukocyte concentration and distribution, which may indicate whether an inflammatory process is occurring. Blood film evaluation may help rule in or out hemoparasites as a cause of potential anemia and identify morphologic changes to erythrocytes that may indicate a cause of anemia.*

  c *Biochemistry profile would allow for the evaluation of organ function and potentially help identify causes of anemia, help refine our differential diagnosis, and suggest further diagnostics.*

  d *Urinalysis is needed for adequate interpretation of any biochemistry profile.*

Hematology

Test	Result	Units	Reference Interval	Units
PCV	34 (0.34)	% (L/L)	35-57 (0.35-0.57)	% (L/L)
Polychromasia:	1+			
RBC Morphology:	RBC morphology appears normal			
nRBC	0	#/100 WBC	0-2	#/100 WBC
WBC Estimate	10,600	#/uL	5,000-15,500	#/uL
Segmented Neturophils	78	%	NA	%
Band Neutrophils	0	%	NA	%
Metamyelocytes	0	%	NA	%
Lymphocytes	11	%	NA	%
Monocytes	9	%	NA	%
Eosinophils	2	%	NA	%
Basophils	0	%	NA	%
Absolute Segmented Neutrophils	8,268	#/uL	2,500-10,750	#/uL
Absolute Band Neutrophils	0	#/uL	0-150	#/uL
Absolute Metamyelocytes	0	#/uL	0	#/uL
Absolute Lymphocytes	1,166	#/uL	850-4,500	#/uL
Absolute Monocytes	954	#/uL	150-1,100	#/uL
Absolute Eosinophils	212	#/uL	50-1,500	#/uL
Absolute Basophils	0	#/uL	0-100	#/uL
Toxic Change	WBC morphology appears normal			
Platelet Estimate	275,000	#/uL	150,000-450,000	#/uL
Platelet Comment	Platelet morphology appears normal			
Total Plasma Protein:	6.3 (63)	g/dL (g/L)	6.0-7.5 (60-75)	g/dL (g/L)
Plasma Color:	Clear			

Case Figure 12.1   Hematologic data. *Absolute leukocyte values are based on WBC estimate and differential count.

e   *Fecal flotation would allow us to support or make GI parasitic infestation less likely as a cause of the patient's clinical signs of anemia.*

f   *Serologic testing for antibodies to* Coccidioides *spp., would either increase or decrease the suspicion for this as a differential.*

3   What low-cost diagnostics could you perform in this patient that might give you similar information to your ideal list?

a   *In this case PCV/TPP, blood film examination, and fecal flotation would be appropriate initial low-cost diagnostics to perform.*

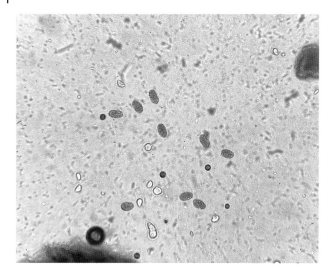

Case Figure 12.2 Fecal flotation (Sheather's sugar solution, 100×).

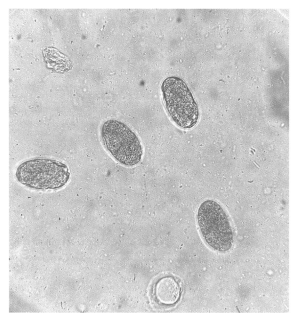

Case Figure 12.3 Fecal direct smear (Sheather's sugar solution, 400×).

Fecal Analysis

Test	Result	Units
Sample Consistency:	Firm, well formed	NA
Sample Color	Dark brown	NA
Fecal Floatation (Sugar Centrifugation)	0–9 Ancylostoma spp., ova identified per low power field	

Case Figure 12.4 Fecal analysis data.

4 What information are you expecting to receive from these diagnostics? In other words, what differential do you expect to rule in or rule out with these diagnostics?

   a *PCV would allow for confirmation of the physical exam findings consistent with anemia (pale pink mucous membranes, slight tachycardia, and tachypnea, etc.).*

   b *TPP may support GI parasite infestation as a differential if the total plasma proteins are decreased.*

   c *Blood film examination will help establish the degree of regeneration if anemia is present. It will also evaluate leukocyte concentration and distribution, which may support inflammation and or stress response and establish platelet concentration.*

   d *Fecal flotation would allow us to support or make GI parasitic infestation less likely as a cause of the patient's clinical signs of anemia.*

5 What results, given the patient's signalment/history/clinical exam findings, would you expect in this patient?

   a *In this patient, a mildly decreased PCV would be expected given the patient's physical exam findings that are consistent with anemia (pale pink mucous membranes, tachycardia, and tachypnea). There may be eosinophilia with or without basophilia if parasitic infestation is present. Other leukogram changes are possible and may be consistent with an inflammatory or stress response. There may be parasite ova found on the fecal flotation given the patient's history and lack of routine anthelminthic administration.*

Diagnostic Result Interpretation Questions

1 Given the diagnostic results, what abnormalities do you identify? What is your interpretation of these findings?

2 Since this patient has a hookworm infestation, why are the stools normal instead of diarrheic?

3 Since this patient has a parasitic infection, why is there no evidence of eosinophilia or basophilia? If we were to see eosinophilia/basophilia, could we for sure attribute that to the parasitic infection?

4 Why is anemia most commonly associated with hookworms as opposed to other common parasites (i.e. roundworm or whipworms)?

5 In this case, what is/are the top differential diagnoses based on the current diagnostic data?

Diagnostic Result Interpretation Answers

1 Given the diagnostic results, what abnormalities do you identify? What is your interpretation of these findings?

    a *There is mild anemia with evidence of a mild regenerative response (1+ polychromasia). The leukogram shows no abnormalities. Fecal flotation reveals the presence of* Ancylostoma *spp. ova consistent with hookworm infestation.*

2 Since this patient has a hookworm infestation, why are the patient's stools normal?

    a *Gastrointestinal parasite infestations do not always cause diarrhea in patients with clinical disease from parasitism. For this reason, fecal examination should be performed four times in the first year of life and then at least twice per year thereafter and dogs should receive routine anthelminthic treatments.*

3 Since this patient has a parasitic infection, why is there no evidence of eosinophilia or basophilia? If we were to see eosinophilia/basophilia, could we definitively attribute that to the parasitic infection?

    a *While eosinophilia or basophilia in peripheral blood can be associated with parasitism, not all patients with parasitism will show this finding. The peripheral blood does not always reflect the inflammatory response that is occurring in the tissue. When present, eosinophilia and/or basophilia in the peripheral blood should raise suspicion for parasitic infestation as a differential. There are other causes of this specific leukogram pattern that have to be considered such as allergic responses.*

4 Why is anemia most commonly associated with hookworms as opposed to other common parasites (i.e. roundworm or whipworms)?

    a *Hookworms are hematophagous parasites; therefore, high parasite burdens can lead to enough collective blood loss through parasite consumption that patients may become anemic. Roundworms are not typically associated with hemorrhage and subsequent anemia, rather they compete with the host for nutrition and are associated with failure to thrive. Whipworm infestation can result in GI hemorrhage; however, only severe infestations cause anemia in adult dogs. In addition, hookworms consume*

significantly higher amounts of blood from the host compared with whipworms. Although not present in this case, hookworm infestation can result in iron deficiency and subsequent anemia in puppies. Iron deficiency in puppies is associated with a microcytic, hypochromic, variably regenerative anemia with associated hypoproteinemia.

5 In this case, what is/are the working diagnoses in this case based on the current diagnostic data?

    a *In this case, the primary differential is hookworm infestation. We cannot entirely rule out co-infestation with another gastrointestinal parasite such as whipworms due to their intermittent ova shedding patterns.*

13 Case #13

13.1 Signalment

Duckie, 3-year-old, a spayed female Australian Cattle Dog

13.2 History

Duckie is a working dog on a cattle ranch in Southern Arizona. The owners report she is current on vaccination but does not receive any medications. The original veterinarian could not determine a cause of Duckie's diarrhea. They originally performed a fecal flotation, CBC, biochemistry, and UA. All of these are reportedly "normal" but the original veterinarian's office is closed and you are unable to obtain records. No medications were prescribed, only a bland diet. Duckie's diarrhea continued with the diet change.

13.3 Presentation

Duckie is presented to you for examination and a second opinion due to chronic diarrhea.

13.4 Physical Exam Findings

Temp: 101.4°F (38.6°C), HR: 100, RR: 32, MM: Pink, CRT: <2 seconds, Hydration status: <5% Dehydrated, BCS: 4/9

    Cardiopulmonary: No murmurs ausculted, strong synchronous pulses, lungs auscult normally

    Abdomen: No abnormalities identified.

    Lymph: No abnormalities identified.

    HEENT: No abnormalities identified.

    Urogenital: No abnormalities identified.

    Integument: No abnormalities identified.

Neurologic: No abnormalities identified.
Musculoskeletal: No abnormalities identified.

Initial Data (History/Signalment/Physical Exam) Questions

1 Given the clinical data, what is the differential diagnosis?

2 What diagnostics ideally would you like to perform (given no resource boundaries) and why?

3 What low-cost diagnostics could you perform in this patient that might give you similar information to your ideal list?

4 What information are you expecting to receive from these diagnostics? In other words, what differential do you expect to rule in or rule out with these diagnostics?

5 What results, given the patient's signalment/history/clinical exam findings, would you expect in this patient?

Initial Data (History/Signalment/Physical Exam) Answers

1 Given the clinical data, what is the differential diagnosis?
   a *The primary differentials for this case are GI parasitic infestation, inflammatory bowel disease, and other secondary gastrointestinal diseases.*

2 What diagnostics ideally would you like to perform (given no resource boundaries) and why?
   a *Ideally a CBC, biochemistry profile, urinalysis, and fecal flotation should be performed. An anthelminthic trial should be performed as well.*
   b *Repeating the diagnostics performed originally would be ideal to establish a baseline for this patient at this time and help direct further diagnostics.*
   c *A deworming trial is beneficial to perform in any patient with diarrhea; this is an inexpensive diagnostic and GI parasites are not always identified via fecal flotation.*

3 What low-cost diagnostics could you perform in this patient that might give you similar information to your ideal list?

   a *PCV/TPP, blood film evaluation, and fecal flotation would be appropriate initial low-cost diagnostics to perform*

4 What information are you expecting to receive from these diagnostics? In other words, what differential do you expect to rule in or rule out with these diagnostics?
   a *PCV would allow evaluation for the presence of anemia.*
   b *TPP may support the possibility of GI disease if total plasma protein is decreased.*
   c *Blood film examination will evaluate leukocyte concentration and distribution, which may support an inflammatory response. Blood film examination will also allow evaluation of platelet density.*
   d *There may be parasite ova found on the fecal flotation given the patient's history and lack of routine anthelminthic administration.*

5 What results, given the patient's signalment/history/clinical exam findings, would you expect in this patient?
   a *In this patient, mild anemia, hypoproteinemia, inflammatory leukogram changes, or positive fecal flotation may be seen.*

Diagnostic Result Interpretation Questions

1 Given the diagnostic results, what abnormalities do you identify? What is your interpretation of these findings?

2 What are broad mechanisms by which these abnormalities occur?

3 In this case, what is/are the top differential diagnoses based on the current diagnostic data?

4 What diagnostic results are most supportive for each of the differential diagnoses?

5 What additional diagnostics would you need to confirm/refute the top differentials for this case?

Hematology

Test	Result	Units	Reference Interval	Units
PCV	51 (0.51)	% (L/L)	35-57 (0.35-57)	% (L/L)
RBC Comment	RBC morphology appears normal			
nRBC	0	#/100 WBC	0-2	#/100 WBC
WBC Estimate	10620	#/uL	5,000-15,500	#/uL
Segmented Neturophils	61	%	NA	%
Band Neutrophils	0	%	NA	%
Metamyelocytes	0	%	NA	%
Lymphocytes	10	%	NA	%
Monocytes	9	%	NA	%
Eosinophils	10	%	NA	%
Basophils	10	%	NA	%
Absolute Segmented Neutrophils	6478.2	#/uL	2,500-10,750	#/uL
Absolute Band Neutrophils	0	#/uL	0-150	#/uL
Absolute Metamyelocytes	0	#/uL	0	#/uL
Absolute Lymphocytes	1062	#/uL	850-4,500	#/uL
Absolute Monocytes	955.8	#/uL	150-1,100	#/uL
Absolute Eosinophils	1062	#/uL	50-1,500	#/uL
Absolute Basophils	1062	#/uL	0-100	#/uL
Toxic Change	None			
WBC Comment	WBC morphology appears normal			
Platelet Estimate	350,000	#/uL	150,000-450,000	#/uL
Platelet Comment	Rare macroplatelets			
Total Plasma Protein:	6.9 (69)	g/dL (g/L)	6.0-7.5 (65-75)	g/dL (g/L)
Plasma Color:	Clear			

Case Figure 13.1 Hematologic data. *Absolute leukocyte values are based on WBC estimate and differential count.

Diagnostic Result Interpretation Answers

1 Given the diagnostic results, what abnormalities do you identify? What is your interpretation of these findings?

   a *PCV and total plasma protein are within the reference interval, and fecal flotation was negative. Moderate basophilia is present, which is supportive of a parasitic or allergic inflammatory process. Although basophilia in the absence of eosinophilia is uncommon, occasionally this can be seen.*

2 What are broad mechanisms by which these abnormalities occur?

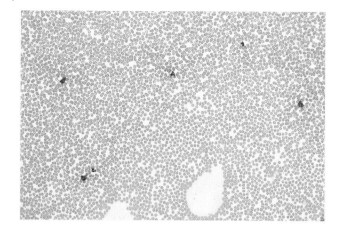

Case Figure 13.2 Blood film (Wrights–Giemsa, 200×).

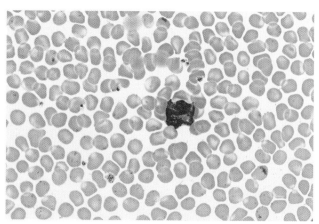

Case Figure 13.4 Blood film (Wrights–Giemsa, 1000×).

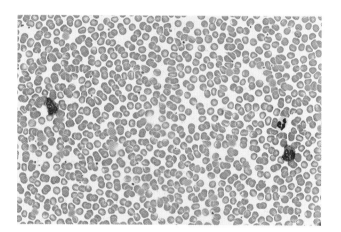

Case Figure 13.3 Blood film (Wrights–Giemsa, 500×).

Fecal Analysis		
Test	**Result**	**Units**
Sample Consistency:	Soft, semiformed	NA
Sample Color	Dark brown	NA
Fecal Floatation (Sugar Centrifugation)	No ova or parasites seen	
Fecal Occult Blood:	Negative	

Case Figure 13.5 Fecal analysis data.

a *Basophilia occurs secondary to increased tissue demand. Basophils help mediate and contribute to chronic inflammatory responses to parasites and allergens. Proinflammatory cytokines released at the site of inflammation stimulate increased basophilopoiesis and increase the number of circulating basophils. Basophilia and eosinophilia are most commonly seen in association with each other. If only one of these leukocytes are increased on hematologic evaluation, this may not necessarily reflect the extent of inflammation that is occurring in the tissue. Therefore, there may be significant eosinophilic inflammation in the tissue that is not reflected in the blood.*

3 In this case, what is/are the top differential diagnoses based on the current diagnostic data?
   a *The primary differentials for this case are GI parasitic infestation or allergen-associated enteropathy.*

4 What diagnostic results are most supportive for each of the differential diagnoses?
   a *Basophilia supports the presence of a parasitic or allergic inflammatory stimulus. A negative fecal flotation supports allergic response over parasitic. However, the clinical signs are not entirely consistent with the allergic process, gastrointestinal manifestations of allergies are commonly accompanied by cutaneous manifestations. Gastrointestinal parasite ova are not always identified in cases of infestation; therefore, parasitic gastrointestinal disease is considered most likely*

5 What additional diagnostics would you need to confirm/refute the top differentials for this case?
   a *A deworming trial is beneficial to perform in any patient with diarrhea; this is an inexpensive diagnostic and GI parasites are not always identified via fecal flotation. If the deworming trial failed to result in improvement of clinical signs, intradermal allergen testing should be pursued as well as abdominal ultrasound.*

14 Case #14

14.1 Signalment

Angel, a 10-year-old spayed female Weimaraner dog

14.2 History

Angel is current on vaccinations, receives a monthly heartworm preventative/anthelminthic combination and an oral ectoparasiticide every three months. She also receives a glucosamine/chondroitin supplement for arthritis. The owners note that she has been slowing down recently. She had a mass removed from her neck about three months ago, which was histologically diagnosed as a high-grade cutaneous mast cell tumor, images of the original cytologic preparation are shown below (see Case Figure 14.1). Her owners also note that yesterday she started vomiting what appears to be coffee grounds, and her stools appear black.

14.3 Presentation

Angel presents for examination due to progressive malaise and acute vomiting.

14.4 Physical Exam Findings

Temp: 102.7°F (39.3°C), HR: 112, RR: 36, MM: Pale Pink, CRT: <2 seconds, Hydration status: <5% Dehydrated, BCS: 6/9

  Cardiopulmonary: No murmurs ausculted, strong synchronous pulses, lungs auscult normally.

  Abdomen: Abdomen is tense on palpation, slightly painful, moderate splenomegaly.

  Lymph: Left axillary lymph node is enlarged (~1.5 cm in diameter).

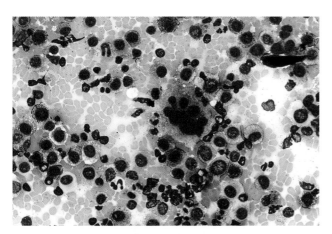

Case Figure 14.1 Cytologic preparation of previously excised mast cell tumor (May Grunwald–Giemsa, 500×).

HEENT: No abnormalities identified.
Urogenital: No abnormalities identified.
Integument: No abnormalities identified.
Neurologic: No abnormal findings.
Musculoskeletal: No abnormalities identified.

Initial Data (History/Signalment/Physical Exam) Questions

1 Given the clinical data, what is the differential diagnosis?

2 What diagnostics ideally would you like to perform (given no resource boundaries) and why?

3 What low-cost diagnostics could you perform in this patient that might give you similar information to your ideal list?

4 What information are you expecting to receive from these diagnostics? In other words, what differential do you expect to rule in or rule out with these diagnostics?

5 What results, given the patient's signalment/history/ clinical exam findings, would you expect in this patient?

Initial Data (History/Signalment/Physical Exam) Answers

1 Given the clinical data, what is the differential diagnosis?
   a *The primary differential would be gastric ulceration, possibly from chronic systemic histamine release, NSAID administration, hyperadrenocorticism, or uremia. Other differentials to consider are gastrointestinal neoplasia unrelated to previous mast cell tumor and coagulopathy.*

2 What diagnostics ideally would you like to perform (given no resource boundaries) and why?
   a *Ideally, a CBC, biochemistry profile, urinalysis, abdominal radiographs, and abdominal ultrasound should be performed.*
   b *CBC will help identify anemia with or without evidence of a regenerative response, evaluate leukocyte concentration and distribution, and estimate platelet concentration. Gastrointestinal ulceration and hemorrhage can result in iron deficiency, depending*

on location and duration of the hemorrhage, CBC may be helpful in identifying this if present. Perforation is a possible sequela of gastrointestinal ulceration, monitoring the leukogram may be beneficial in identifying underlying inflammatory leukogram changes with or without evidence of sepsis.

c Biochemical profile is important to evaluate organ function and ensure that there are no other conditions contributing to this patient's illness.

d Urinalysis is critical for adequate interpretation of any biochemical profile.

e Abdominal radiographs will help screen for metastatic lesions, evidence of perforation, or other disease

processes within the abdomen that are potentially contributing to the patient's clinical signs of pain.

f Abdominal ultrasound will help screen for metastatic lesions, signs of perforation, or other disease processes within the abdomen potentially contributing to the patient's clinical signs of pain.

3 What low-cost diagnostics could you perform in this patient that might give you similar information to your ideal list?

a PCV/TPP, blood film evaluation, BUN, and urinalysis. In this case, the presence of melena eliminates the need to perform a fecal occult blood test.

Hematology				
Test	**Result**	**Units**	**Reference Interval**	**Units**
PCV	32 (0.32)	% (L/L)	35-57 (0.35-0.57)	%
RBC Comment	RBC morphology appears normal			
nRBC	0	#/100 WBC	0-2	#/100 WBC
WBC Estimate	8200	#/uL	5,000-15,500	#/uL
Segmented Neturophils	37	%	NA	%
Band Neutrophils	0	%	NA	%
Metamyelocytes	0	%	NA	%
Lymphocytes	13	%	NA	%
Monocytes	10	%	NA	%
Eosinophils	40	%	NA	%
Basophils	0	%	NA	%
Absolute Segmented Neutrophils	3034	#/uL	2,500-10,750	#/uL
Absolute Band Neutrophils	0	#/uL	0-150	#/uL
Absolute Metamyelocytes	0	#/uL	0	#/uL
Absolute Lymphocytes	1066	#/uL	850-4,500	#/uL
Absolute Monocytes	820	#/uL	150-1,100	#/uL
Absolute Eosinophils	3280	#/uL	50-1,500	#/uL
Absolute Basophils	0	#/uL	0-100	#/uL
Toxic Change	None			
WBC Comment	WBC morphology appears normal			
Platelet Estimate	~150,000	#/uL	150,000-450,000	#/uL
Platelet Comment	Platelet clumping, estimate reflects the minimum number present			

Case Figure 14.2   Hematologic data. *Absolute leukocyte values are based on WBC estimate and differential count.

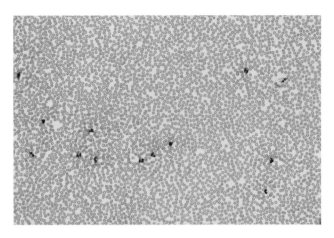

Case Figure 14.3 Blood film (Wrights–Giemsa, 200×).

4 What information are you expecting to receive from these diagnostics? In other words, what differential do you expect to rule in or rule out with these diagnostics?

   a *PCV/TPP will evaluate for anemia and plasma protein status, which may be altered in the presence of gastrointestinal disease.*

   b *Examination of a blood film will evaluate leukocyte concentration, distribution, and platelet density.*

   c *BUN will help establish renal function, and possibly support the presence of gastrointestinal hemorrhage if increased in the presence of adequately concentrated urine.*

   d *Urinalysis will allow for adequate interpretation of BUN in this patient.*

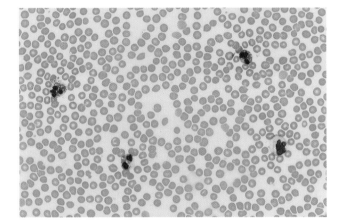

Case Figure 14.4 Blood film (Wrights–Giemsa, 500×).

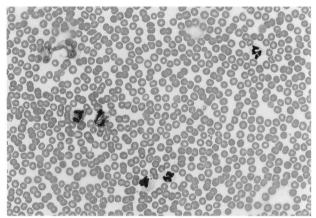

Case Figure 14.5 Blood film (Wrights–Giemsa, 500×).

Chemistry				
Test	**Result**	**Units**	**Reference Interval**	**Units**
Total Plasma Protein:	6.4 (64)	g/dL (g/L)	6.0-7.5 (60-75)	g/dL (g/L)
Plasma Color:	Clear			
BUN (Azostix®):	50-80 (17.85-28.57)	mg/dL (mmol/L)	<30 (10.71)	mg/dL (mmol/L)
USG:	1.035			
Urine Protein:	Negative			
Urine Glucose:	Negative			
Urine Ketone	Negative			
Urine pH:	7.0			
Urine Bilirubin	Negative			
Urine Sediment:	No casts/ cyrstals seen	#/lpf	0-1 Hyaline Casts	#/lpf

Case Figure 14.6 Biochemistry and urinalysis data. Urinalysis sample by cystocentesis.

5 What results, given the patient's signalment/history/clinical exam findings, would you expect in this patient?

   a *In this case, a decreased PCV and increased BUN with adequately concentrated USG are expected given the presence of melena in this patient. Total plasma protein may be decreased or normal. There may be evidence of inflammatory or stress response in the leukogram.*

Diagnostic Result Interpretation Questions

1 Given the diagnostic results, what abnormalities do you identify? What is your interpretation of these findings?

2 Are any of these diagnostic results surprising/unexpected?

3 What are broad mechanisms by which these abnormalities occur?

4 In this case, what is the working diagnosis based on the current diagnostic data?

5 What diagnostic results are most supportive for each of the differential diagnoses?

6 What additional diagnostics would you need to confirm/refute the top differentials for this case?

Diagnostic Result Interpretation Answers

1 Given the diagnostic results, what abnormalities do you identify? What is your interpretation of these findings?

   a *There is a mild anemia with no evidence of regeneration, which is likely secondary to chronic inflammation. Blood loss into the gastrointestinal lumen may also contribute to anemia; this may be acute, and therefore, regeneration is not yet evident.*

   b *Moderate eosinophilia is present and is likely secondary to mast cell disease.*

   c *There is moderate to marked azotemia with adequately concentrated urine specific gravity. In the absence of dehydration, this finding is consistent with hemorrhage into the GI tract.*

2 Are any of these diagnostic results surprising/unexpected?

   a *Eosinophilia was unexpected in this patient but is not surprising since this can occur as a paraneoplastic finding in patients with mast cell tumors.*

3 What are broad mechanisms by which these abnormalities occur?

   a *Anemia is the result of suppression of erythropoiesis by proinflammatory cytokines and gastrointestinal hemorrhage.*

   b *Eosinophilia is the result of cytokines production and release by mast cells. Mast cells produce eosinophilopoietic (i.e. IL-5) and eosinophilotactic (i.e. eotaxin) cytokines, which may lead to eosinophilia in cases of mast cell tumors, where numbers of mast cells are markedly increased.*

   c *Azotemia occurs secondary to increased protein digestion. Hemorrhage into the GI lumen causes digestion of blood components that are rich in proteins, which are then metabolized forming urea and increasing concentrations in the blood.*

4 In this case, what is the working diagnosis based on the current diagnostic data?

   a *The primary differential in this case is mast cell tumor metastasis with secondary GI ulceration and eosinophilia*

5 What additional diagnostics would you need to confirm/refute the top differentials for this case?

   a *GI endoscopy would be ideal to confirm the presence of gastric ulceration and allow for biopsy of any lesions found to further evaluate for neoplasia. Abdominal ultrasound and fine needle aspirates of identified masses, the swollen left axillary lymph node, and spleen would be helpful to identify potential metastatic mast cell disease.*

15 Case #15

15.1 Signalment

Chase, a 2-year-old castrated male Golden Doodle dog

15.2 History

Chase is current on vaccinations, receives a monthly heartworm preventative/anthelminthic combination and an oral ectoparasiticide.

15.3 Presentation

Chase presents as an emergency due to acute onset lethargy, panting, and lateral recumbency. The owners noticed that he is dribbling red-colored urine.

15.4 Physical Exam Findings

Temp: 99.7°F (37.6°C), HR: 156, RR: 88, MM: Pale, CRT: <2 seconds, Hydration status: <5% Dehydrated, BCS: 5/9

Cardiopulmonary: On auscultation of the heart, there is a slight (Grade 1–2/6) systolic murmur. Cardiac rhythm is normal, and pulses are strong and synchronous. On auscultation, the lungs have normal sounds in all lung fields.

Abdomen: Abdomen is tense on palpation, slightly painful, moderate splenomegaly.

Lymph: No abnormalities identified.

HEENT: No abnormalities identified.

Urogenital: No abnormalities identified.

Integument: No abnormalities identified.

Neurologic: Patient is extremely lethargic, is reluctant to ambulate but will if stimulated enough, normal conscious proprioceptive responses and nociceptive responses. A brief cranial nerve exam is within normal limits.

Musculoskeletal: No abnormalities identified.

Initial Data (History/Signalment/Physical Exam) Questions

1 Given the clinical data, what is the differential diagnosis?

2 What diagnostics ideally would you like to perform (given no resource boundaries) and why?

3 What low-cost diagnostics could you perform in this patient that might give you similar information to your ideal list?

4 What information are you expecting to receive from these diagnostics? In other words, what differential do you expect to rule in or rule out with these diagnostics?

5 What results, given the patient's signalment/history/clinical exam findings, would you expect in this patient?

6 What questions would be important to ask an owner in this case?

Initial Data (History/Signalment/Physical Exam) Answers

1 Given the clinical data, what is the differential diagnosis?
   a *The primary differentials in this case are acute hemolytic anemia, toxin ingestion, coagulopathy, cardiovascular disease, cystitis with secondary endotoxemia, or rhabdomyolysis secondary to myopathy.*

2 What diagnostics ideally would you like to perform (given no resource boundaries) and why?
   a *CBC, biochemistry profile, and urinalysis would be appropriate initial diagnostics.*
   b *CBC will provide information that may clarify the origin of anemia in this patient, assess for regeneration, leukocyte concentration and distribution, and platelet mass. Evaluation of the blood film performed with the CBC will help identify the cause of anemia in this patient. Evaluation of plasma color in conjunction with urinalysis findings would allow differentiation between myoglobinuria and hemoglobinuria.*
   c *Biochemistry profile will allow for evaluation of organ function to identify the potential inciting causes of the patient's clinical signs.*
   d *Urinalysis is critical for interpretation of any biochemical profile. In addition, urine color and other characteristics are critical to identifying the cause of this patient's illness (i.e. distinguishing myoglobinuria vs. hemoglobinuria).*

3 What low-cost diagnostics could you perform in this patient that might give you similar information to your ideal list?
   a *PCV/TPP, blood film evaluation, BUN, and urinalysis would be appropriate initial low-cost diagnostics to perform in this case.*

4 What information are you expecting to receive from these diagnostics? In other words, what differential do you expect to rule in or rule out with these diagnostics?
   a *PCV/TPP will confirm the presence of anemia and allow for evaluation of the plasma color. Total plasma protein may help eliminate hemorrhage as a potential cause of anemia in this patient.*
   b *Blood film examination will allow evaluation of erythrocyte morphology and help confirm that hemolytic anemia is present (i.e. presence of ghost cells, Heinz bodies, eccentrocytes, etc.). Evaluation*

Micro-Hematocrit Capillary Tube Reader
Permits Reading of Packed Cell
Volume Directly in Percentage
For In Vitro Diagnostic Use

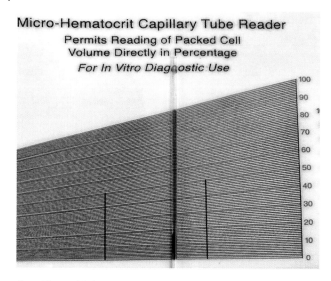

Case Figure 15.1 Hematocrit tube gross image 1.

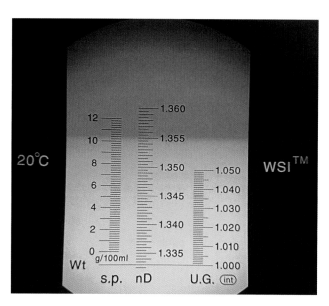

Case Figure 15.3 Refractometry measurement of total plasma protein.

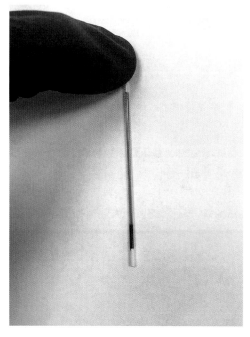

Case Figure 15.2 Hematocrit tube gross image 2.

of the blood film may also aid in identifying potential causes of hemolysis (i.e. oxidative injury, erythroparasites).

c *BUN is important to evaluate in cases of hemolytic anemia, especially when intravascular origin is suspected because of the risk for acute kidney injury in these patients.*

d *Urinalysis is important to evaluate to confirm the cause of pigmenturia. Evaluation of sediment for*

erythrocytes is necessary to rule in or out hematuria. Concurrent evaluation of the plasma color and urine after centrifugation will assist in differentiating myoglobinuria from hemoglobinuria.

5 What results, given the patient's signalment/history/ clinical exam findings, would you expect in this patient?

a *Given the critical presentation of this patient, moderate to marked anemia can be expected. Pigmenturia in the presence of anemia is suggestive of intravascular hemolysis. The blood film may reveal evidence of hemolysis. It is expected to see a positive heme reaction on urinalysis considering the gross urine appearance. Evidence of renal injury may be indicated by an increased BUN and isosthenuria.*

6 What questions would be important to ask an owner in this case?

a *Is there potential that the patient could have ingested anything out of the ordinary? Is ingestion of onions, garlic, acetaminophen, coins, rat poison, pesticides, and other drugs or toxins possible?*

The owners report that ingestion of coins and garlic are not possible; however, they did eat liver and onions for dinner last night and cannot rule out the possibility that their children shared with Chase. In addition, one of the owners accidentally spilled a bottle of acetaminophen on the floor. They thought they cleaned all the pills up but did not know how many were in the bottle before it was spilled.

Hematology

Test	Result	Units	Reference Interval	Units
PCV	17 (0.17)	% (L/L)	35-57 (0.35-0.57)	% (L/L)
RBC Comment:	3+ Heinz bodies, 2+ Eccentrocytes, 2+ Ghost cells			
WBC Estimate	13,400	#/uL	5,000-15,500	#/uL
Segmented Neturophils	77	%	NA	%
Band Neutrophils	0	%	NA	%
Metamyelocytes	0	%	NA	%
Lymphocytes	12	%	NA	%
Monocytes	8	%	NA	%
Eosinophils	3	%	NA	%
Basophils	0	%	NA	%
Absolute Segmented Neutrophils	10,318	#/uL	2,500-10,750	#/uL
Absolute Band Neutrophils	0	#/uL	0-150	#/uL
Absolute Metamyelocytes	0	#/uL	0	#/uL
Absolute Lymphocytes	1,608	#/uL	850-4,500	#/uL
Absolute Monocytes	1,072	#/uL	150-1,100	#/uL
Absolute Eosinophils	402	#/uL	50-1,500	#/uL
Absolute Basophils	0	#/uL	0-100	#/uL
Toxic Change	WBC morphology appears normal			
Platelet Estimate	400,000	#/uL	150,000-450,000	#/uL
Platelet Comment	Platelet morphology appears normal			

Case Figure 15.4 Hematologic data. *Absolute leukocyte values are based on WBC estimate and differential count.

Case Figure 15.5 Blood film (Wrights–Giemsa, 200X *Blood film courtesy of Dr. Jennifer Bouschor, DVM, PhD, DACVP).

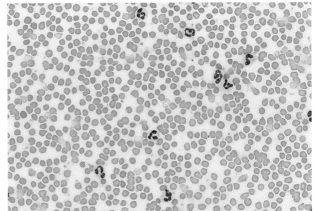

Case Figure 15.6 Blood film (Wrights–Giemsa, 500X *Blood film courtesy of Dr. Jennifer Bouschor, DVM, PhD, DACVP).

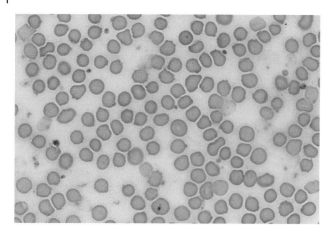

Case Figure 15.7 Blood film (Wrights–Giemsa, 1000X *Blood film courtesy of Dr. Jennifer Bouschor, DVM, PhD, DACVP).

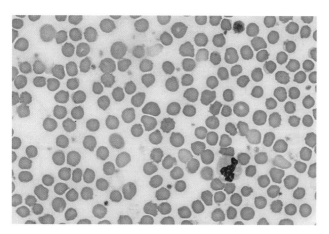

Case Figure 15.8 Blood film (Wrights–Giemsa, 1000X *Blood film courtesy of Dr. Jennifer Bouschor, DVM, PhD, DACVP).

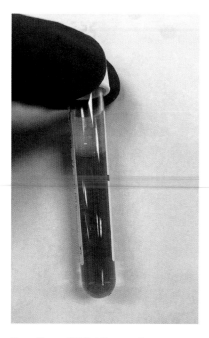

Case Figure 15.9 Gross urine appearance, postcentrifugation.

Diagnostic Result Interpretation Questions

1 Given the diagnostic results, what abnormalities do you identify? What is your interpretation of these findings?

2 What are broad mechanisms by which these abnormalities occur?

3 Why is this patient's total plasma protein moderately increased at 10.2 g/dL?

4 What are the most common causes of this type of hemolytic anemia in dogs?

5 In this case, what is/are the top differential diagnoses based on the current diagnostic data?

6 What additional diagnostics would you need to confirm/refute the top differentials for this case?

Diagnostic Result Interpretation Answers

1 Given the diagnostic results, what abnormalities do you identify? What is your interpretation of these findings?
a *Moderate anemia with significant erythrocyte morphology changes consistent with acute intravascular hemolysis (eccentrocytes, Heinz bodies, and ghost cells).*
b *The hemolyzed plasma, red urine, positive heme reaction, and absence of erythrocytes in the urine sediment confirms hemoglobinuria and supports the presence of acute intravascular hemolysis and hemoglobinemia.*
c *Azotemia with no evidence of dehydration and inadequately concentrated urine may be indicative of renal origin. This may indicate acute kidney injury secondary to hemoglobinemia and hemoglobinuria. A serum creatinine is required to confirm azotemia due to decreased GFR of renal origin.*

2 What are broad mechanisms by which these abnormalities occur?
a *Anemia in this case is due to significant oxidative erythrocyte injury and erythrocyte lysis within the vascular space (intravascular hemolysis).*
b *Heinz bodies and eccentrocytes both form secondary to oxidative injury. Heinz bodies form due to*

Chemistry

Test	Result	Units	Reference Interval	Units
Total Plasma Protein:	10.4 (104)	g/dL (g/L)	6.0-7.5 (60-75)	g/dL (g/L)
Plasma Color:	2+ Hemolysis (Red)			
BUN (Azostix®):	30-40 (10.71-14.28)	mg/dL (mmol/L)	<30 (10.71)	mg/dL (mmol/L)
Blood Glucose:	130 (7.2)	mg/dL (mmol/L)	65-200 (3.6-11.1)	mg/dL (mmol/L)
Urine Color:	Rose			
USG:	1.020			
Urine Protein:	Negative			
Urine Glucose:	Negative			
Urine Ketone:	Negative			
Urine Heme:	3+			
Urine pH:	7.0			
Urine Bilirubin	Negative			
Urine Sediment:	No sediment present after centrifugation	#/lpf	0-1 Hyaline Casts	#/lpf

Case Figure 15.10   Biochemistry and urinalysis data. Urinalysis sample by cystocentesis.

hemoglobin crystallization. Eccentrocytes form due to fusion of erythrocyte cell membranes.

c *Hemoglobinuria is due to the presence of free hemoglobin in the blood (hemoglobinemia). Hemoglobinemia in this case is the result of intravascular hemolysis and subsequent release of hemoglobin. Intravascular hemolysis can quickly overwhelm the haptoglobin scavenging mechanism resulting in hemoglobinemia. Unbound hemoglobin easily passes into the glomerular filtrate because of its small size, and ultimately is excreted.*

d *Azotemia occurs secondary to hemoglobin induced renal injury. Iron within the hemoglobin molecule is a major contributor to nephrotoxicity. Iron promotes free radical formation, which damages cells in the nephron leading to renal injury.*

3 Why is this patient's total plasma protein moderately increased at 10.2 g/dL?

a *The increased total plasma protein is artifactual. Hemolysis or hemoglobinemia will artificially increase the total plasma protein measurement by refractometry. Refer to Case Figure 15.3 and note the red hue to the refractometry measurement.*

4 What are the most common causes of this type of hemolytic anemia in dogs?

a *In dogs, the most common causes of intravascular hemolysis are onion, garlic, acetaminophen, and zinc ingestion. Less commonly, patients with copper storage disease may develop intravascular hemolytic anemias.*

5 In this case, what is/are the working diagnosis based on the current diagnostic data?

a *The primary differentials in this case are onion toxicity or acetaminophen toxicity. Although the owners did not give any direct evidence of onion or acetaminophen ingestion, these are the only toxicants that the patient could have ingested. It is possible that the owners did not find all of the acetaminophen tablets spilled. It is also entirely possible that the client's children fed the patient liver and onions. Garlic or zinc containing coin ingestion cannot be entirely ruled out but are considered less likely.*

6 What additional diagnostics would you need to confirm/refute the top differentials for this case?

a *In this case, the clinical and current laboratory findings are sufficient to support the presence of acute intravascular hemolytic anemia. Abdominal radiographs should be performed to ensure that there are no coins within the patient's gastrointestinal tract.*

References

1 Goddard, A. et al. (2008). Prognostic usefulness of blood leukocyte changes in canine Parvoviral enteritis. *Journal of Veterinary Internal Medicine* 22 (2): 309–316.

2 Cudney, S.E., Wayne, A.S., and Rozanski, E.A. (2021). Diagnostic utility of abdominal ultrasonography for evaluation of dogs with nontraumatic hemoabdomen: 94 cases (2014–2017). *Journal of the American Veterinary Medical Association* 258 (3): 290–294.

Index